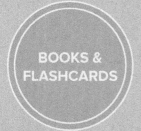
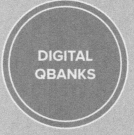
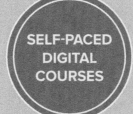
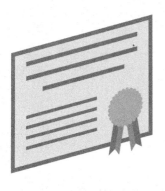
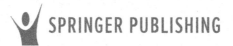

FNP AND AGNP CERTIFICATION EXPRESS REVIEW

FNP AND AGNP CERTIFICATION EXPRESS REVIEW

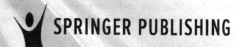

SPRINGER PUBLISHING

Springer Publishing Company, LLC
11 West 42nd Street, New York, NY 10036
www.springerpub.com

Acquisitions Editor: Suzanne Toppy
Compositor: diacriTech

ISBN: 978-0-8261-5972-4
ebook ISBN: 978-0-8261-5973-1
DOI: 10.1891/9780826159731

Printed by BnT

The author and the publisher of this Work have made every effort to use sources believed to be reliable to provide information that is accurate and compatible with the standards generally accepted at the time of publication. Because medical science is continually advancing, our knowledge base continues to expand. Therefore, as new information becomes available, changes in procedures become necessary. We recommend that the reader always consult current research and specific institutional policies before performing any clinical procedure or delivering any medication. The author and publisher shall not be liable for any special, consequential, or exemplary damages resulting, in whole or in part, from the readers' use of, or reliance on, the information contained in this book. The publisher has no responsibility for the persistence or accuracy of URLs for external or third-party Internet websites referred to in this publication and does not guarantee that any content on such websites is, or will remain, accurate or appropriate.

Library of Congress Control Number: 2021909866

Contact sales@springerpub.com to receive discount rates on bulk purchases.

Publisher's Note: New and used products purchased from third-party sellers are not guaranteed for quality, authenticity, or access to any included digital components.

Printed in the United States of America.

CONTENTS

PREFACE

If you have purchased this *Express Review*, you are likely well into your exam prep journey to certification. This book has been designed to be a high-speed review—a last-minute gut check before your exam day. We created this review, which is a quick summary of the key topics you'll encounter on the exam, to supplement to your certification preparation studies. We encourage you to use it in conjunction with other study aids to ensure you are as prepared as possible for the exam.

This book follows the American Academy of Nurse Practitioners Certification Board's (AANPCB) and American Nurses Credentialing Center's (ANCC) most recent exam content outlines and uses a succinct, bulleted format to highlight what you need to know. The aim of this book is to help you solidify your retention of information in the month or so leading up to your exam. It is written by certified nurse practitioners who are familiar with the exam and the content you need to know. Special features appear throughout the book to call out important information, including the following:

- **Complications:** Problems that can arise with certain disease states or procedures
- **Clinical Pearls:** Additional patient care insights and strategies for knowledge retention
- **Alerts:** Need-to-know details on how to handle emergency situations or when to transfer care
- **Pop Quizzes:** Critical-thinking questions to test your ability to synthesize what you learned (answers in Chapter 17)
- **List of Abbreviations:** A useful appendix to help guide you through the alphabet soup of clinical terms

We know life is busy. Being able to prepare for your exam efficiently and effectively is paramount, which is why we created this *Express Review*. You have come to the right place as you continue on your path of professional growth and development. The stakes are high, and we want to help you succeed. Best of luck to you on your certification journey. You've got this!

PASS GUARANTEE

If you use this resource to prepare for your exam and you do not pass, you may return it for a refund of your full purchase price. To receive a refund, you must return your product along with a copy of your original receipt and exam score report. Product must be returned and received within 180 days of the original purchase date. Excludes tax, shipping, and handling. One offer per person and address. Refunds will be issued within eight weeks from acceptance and approval. This offer is valid for US residents only. Void where prohibited. To begin the process, please contact customer service at CS@springerpub.com.

1

GENERAL EXAMINATION INFORMATION

OVERVIEW

- In this chapter, we will review the examination information for certification as a family or adult-gerontology primary care nurse practitioner through the AANPCB and the ANCC. While the blueprints for the exams administered by these certifying bodies differ significantly, we have organized this book by organ system, as most students study using this methodology.

AANPCB CERTIFICATION

- The AANPCB has been certifying nurse practitioners since 1993 to validate nurse practitioners' achievements in education, knowledge, and professional expertise.
- The eligibility and requirements for certification are posted on its website at www.aanpcert.org/certs/qualifications.
- Once certified, family nurse practitioners will receive the FNP-C credential and adult-gerontology primary care nurse practitioners will receive the A-GNP credential.
- Because information changes from time to time, the best source of information about eligibility, application process, fees, scheduling, test site information, and other details about the exam is in the candidate handbook. You can view this on the AANPCB website.

About the Examinations

- Both computer-based examinations contain 150 multiple-choice format questions. Fifteen questions are pretest questions that are not scored. Your score is based on 135 questions, but you will take all 150 questions to complete the exam. The exams are not adaptive, which means the questions will not get easier or more difficult based on how you answer the questions.
- AANPCB provides test blueprints with percentages in each domain category. Detailed test blueprints are provided on their website.
- Test-taking tips can be accessed on the AANPCB's website with recommendations for your study plan. Information about practice testing is also available.
- If you have used accommodations for testing in the past and think you may need them for this exam, complete the special accommodations request form application on the AANPCB website and fax to the testing center.
- You will have a 120-day window to take the examination after you apply.

How to Apply

- Applications to take the certification exam are accepted online and by mail. If you choose to apply online, have PDFs of supporting documentation ready to upload. You are eligible for a $75 discount on the certification exam if you become an AANP member at the time of application.

How to Contact AANPCB

Website: www.aanpcert.org
Email: certification@aanpcert.org
Email Official Transcripts to: transcripts@aanpcert.org

Certification Administration: (512) 637-0500
Toll-free Number: (855) 822-6727
Fax: (512) 637-0540 or (512) 637-0334

Mailing Address:	Street Address:
P.O. Box 12926	2600 Via Fortuna, Suite 240
Austin, TX 78711-2926	Austin, TX 78746-7006

ANCC CERTIFICATION

- The ANCC has been validating nursing expertise since 1990. Their certification offers a valid and reliable assessment of the entry-level clinical knowledge and skills of nurse practitioners. The eligibility and requirements for certification as an family or adult-gerontology primary care nurse practitioner are posted on its website at www.nursingworld.org.
- Once certified, family nurse practitioners will receive the FNP-BC credential and adult-gerontology primary care nurse practitioners will receive the AGPCNP-BC credential.
- You can review the website which provides information about eligibility, the application process, fees, scheduling, testing site information, and other pertinent information. Because this information changes from time to time, the ANCC website is your most reliable and up-to-date resource for these details.

About the Examinations

- The computer-based examinations contain 175 multiple-choice and alternate item format questions. Alternate item formats include multiple response items, hot spots, and drag and drop. Twenty-five questions are pretest questions that are not scored. Your score is based on 150 questions. You will take all 175 questions to complete the exam. These exams are not adaptive.
- ANCC provides test content outlines with an explanation of examination content. Visit the ANCC website for the most current blueprint details.
- The exam handbooks contain recommendations to prepare for the certification examination.
- You will have a 90-day window to take the examination after you apply.
- If you have used accommodations for testing in the past and think you may need them for this exam, review the instructions in the testing handbook on the procedural steps.

How to Apply

- Applications to take the certification exam are accepted online. If you become a member of the American Nurses Association, you will receive a discounted testing price.

How to Contact ANCC

Website: www.nursingworld.org/our-certifications/
Email: aprnvalidation@ana.org

Toll-free Number: (800) 284-2378

ANCC Certification Registration
8515 Georgia Ave, Suite 400
Silver Spring, MD 20910-3412

2

PHARMACOLOGY REVIEW

See Table 2.1 for contraindications, precautions, and drug interactions.

ANALGESICS OVERVIEW

- Analgesics are pharmacologic agents used to manage acute and chronic pain in primary care that arises from a variety of causes. They are prescribed as an adjunct to nonpharmacological strategies in a comprehensive pain management plan.

General Guidelines

History and Physical
- Obtain a detailed history of pain, including past treatments, consultations, and diagnostics.
- Perform a depression, substance use, and suicidality screen.
- Calculate fall risk.
- Discuss the pain's impact on functional health and coping.
- Review pertinent medical records.
- Perform a musculoskeletal, neurologic, and focused exam of the painful site.
- Obtain an allergy profile.
- Review analgesic medication options and compare to the patient's current medication profile and comorbidities. Minimize the risk of CNS toxicity, cumulative sedation, falls, and hepatorenal injury when selecting the analgesic agent.

Planning/Interventions
- Prescribe nonpharmacological strategies appropriate for the patient's condition.
- Provide therapeutic exercise and activity instructions for acute or chronic pain.
- Discuss the benefits of tai chi, yoga, massage, spinal manipulation, and acupuncture, if appropriate for the patient's condition.
- Provide referrals for CBT and physical therapy as needed.

ACETAMINOPHEN

Mechanism of Action

- The specific mechanism of action is unknown, but acetaminophen may work peripherally to block pain impulse and inhibit prostaglandin synthesis in the CNS.

Indications

- First-line agent for mild to moderate pain (acute or chronic) or as an adjunct to restorative therapies, complementary and integrative health, and behavioral health approaches in chronic pain

Commonly Prescribed Medications

- Acetaminophen (oral, rectal, and injectable)
- Paracetamol, acetaminophen XR (oral)

Diagnostic Testing

Baseline
- BMP, CBC, and/or LFTs in suspected hepatorenal impairment

Follow-Up
- Check BMP, CBC, LFTs in suspected hepatorenal impairment.
- Obtain serum acetaminophen level in suspected toxicity.

NONSTEROIDAL ANTI-INFLAMMATORY DRUGS

Mechanism of Action

- Inhibit prostaglandin synthesis by inhibiting COX-1 and COX-2

Indications

- First-line agent for mild to moderate pain (acute or chronic), especially with inflammatory syndromes, or as an adjunct to restorative therapies, complementary and integrative health, and behavioral health approaches in chronic pain

Commonly Prescribed Medications

- Ibuprofen (oral and injectable)
- Diclofenac (oral, topical, and injectable)
- Diflunisal, etodolac, fenoprofen, indomethacin (oral, topical, and injectable)
- Ketorolac (oral and injectable)
- Meloxicam (oral and injectable)
- Naproxen, nabumetone, piroxicam (oral)

Diagnostic Testing

Baseline
- BMP and LFTs in suspected hepatorenal impairment
- CBC in suspected anemia

Follow-Up
- Check BMP and LFTs in suspected hepatorenal impairment.
- Obtain CBC in suspected anemia.

COX-2 INHIBITORS

Mechanism of Action

- Inhibit prostaglandin synthesis by inhibiting COX-2

Indications

- Acute or chronic pain observed in OA, RA, ankylosing spondylitis, acute pain, primary dysmenorrhea
- Prescribed in place of NSAIDs but can be prescribed in addition to acetaminophen

Commonly Prescribed Medications

- Celecoxib (oral)

Diagnostic Testing

Baseline
- BMP and LFTs in suspected hepatorenal impairment
- CBC in suspected anemia

Follow-Up
- Check BMP and LFTs in suspected hepatorenal impairment.
- Obtain CBC in suspected anemia.

SEROTONIN NOREPINEPHRINE REUPTAKE INHIBITORS

Mechanism of Action
- May enhance descending inhibitor pain pathways by inhibiting the uptake of serotonin and norepinephrine

Indications
- First-line therapy for neuropathic pain; second-line therapy in osteoarthritis
- Considered in chronic musculoskeletal pain, fibromyalgia, non-neuropathic, noncancer pain

Commonly Prescribed Medications
- Duloxetine, venlafaxine (oral)

Diagnostic Testing

Baseline
- BMP to assess baseline electrolytes and LFTs to evaluate for hepatic impairment
- 12-lead EKG in older adults to evaluate QT interval
- Screening for underlying HTN

Follow-Up
- BMP to identify hyponatremia in older adults and LFTs for hepatic impairment

GABA ANALOG

Mechanism of Action
- Antinociceptive that binds to alpha-2 delta subunit in CNS, which reduces pro-nociceptive neurotransmitters

Indications
- Second-line therapy for neuropathic pain, fibromyalgia

Commonly Prescribed Medications
- Gabapentin, pregabalin (oral)

Diagnostic Testing

Baseline
- BMP and LFTs in suspected hepatorenal impairment
- CBC in suspected pancytopenia
- 12-lead EKG to evaluate PR interval if needed

Follow-Up
- Check BMP and LFTs in suspected hepatorenal impairment.
- Check CBC with suspected pancytopenia.
- Obtain 12-lead EKG in suspected conduction defect.

MUSCLE RELAXANTS

Mechanism of Action

- *Baclofen*: GABA agonist that reduces spasticity possibly through reflex inhibition
- *Tizanidine*: Central alpha-2-adrenergic receptor agonist that reduces spasticity by increasing presynaptic inhibition of motor neurons
- *Dantrolene*: Peripherally acting muscle relaxant that reduces spasticity
- *Methocarbamol*: CNS depressant with antispasmodic properties

Indications

- Spasticity (baclofen, dantrolene, tizanidine)
- Muscle spasm (cyclobenzaprine, methocarbamol)

Commonly Prescribed Medications

- *Anti-spasticity agents*: Baclofen (oral, intrathecal), dantrolene (oral and parenteral), tizanidine (oral)
- *Antispasmodic*: Cyclobenzaprine, methocarbamol (oral and parenteral)

Diagnostic Testing

Baseline
- BMP and LFTs in suspected hepatorenal impairment
- CBC if anemia is suspected

Follow-Up
- Check BMP and LFTs in suspected hepatorenal impairment.
- Obtain CBC if anemia is suspected.

CAPSAICIN CREAM/PATCH

Mechanism of Action

- Topical TRPV1 agonist

Indications

- Temporary relief of neuropathic and skeletal muscle pain
- Capsaicin 8% patch is an office procedure for neuropathic pain and can last up to 3 months.

Commonly Prescribed Medications

- Methyl salicylate gel patch, capsaicin patch (topical)

Diagnostic Testing

Baseline
- BP

Follow-Up
- Monitor for an increase in BP for in-office prescription therapy.

LIDOCAINE PATCH OTC

Mechanism of Action

- Local anesthetic

Indications

- Relief of postherpetic neuralgia
- Lidocaine 5% available by prescription

Commonly Prescribed Medications

- Lidocaine 4% or 5% (topical)

Diagnostic Testing

Baseline
- None

Follow-Up
- None

OPIOID AGONIST (SCHEDULE IV)

Mechanism of Action

- Centrally acting synthetic opioid

Indications

- Moderate to severe acute and chronic pain

Commonly Prescribed Medications

- Tramadol hydrochloride (schedule IV; oral)

Diagnostic Testing

Baseline
- BMP and LFTs in suspected hepatorenal impairment

Follow-Up
- BMP and LFTs in suspected hepatorenal impairment

OPIOIDS (SCHEDULES II–III)

Mechanism of Action

- Centrally acting synthetic opioid

Indications

- Moderate to severe acute pain
- Prescribed for chronic pain only according to state and federal guidelines to decrease dependence and abuse

Commonly Prescribed Medications

- *Schedule II*: Hydrocodone, methadone, hydromorphone (oral and parenteral), meperidine (oral and parenteral), oxycodone, fentanyl (intranasal, parenteral, transdermal, transmucosal)
- *Schedule III*: Acetaminophen with codeine (oral)

Diagnostic Testing

Baseline
- BMP and LFTs in suspected hepatorenal impairment

Follow-Up
- BMP and LFTs in suspected hepatorenal impairment

Table 2.1 Analgesic Agents

Class	Contraindications/Precautions/Adverse Effects	Drug Interactions
Acetaminophen	• Hold in patients with allergy or liver failure. • Monitor for hepatotoxicity, nephrotoxicity at high doses. Max dose in 24 hr is 3 g/d. • Use caution with G6PD deficiency, or hepatic or renal impairment. • Use caution with alcohol consumption. • Do not prescribe in combination with other drugs containing acetaminophen.	• Use caution when prescribing with other hepatotoxins and nephrotoxins especially pexidartinib or pretomanid. • Acetaminophen decreases the effects of warfarin, imatinib, lixisenatide. • Acetaminophen increases the level of levonorgestrel, tinidazole, tazemetostat, lomitapide, dapsone, and busulfan.
NSAIDs	• Hold with an allergy to aspirin, other NSAIDs. • Hold with active bleeding. • Use caution in asthma, HF, pancytopenia, PUD/GERD, SLE, inflammatory bowel disease. • Monitor for hyperkalemia if administered with ACEIs, ARBs, oral contraceptives. • Monitor for nephrotoxicity, hepatotoxicity. • Monitor during MI, stroke, DVT/PE, HTN, ASCVD, CABG/PCI. • May cause tinnitus and edema. • Give with food to avoid GI distress.	• Increased risk of bleeding when taken with COX-2 inhibitors, anticoagulants, aspirin, antiplatelets, and thrombolytics. • Coadministration with lithium can cause toxicity. • NSAIDs decrease the effect of spironolactone, ACIs, ARBs, beta blockers, and triamterene and increase potassium. • Coadministration with digoxin, oral contraceptives containing drospirenone and NSAIDs increases potassium. • NSAIDs decrease the effect of terazosin furosemide in presence of renal damage. • Clomipramine, cyclosporine, dexamethasone, mesalamine increase toxicity. • Coadministration with Quinolones increase seizures. • SNRI, chlorpropamide, trazodone, azoles, nateglinide, HCTZ, furosemide increases the effect of NSAIDs.

Class	Contraindications/Precautions/Adverse Effects	Drug Interactions
Lidocaine patch	• Allergy to lidocaine or equivalent • Seizures in overdose	• *Caution in coadministration with antiarrhythmics*: Disopyramide, flecainide, mexiletine, moricizine, procainamide, propafenone, quinidine, or tocainide.
SNRIs	• Monitor for suicidality, serotonin syndrome, or activation of mania/hypomania. • Avoid use in patients with GFR <30 mL/min, cirrhosis, or MAOIs. • Monitor for falls, orthostatic hypotension. • Monitor for hyponatremia, hypertension, urinary retention. • Wean off slowly to avoid abrupt withdrawal syndrome.	• Wait 14 days before starting MAOIs. • Serotoninergic drugs (MAOIs, TCAs, St. John's wort, buspirone, triptans, tryptophan, lithium, fentanyl, tramadol, amphetamine) increase the risk of serotonin syndrome. • CYP1A2 and CYP2D6 inhibitors increase drug concentration. • Use with NSAIDs, ASA, or warfarin can increase the risk of bleeding.
GABA analogs	• Hold in patients with allergy, respiratory depression, angioedema, AV block. • Hold for myopathy and check CK. • Monitor for thrombocytopenia, renal failure, especially in older adults. • Use caution with antiarrhythmics. • Monitor for dizziness, somnolence, encephalopathy, and accidental injury. • Peripheral edema, weight gain, blurred vision may occur. • Wean off slowly to avoid abrupt withdrawal syndrome.	• Coadministration with opioids, benzodiazepine, muscle relaxants, or antihistamines increases the risk for respiratory depression. • Coadministration with alcohol, antihistamines, ACEIs, barbiturates, everolimus, TCAs, BZ, SSRIs, SNRIs, MAOIs, trazodone, opioids, bupropion, buspirone, chlordiazepoxide, or zolpidem increases the toxicity or effect of the other.
Muscle relaxants	• Hold tizanidine in patients taking potent inhibitors of CYP1A2 such as fluvoxamine or ciprofloxacin. • Monitor for syncope and hypotension, hepatotoxicity, psychotic behavior. • Caution patients with renal/hepatic impairment, somnolence, or dizziness that muscle relaxants can increase the risk for injury. • Wean off slowly to avoid abrupt withdrawal syndrome.	• *Tizanidine is contraindicated in potent CYP1A2 inhibitors*: Atazanavir, fluvoxamine, ciprofloxacin, enoxacin, oral contraceptives. • Tizanidine levels are decreased by barbiturates, smoking, primidone, rifampin, azoles. • Tizanidine levels are increased by weak and moderate CYP1A2 inhibitors: cimetidine, macrolides, INH, mexiletine, zileuton, peginterferon, verapamil. • Tizanidine levels are increased by SSRIs, ARBs, ACEIs, beta blockers, alpha blockers, and spironolactone. • Additive effect with clonidine or methyldopa.

(continued)

Table 2.1 Analgesic Agents (*continued*)

Class	Contraindications/Precautions/ Adverse Effects	Drug Interactions
Opioid agonists	• Risk of addiction (REMS). • Hold with impaired LOC, respiratory depression, acute asthma/ decompensated COPD, and Cor pulmonale. • Monitor for excess sedation hypotension and risk for injury/ trauma. • Do not prescribe with other sedating agents. • Use caution in patients with hepatic and renal impairment. • Monitor for adrenal insufficiency, GI distress, constipation, urinary retention, depression, and accidental poisoning in children. • Adults and newborns are at risk for abrupt withdrawal syndrome.	• Use caution with use of cytochrome P450 3A4 inducers, 3A4 inhibitors, or 2D6 inhibitors. • Increased sedation can occur with benzodiazepine, muscle relaxants, barbiturates, trazodone, opioids, and antihistamines. • Increased risk for seizure with coadministration of SSRI, SNRI, 5-HT3 antagonists TCA, and MAOIs.
Opioids	• Schedules II–IV opioids have potential for risk abuse with schedule II having the highest risk for addiction/abuse (REMS). • Hold with impaired LOC, respiratory depression, acute asthma/ decompensated COPD and Cor pulmonale, or ileus. • Use caution in patients with seizure history. • Monitor for excess sedation, hypotension, and risk for injury/ trauma. • Do not prescribe with other sedating agents. • Use caution in patients with hepatic and renal impairment. • Monitor for adrenal insufficiency, GI distress, constipation, urinary retention, depression, and accidental poisoning in children. • Adults and newborns are at risk for abrupt withdrawal syndrome.	• Use of opioids that undergo phase 1 metabolism with a CYP3A4 inhibitor, such as macrolide antibiotics, azole-antifungal agents, or protease inhibitors, may increase plasma concentrations of opioids. • *Concomitant use with a CYP3A4 inducer*: Rifampin, carbamazepine, and phenytoin, or discontinuation of an inhibitor can lead to withdrawal symptoms.

Note: All agents would be contraindicated in the presence of hypersensitivity to the medication or one of its components.

ANXIOLYTICS AND ANTIDEPRESSANTS

Table 2.2, which provides contraindications, precautions, and drug interactions for anxiolytics and antidepressants, can be found at the end of this section.

ANXIOLYTICS OVERVIEW

- Acute symptoms of anxiety and panic disorder can be managed pharmacologically with benzodiazepine (short-term clonazepam) or hydroxyzine according to the patient's risk profile and preferences.
  - Note that risk for suicidality and accidental overdose needs to be considered when prescribing benzodiazepines.
  - Hydroxyzine can be considered an alternative agent while titrating on an antidepressant for GAD.
- Initiate SSRI or SNRI as first-line therapy in combination with CBT. Consider alternative medications if features of OCD, PTSD, insomnia, or comorbid conditions are present. Consider prescribing the following agents according to comorbid condition:
  - *SSRI*: GAD, SAD, panic disorder, OCD, or PTSD.
  - *SNRI*: GAD, SAD, panic disorder, or PTSD.
  - *TCA*: Clomipramine for OCD.
  - *Buspirone*: GAD.
- Agents utilized as an adjunct:
  - *GABA analog*: Pregabalin or topiramate for GAD.
  - *Beta blocker*: Propranolol, off-label for acute panic disorder.
  - *Hydroxyzine*: GAD.
  - *Alpha-2 antagonist*: Mirtazapine is a tetracyclic antidepressant used off-label for insomnia, which may be present in anxiety. Refer to psychiatry for use in children and adolescents with comorbid insomnia.

ANTIDEPRESSANTS OVERVIEW

- Depression is managed with psychotherapy and medication. Consider the comorbid mental health disorders when selecting initial or adjunct antidepressant therapy in the adult:
  - SSRIs are first-line therapy. An SNRI can be considered in comorbid pain or anxiety and should be titrated every 1 to 2 weeks based on patient response.
  - Bupropion (NDRI) can augment therapy if there is a partial response to SSRI. Consider adding bupropion especially if the patient requires intervention for tobacco cessation.

General Guidelines

- All patients being treated with antidepressants should be monitored closely for clinical worsening, suicidality, and unusual changes in behavior, especially when therapy is initiated or changed.
- All patients being treated with antidepressants should be weaned and not stopped abruptly. Acute withdrawal symptoms include flu-like syndrome, insomnia, nausea, and irritability.
- Many antidepressants may cause QT prolongation when another drug is added. Instruct the patient to inform all providers of antidepressant use.

SELECTIVE SEROTONIN REUPTAKE INHIBITORS

Mechanism of Action

- Inhibit reuptake of serotonin

Indications

- First-line therapy for anxiety and depression as an alternative to SNRI.
- Fluoxetine is a first-line agent in children and adolescents, but sertraline, citalopram, and escitalopram can be considered.
- Cannot be combined with MAOIs, SNRIs, TeCAs.

Commonly Prescribed Medications

- Fluoxetine, sertraline, citalopram, escitalopram, paroxetine (oral)

Diagnostic Testing

Baseline

- BMP, LFTs to assess baseline electrolytes and evaluate for hepatic impairment
- 12-lead EKG in older adults to evaluate QT interval
- Screening for underlying HTN

Follow-Up

- BMP, LFTs to identify hyponatremia in older adults and with hepatic impairment

SEROTONIN NOREPINEPHRINE REUPTAKE INHIBITORS

Mechanism of Action

- Inhibit reuptake of serotonin and norepinephrine

Indications

- First-line therapy for anxiety and depression as an alternative to SSRI
- Duloxetine preferred as first-line agent in children age >7 years for anxiety
- Can be considered as a second-line agent if SSRI fails
- Cannot be combined with MAOIs, SSRIs, TeCAs

Commonly Prescribed Medications

- Duloxetine, venlafaxine (oral)

Diagnostic Testing

Baseline

- BMP, LFTs to assess baseline electrolytes and evaluate for hepatic impairment
- 12-lead EKG in older adults to evaluate QT interval
- Screening for underlying HTN

Follow-Up

- BMP, LFTs to identify hyponatremia in older adults and hepatic impairment

NOREPINEPHRINE DOPAMINE RECEPTOR INHIBITORS

Mechanism of Action

- Weak inhibitors of the neuronal reuptake of norepinephrine and dopamine but do not inhibit monoamine oxidase

Indications

- Second-line therapy for MDD or as an adjunct to SSRI or SNRI
- Can be considered first-line therapy in patients requiring assistance with tobacco cessation

Commonly Prescribed Medications

- Bupropion hydrochloride (oral)

Diagnostic Testing

Baseline
- BMP and LFTs in suspected hepatorenal impairment
- CBC in suspected pancytopenia

Follow-Up
- BMP and LFTs in suspected hepatorenal impairment
- CBC in suspected pancytopenia

TRICYCLIC ANTIDEPRESSANTS

Mechanism of Action

- Inhibit serotonin uptake and may inhibit norepinephrine
- Strong anticholinergic and sedation effect

Indications

- Can be considered as a third-line agent if SSRI or SNRI fails
- Is an alternative class to SSRI or SNRI with comorbid OCD
- TCAs not to be prescribed for children and adolescents with anxiety or depression
- Cannot be prescribed with TeCAs or MAOIs
- Distributed in breast milk

Commonly Prescribed Medications

- Amitriptyline, clomipramine, imipramine, desipramine (oral)

Diagnostic Testing

Baseline
- BMP to assess electrolytes
- CBC in suspected hematopoietic dysfunction

Follow-Up
- Obtain 12-lead EKG to evaluate QT interval with syncope or palpitations.
- Check BMP to evaluate for SIADH.
- Check CBC in suspected pancytopenia.

AZAPIRONES

Mechanism of Action

- Believed to enhance dopamine and suppress serotonin through a subtype serotonin receptor

Indications

- Third-line therapy in GAD for short-term use or alone
- Cannot be prescribed with MAOIs, antipsychotics, or other serotonergic agents
- Refer to psychiatry in prescribing with SSRI or SNRI for short-term use with careful supervision

Commonly Prescribed Medication

- Buspirone hydrochloride (oral)

Diagnostic Testing

Baseline
- BMP and LFTs with suspected hepatorenal dysfunction

Follow-Up
- BMP and LFTs with suspected hepatorenal dysfunction

BENZODIAZEPINES

Mechanism of Action

- Sedation and reduction of panic by enhancing GABA in the CNS

Indications

- Second-line medications used as an adjuvant to SSRI or SNRI for short-term use in anxiety and panic disorders
- Should be prescribed in scheduled doses to prevent abuse/addiction

Commonly Prescribed Medications

- Alprazolam, chlordiazepoxide, clonazepam, flurazepam, temazepam (oral)
- Diazepam (oral, rectal, parenteral)
- Lorazepam (oral, parenteral)
- Midazolam (parenteral)

Diagnostic Testing

Baseline
- None

Follow-Up
- Toxicology screen in suspected overdose

ANTIHISTAMINES

Mechanism of Action

- Antihistamine with anxiolytic effect

Indications

- Is a second-line therapy added as an adjunct to SSRI or SNRI when initially titrating
- Can be prescribed as needed for panic
- Has a low abuse potential
- Not to be used in early pregnancy or lactation

Commonly Prescribed Medications

- Hydroxyzine (oral and parenteral)

 POP QUIZ 2.1

A 58-year-old male with a history of depression and osteoarthritis in both knees presents to the primary care provider to discuss pain management and increased anhedonia. He reports that his knee pain disturbs his sleep and no longer responds to NSAIDs and acetaminophen. The pain has caused him to stop exercising, which he previously used to improve his mood, and he has noticed that his depression has increased in the recent past. What medications should be prescribed to address the patient's concerns?

Diagnostic Testing

Baseline
- None

Follow-Up
- Use 12-lead EKG to evaluate QT interval with syncope or palpitations.
- See Table 2.2 for contraindications, precautions, and drug interactions for antidepressants and anxiolytics.

Table 2.2 Anxiolytics and Antidepressants		
Class	**Contraindications/Precautions/ Adverse Effects**	**Drug Interactions**
SSRIs	• Monitor for suicidality, serotonin syndrome, and activation of mania/hypomania. • Avoid use in patients with cirrhosis. • Avoid use with MAOIs. • Monitor for falls and orthostatic hypotension. • Monitor for hyponatremia.	• Wait 14 days before starting MAOIs. • Serotoninergic drugs (TCAs, SNRI, St. John's wort, Buspirone, triptans, tryptophan, lithium, fentanyl, tramadol, amphetamine) increase the risk of serotonin syndrome. • CYP2D6 inhibitors increase drug concentration. • Pimozide and thioridazine prolong the QT interval. • NSAIDs, ASA, and warfarin can increase the risk of bleeding.
SNRIs	• Monitor for suicidality, serotonin syndrome, or activation of mania/hypomania. • Avoid use in patients with GFR <30 mL/min, cirrhosis, or MAOIs. • Monitor for falls and orthostatic hypotension. • Monitor for hyponatremia, hyperglycemia in DM, hypertension, and urinary retention. • Wean off slowly to avoid abrupt withdrawal syndrome.	• Wait 14 days before starting MAOIs. • Serotoninergic drugs (MAOIs, TCAs, SSRIs, St. John's wort, Buspirone, triptans, tryptophan, lithium, fentanyl, tramadol, amphetamine) increase the risk of serotonin syndrome. • CYP1A2 and CYP2D6 inhibitors increase drug concentration. • NSAIDs, ASA, and warfarin can increase the risk of bleeding.
NDRIs	• Do not administer with MAOIs or patients with seizures, angle-closure glaucoma, or uncontrolled hypertension and ASCVD. • Monitor for seizure, suicidality, mania, psychosis, serotonin syndrome, rhabdomyolysis. • Monitor hepatorenal function, pancytopenia, and PT/INR, and adjust the dose.	• Decreased doses of bupropion may be required when prescribed with CYP2B6 inhibitors. • Decreased doses of TCA, SSRI, SNRI, antipsychotics, beta blockers, and type 1C antiarrhythmics may be required when prescribed with bupropion. • Increased doses of bupropion required when administered with CYP2B6 inducers. Coadministration with digoxin may decrease plasma digoxin levels.

(continued)

Table 2.2 Anxiolytics and Antidepressants (*continued*)

Class	Contraindications/Precautions/ Adverse Effects	Drug Interactions
TCAs	• Monitor for suicidality, serotonin syndrome, and mania. • Avoid in patients with BPH with retention, Graves' disease, renal insufficiency, glaucoma, epilepsy, or cirrhosis. • Monitor for sedation, seizures, and risk for injury from the orthostatic effect. • Monitor for rash. • Monitor for SIADH, pancytopenia, hypertension, urinary retention, and erectile dysfunction. • Wean off slowly to avoid abrupt withdrawal syndrome. • Avoid in geriatric patients due to anticholinergic effects.	• Wait 14 days before starting MAOIs. • Serotoninergic drugs (MAOIs, SNRIs, SSRIs, St. John's wort, buspirone, triptans, tryptophan, lithium, fentanyl, tramadol, amphetamine) increase the risk of serotonin syndrome. • CYP1A2 and CYP2D6 inhibitors increase drug concentration. • NSAIDs, ASA, and warfarin can increase the risk of bleeding.
Benzodiazepines	• This class of drugs has a high risk for abuse and addiction. • Hold the medication in severe liver disease, acute angle glaucoma. • Monitor for suicidality, respiratory depression, hypotension, and syncope especially if taking other centrally acting agents. • Use increases risk for injury related to impaired judgment and psychomotor performance. • Use with caution in patients with seizures, renal impairment, porphyria. • Wean slowly to avoid risk for abrupt withdrawal. • Avoid in geriatric patients and patients with a neurodegenerative cognitive disease.	• The CNS-depressant effect may be potentiated by alcohol, narcotics, barbiturates, nonbarbiturate hypnotics, antianxiety agents, the phenothiazine, thioxanthene, and butyrophenone classes of antipsychotic agents, MAOIs, tricyclic antidepressants, and other anticonvulsant drugs. • P450 3A inhibitors can increase the effect of the drug.
Azapirones	• Hold if patient is taking MAOIs or haloperidol. • Hold for patients with severe hepatic and renal impairment. • Increased risk for sedation when combined with other sedating agents. • Monitor for risk for injury due to impaired judgment/motor performance when initiated. • Will not block withdrawal symptoms of benzodiazepines.	• Coadministration with MAOIs or haloperidol is contraindicated. • Buspirone is metabolized by CYP3A4. Its drug levels are increased with cimetidine, diltiazem, verapamil, erythromycin, grapefruit juice, itraconazole, and nefazodone.
Antihistamines	• Hold in patients with a prolonged QT interval. • Monitor for worsened CNS depression with concurrent use with CNS depressants. • Monitor for QT prolongation. • Can cause rash, dry mouth. • Monitor for sedation, injury from impaired motor performance. • Avoid in geriatric patients and patients with a neurodegenerative cognitive disease.	• Hydroxyzine may potentiate meperidine, barbiturates, and other CNS depressants. • Monitor closely when prescribed with classes IA and III antiarrhythmics medications that prolong the QT interval.

Note: All agents are contraindicated in the presence of hypersensitivity to the medication or one of its components.

ANTI-INFECTIVE MEDICATIONS

ANTIBIOTICS

Overview

- Antibiotic classes used in primary care include penicillin, beta lactamases, cephalosporins, macrolides, quinolones, tetracyclines, aminoglycosides, and the phosphoric acid derivative fosfomycin. Evolving drug resistance is reducing the availability of efficacious agents.
- According to the CDC, outpatient antibiotics are often prescribed unnecessarily for respiratory conditions. Specifically, fluoroquinolones have been unnecessarily prescribed in UTIs, colds, and bronchitis.
  - In 2018, the FDA warned against prescribing quinolones when there are other alternatives, due to an increase in resistance and aortic rupture.
  - Moreover, they observed that the antibiotic course for sinus infections was longer than recommended.
- The CDC observed that clinicians caring for children prescribed azithromycin when amoxicillin was indicated in 18% of cases. They made the recommendation for improved prescribing, which are outlined in Table 2.3.

Table 2.3 CDC Outpatient Antibiotic Recommendations

Acute bronchitis	• In patients without comorbidities, provide a delayed prescription and symptomatic care.

Adult uncomplicated sinusitis	• Prescribe antibiotics for a 5- to 7-day course if the following IDSA criteria for uncomplicated infection are present:
	  • No risk of antibiotic-resistant infection
	  • No signs of infection spreading beyond the sinuses
	  • Started to get better in a few days on antibiotics

Pediatric bacterial otitis media, sinusitis, and strep pharyngitis	• *Otitis media:* Prescribe amoxicillin if not received in the past 30 days, otherwise amoxicillin with clavulanic acid. In non-type 1 PCN allergy, prescribe cefdinir, cefuroxime, or ceftriaxone. • *Acute sinusitis:* Prescribe amoxicillin with or without clavulanic acid. • *Strep pharyngitis:* Prescribe amoxicillin or penicillin V. In non-type 1 PCN allergy, prescribe cephalexin, cefadroxil, or macrolide.
Viral URI	• Recommends watchful waiting. Give a delayed prescription with symptomatic care instructions and follow-up in 48 hr.
Bronchiolitis	• Recommends watchful waiting over the course. It will worsen over 2–5 days before improving. Nasal aspiration is the mainstay.
Uncomplicated UTI in adult	• Prescribe fosfomycin in a single dose, OR nitrofurantoin 5–7 days, OR TMP-SMX for 3 days. Reserve quinolone use.
Child with confirmed bacterial UTI	• Prescribe TMP-SMX, amoxicillin and clavulanic acid, or cephalosporin agent • Refer UTIs to urology if obstructive uropathy is suspected.

Drug Resistance in Common Organisms

- Inactivation, beta-lactamase resistance, carbapenem resistance, extended spectrum beta-lactamase resistance, and multidrug resistance occur in many microorganisms. Developments in antibiotic resistance are continually evolving. Antibiotic stewardship is key to management. See Alert.
- ESKAPE organisms (highly virulent, prevalent with evolving resistance):
  - *Enterococcus faecium*: Beta lactamase, vancomycin
  - *Staphylococcus aureus*: Methicillin, vancomycin
  - *Klebsiella pneumoniae*: Beta-lactamase, carbapenem, extended spectrum beta lactamases
  - *Acinetobacter baumannii*: Multidrug resistance
  - *Pseudomonas aeruginosa*: Multidrug resistance
  - *Enterobacter* spp.: Multidrug resistance

General Guidelines

- Follow CDC core elements for antibiotic stewardship, which include infection prevention, screening, and reporting.
- Initiate transmission-based precautions in addition to standard precautions using appropriate PPE in suspect infections.
- Employ routine cleaning and disinfection of environmental surfaces and reusable medical equipment.
- Maintain an updated list of diseases reportable to the public health authority.
- Disseminate hygiene and cleaning instructions for prevention of contact transmission of resistant organisms (e.g., CA-MRSA) in high-risk community settings: Congregate housing, schools, sports facilities, and day care and older adult care facilities.
- Obtain cultures in suspect infections and submit resistant isolates to the health department.
- Follow clinical and treatment guidelines, consider fungal infections for respiratory infections that do not respond to antibiotics (valley fever, histoplasmosis, blastomycosis), monitor for s/s sepsis, perform appropriate diagnostic testing, and optimize TB therapy.

 ALERT

CDC Core Elements for Outpatient Antibiotic Stewardship Checklist

- Display commitment to antibiotic stewardship.
- Use evidence-based diagnostics criteria and treatment.
- Use delayed prescribing or watchful waiting when appropriate.
- Self-evaluate prescribing practicing in antimicrobial therapy.
- Participate in continuing education.
- Educate patients about risks with antibiotic use.

Drug Contraindications

- PCN allergy can be type 1 or non-type 1. Cephalosporins may be prescribed in non-type 1 hypersensitivity.
- Many anti-infective agents are substrates, inhibitors, or inducers of cytochrome P450 enzymes. Use an evidence-based reference to compare the anti-infective to a drug interaction chart such as the Flockhart Table: drug-interactions.medicine.iu.edu/MainTable.aspx
- Antibiotic exposure is the primary risk factor for *Clostridium difficile* colitis. Infection is more common in cephalosporins, fluoroquinolones, aminopenicillins, and clarithromycin but can occur with any antibiotic. Assess for risk of *Clostridium difficile* colitis in all patients complaining of diarrhea.
- See Table 2.4 for antibiotic contraindications, precautions, and interactions.

CEPHALOSPORINS

Mechanism of Action

- Inhibit cell wall synthesis

Indications

Eradicate gram-positive and gram-negative bacteria according to specific generation and agent. Assess for the likelihood of resistance with suspected ESKAPE organism and refer to individual agent for preferred agent within class based on suspected organism.
- *First generation*: Proteus, Escherichia coli, Klebsiella: Methicillin-sensitive Staphylococcus, Streptococci
  - Gram-negative effect < gram positive effect
- *Second generation*: Haemophilus influenzae, Enterobacter aerogenes, and some Neisseria, Proteus, some Escherichia coli, Enterobacter, Klebsiella, Staphylococci, Streptococcus pneumoniae, Streptococcus pyogenes
  - Gram-negative effect > gram positive effect
- *Third generation*: Haemophilus influenzae, and Escherichia coli, Neisseria spp., Proteus, Pseudomonas, Enterobacteriaceae, Citrobacter, Klebsiella, Serratia, Acinetobacter, Moraxella catarrhalis, Clostridium
  - Gram-negative effect > gram-positive effect
  - Treats gram-negative organisms resistant to first- or second-generation cephalosporins
- *Fourth generation*: Most gram-positive + cocci, most gram-negative organisms including Serratia, Pseudomonas, and Enterobacter
- *Fifth generation*: MRSA, gram-positive and gram-negative bacteria
- *Beta-lactam inhibitors*: Ceftazidime–avibactam for pseudomonas in cystic fibrosis

Commonly Prescribed Medications

- *First generation*: Cephalexin, cefadroxil (oral); cefazolin (parenteral)
- *Second generation*: Cefaclor, cefprozil (oral); cefuroxime (oral and parenteral); cefotetan and cefoxitin (parenteral)
- *Third generation*: Cefdinir, cefditoren, cefixime, cefpodoxime, ceftibuten (oral); cefoperazone, cefotaxime, ceftazidime, ceftizoxime, ceftriaxone (parenteral)
- *Fourth generation*: Cefepime cefpirome (parenteral)
- *Fifth generation*: Ceftaroline fosamil (parenteral)
- *Cephalosporin + beta-lactam inhibitor*: Ceftazidime/avibactam, ceftolozane/tazobactam (parenteral)

Diagnostic Testing

Baseline
- Obtain c/s immunoassay for causative organisms based on history and physical exam, as indicated.
- Check BMP and LFTs in suspected hepatorenal impairment.
- Obtain CBC in suspected hemopoietic dysfunction.

Follow-Up
- Monitor sensitivity report to adjust empiric therapy.
- Check BMP and LFTs in suspected hepatorenal impairment.
- Obtain CBC in suspected hemopoietic dysfunction.
- Monitor renal function when antibiotics are administered with aminoglycosides and diuretics.
- *NOTE*: May cause false-positive glucose reaction in urine.

MACROLIDES

Mechanism of Action

- Bind to the 23S rRNA of the 50S ribosomal subunit of susceptible microorganisms inhibiting bacterial protein synthesis

Indications

- Gram-positive and gram-negative chlamydia and mycobacteria
- Common substitute for penicillin type I hypersensitivity
- *Staphylococcus aureus, Streptococcus agalactiae, Streptococcus pneumoniae, Streptococcus pyogenes, Haemophilus ducreyi, Haemophilus influenzae, Moraxella catarrhalis, Neisseria gonorrhoeae, Chlamydophila pneumoniae, Chlamydia trachomatis, Mycoplasma pneumoniae, Bordetella pertussis, Legionella pneumophila*

Commonly Prescribed Medications

- Clarithromycin, fidaxomicin (oral)
- Erythromycin, azithromycin, (oral, ophthalmic, parenteral)
- Azithromycin, clarithromycin, erythromycin (topical)

Diagnostic Testing

Baseline
- C/s, immunoassay for causative organism based on history and physical exam, as indicated
- 12-lead EKG to evaluate QT interval
- BMP and LFTs in suspected hepatorenal impairment
- CBC in suspected hemopoietic dysfunction

Follow-Up
- Monitor sensitivity report to adjust empiric therapy.
- Check BMP and LFTs in suspected hepatorenal impairment.
- Obtain CBC in suspected hemopoietic dysfunction.
- Obtain 12-lead EKG to assess QT interval if irregular rhythm suspected.

PENICILLINS

Mechanism of Action

- Inhibition of cell wall synthesis for gram-positive and some gram-negative bacteria and spirochetes

Indications

- *Natural penicillin*: Streptococci, *pneumococci*, and *staphylococci* that do not produce penicillinase or beta lactamase
- *Semisynthetic/penicillinase-resistant penicillins*: Gram-positive organisms that produce penicillinase and are sensitive to methicillin
- *Aminopenicillins (broad-spectrum)*: Gram-positive and some gram-negative microorganisms that do not produce beta lactamase
- *Extended spectrum penicillin*: Gram-positive skin flora and gram-negative pseudomonas, no beta-lactamase resistance
- *Beta-lactam inhibitors (combined with aminopenicillins or extended-spectrum penicillins)*: Gram-negative and some gram-positive microorganisms that produce beta lactamase

Commonly Prescribed Medications

- *Natural penicillins*: Penicillin VK; penicillin G (parenteral)
- *Semisynthetic penicillinase-resistant penicillins*: Dicloxacillin; oxacillin (parenteral); nafcillin (parenteral)
- *Aminopenicillins*: Amoxicillin; ampicillin (parenteral)
- *Extended-spectrum penicillin*: Piperacillin and ticarcillin (parenteral)
- *Beta-lactam inhibitors (in combination with penicillin)*: Clavulanate (oral and parenteral), sulbactam (parenteral), tazobactam (parenteral)

Diagnostic Testing

Baseline
- Perform skin testing for allergy if type I hypersensitivity is suspected and agent is preferred.
- Obtain c/s, U/A, or rapid immunoassay for causative organisms based on history and physical.
- Check BMP and LFTs in suspected hepatorenal impairment.
- Obtain CBC in suspected hemopoietic dysfunction.

Follow-Up
- Monitor sensitivity report to adjust empiric therapy.
- Check BMP and LFTs in suspected hepatorenal impairment.
- Obtain CBC in suspected hemopoietic dysfunction.

QUINOLONES

Mechanism of Action
- Inhibit enzymes required for bacterial DNA replication

Indications
- Gram-positive and gram-negative bacteria, including *Bacillus anthracis, Enterococcus, MS Staphylococcus, Streptococcus pneumoniae, Streptococcus pyogenes, Haemophilus influenzae, Escherichia coli, Proteus, Klebsiella, Pseudomonas, Salmonella, Serratia, Shigella, Yersinia, Morganella, Moraxella catarrhalis, Neisseria gonorrhoeae, Campylobacter, Citrobacter*

Commonly Prescribed Medications
- Gemifloxacin, ofloxacin (oral)
- Ciprofloxacin, delafloxacin, levofloxacin, moxifloxacin, (oral and parenteral)
- Besifloxacin, ciprofloxacin, gatifloxacin, levofloxacin, moxifloxacin, ofloxacin (ophthalmic)
- Ciprofloxacin, ofloxacin (otic)

Diagnostic Testing

Baseline
- Obtain c/s, based on history and physical exam, as indicated.
- Obtain 12-lead EKG to evaluate QT interval if at risk for irregular heart rhythm.
- Check BMP and LFTs in suspected hepatorenal impairment.
- Obtain CBC in suspected hemopoietic dysfunction.

Follow-Up
- Monitor sensitivity report to adjust empiric therapy.
- Check BMP and LFTs in suspected hepatorenal impairment.
- Obtain CBC in suspected hemopoietic dysfunction.
- Obtain 12-lead EKG to assess QT interval in suspected irregular rhythm.

SULFONAMIDES

Mechanism of Action
- Inhibit biosynthesis of nucleic acids and proteins essential to many bacteria

Indications
- *Gram-positive cocci: Streptococcus pneumoniae, MRSA*
- *Gram-negative: Proteus, Escherichia coli, Enterobacter, Klebsiella, Haemophilus influenzae, Morganella, Shigella, Pneumocystis jiroveci*

Commonly Prescribed Medications

- TMP-SMX (oral and parenteral)
- Sulfacetamide (ophthalmic)
- Erythromycin/sulfisoxazole (oral combination for pediatrics)

Diagnostic Testing

Baseline
- C/s based on history and physical exam, as indicated.
- BMP and LFTs in suspected hepatorenal impairment.
- CBC in suspected hemopoietic dysfunction.
- Folic acid in suspected folate deficiency.

Follow-Up
- Monitor sensitivity report to adjust empiric therapy.
- Check BMP and LFTs in suspected hepatorenal impairment.
- Obtain CBC in suspected hemopoietic dysfunction.
- Check folic acid in suspected folate deficiency.

TETRACYCLINES

Mechanism of Action

- Inhibit protein synthesis by blocking 30S ribosome subunit, preventing bacteria from growing

Indications

- Consider for gram-positive and gram-negative bacteria, chlamydia, mycoplasma, protozoans, or rickettsia. Alternative for syphilis in patients with PCN allergy. Consider doxycycline or minocycline for community-acquired MRSA.

Commonly Prescribed Medications

- Demeclocycline, sarecycline (oral)
- Eravacycline (parenteral)
- Doxycycline, minocycline, omadacycline (oral and parenteral)
- Tetracycline (oral, ophthalmic, and topical)

Diagnostic Testing

Baseline
- Obtain c/s, immunoassay for a causative organism (i.e., RPR, tick-borne diseases) based on history and physical as indicated.
- Check BMP and LFTs in suspected hepatorenal impairment.
- Obtain CBC in suspected hemopoietic dysfunction.

Follow-Up
- Monitor sensitivity report to adjust empiric therapy.
- Check BMP and LFTs in suspected hepatorenal impairment.
- Obtain CBC in suspected hemopoietic dysfunction.

Table 2.4 Antibiotics

Class	Contraindications/Precautions/ Adverse Effects	Drug Interactions
Cephalosporins	• Hold in patients with type 1 allergy to PCN, beta-lactam inhibitors, and cephalosporins. • Monitor for CDAD, hepatotoxicity, serum sickness-like reactions, candidiasis, pancytopenia, and rash. • Use caution in patients with renal impairment. • Positive direct Coombs test is a contraindication.	• Monitor for increased bleeding with warfarin. Monitor renal function with other antibiotics and agents that can cause renal toxicity.
Macrolides	• Hold in patients with allergy and QT prolongation. • Monitor for rash, hepatotoxicity, jaundice, and thrombocytopenia. • Monitor for GI distress and CDAD. • Watch for exacerbation of myasthenia gravis. • Watch for anemia and leukopenia in pediatric patients.	• *Nelfinavir*: Monitor for increased liver function tests and hearing impairment. • *Warfarin*: Monitor for increased prothrombin time. • Macrolides are strong P450 inhibitors. Monitor when administering with other P450 inhibitors.
Penicillins	• Hold in patients with type 1 allergy to PCN, beta lactam inhibitors or cephalosporins, and methicillin-resistant bacteria. • Monitor for CDAD, hepatotoxicity, rash, hemolytic anemia, and renal impairment. • Use caution with history of atopy, cystic fibrosis.	• Tetracyclines decrease effect. • Medication may interfere with BCG, cholera and typhoid immunizations, and oral contraceptives.
Quinolones	• Hold in patients with allergy, QT prolongation, fluoroquinolone resistance, and known myasthenia gravis. • May cause aortic dissection in patients with aortic aneurysm or increased risk (Marfan syndrome, PAD, HTN). • Monitor for ruptured tendon, arthropathy. • Monitor for rash, peripheral neuropathy, seizures, increased ICP, tremors, nephritis, hepatitis, pancytopenia, CDAD, and photosensitivity.	• There is an increased risk of seizures with theophylline, phenytoin. • May increase levels of digoxin, sildenafil, and duloxetine. • Increase serum drug concentration of CYP1A2 substrates (methylxanthines, caffeine, tizanidine, ropinirole, clozapine, olanzapine, and zolpidem). • Increase risk of torsades de pointes with any agents such as amiodarone, TCAs, procainamide, quinidine, sotalol terfenadine, or any medications that prolong the QT interval.

(continued)

Table 2.4 Antibiotics (*continued*)

Class	Contraindications/Precautions/Adverse Effects	Drug Interactions
Sulfonamides	• Hold in patients with allergy, G6PD deficiency, history of drug-induced thrombocytopenia, liver disease, and renal insufficiency. • Monitor for rash, pancytopenia, and CDAD. • Monitor for hyperkalemia, hypoglycemia, hyponatremia. • Use with caution in patients with impaired renal or hepatic dysfunction, folate deficiency, bronchial asthma, CKD, and thyroid disease.	• Use caution with the administration of drugs that are substrates of CYP2C8 (TZDs) and 2C9 (phenytoin, SU) or OCT2 (metformin). • Increased risk of thrombocytopenia with thiazide diuretics. • *Warfarin (CYP2C9)*: Monitor for increased prothrombin time. • Increase risk of adverse effects with cyclosporine, digoxin, pyrimethamine, TCAs, ACEI
Tetracyclines	• Hold in patients with allergy, patients who are pregnant and lactating, children age <8 years, and patients with esophageal irritation. • Monitor for GI distress, teeth discoloration, rash, renal toxicity, hepatotoxicity, hemolytic anemia, pancytopenia, and lupus-like syndrome.	• PCN decreases effect. • Oral contraceptives are less effective. • Doxycycline, a tetracycline derivative, lowers serum levels of carbamazepine, phenytoin, thus increasing seizure risk. • Anticoagulants may require downward adjustment. • Antacids impair absorption.

ANTIFUNGALS

Overview

- Antifungals are used to treat mycotic infections. Common infections treated in primary care include oropharyngeal and vaginal candidiasis, onychomycosis, and tinea infections.
- Common antifungal categories used in primary care include polyenes, azoles, and allylamines.
- Careful attention is warranted in patients who are immunocompromised by maturation, disease, medication, or procedures. Oral and gastrointestinal candidiasis can progress to candidemia and can become invasive, causing multisystem organ involvement.
- Drug resistance has emerged in many antifungal categories. Multidrug-resistant *Candida auris* has been isolated in acute care hospitals and long-term care facilities. Discharged patients who have central lines are at the highest risk for this infection. Immunocompromised patients who present in primary care with suspected *Candida auris* fungal infection and signs of systemic illness require hospitalization for management.
- *Candida auris* spreads from contaminated surfaces and requires specialized lab handling. If suspected, thorough environmental cleaning is required in compliance with public health standards.

General Guidelines

- Use the Flockhart chart to assess medication profile when prescribing an azole.
- Prescribe antifungal drugs appropriately and document the dose, duration, and indication for every antifungal prescription.

- Test for antifungal resistance in patients with an invasive disease who are not improving with first-line antifungal drugs.
- Be aware of resistance patterns, including antifungal resistance, in the facility and community.
- Table 2.5 provides information on contraindications, precautions, and interactions.

ALLYLAMINE DERIVATIVES

Mechanism of Action

- Inhibit biosynthesis of ergosterol, an essential component of the fungal cell membrane, via inhibition of the squalene epoxidase enzyme

Indications

- Dermatophytosis, tinea

Commonly Prescribed Medications

- Butenafine (topical)
- Terbinafine (oral and topical)

Diagnostic Testing

Baseline
- Fungal culture
- LFTs in suspected hepatic impairment
- CBC in suspected hemopoietic dysfunction
- 12-lead EKG in suspected irregular heart rhythm

Follow-Up
- Perform antifungal susceptibility testing if no response to therapy.
- Check LFTs in suspected hepatic impairment.
- Obtain CBC in suspected hemopoietic dysfunction.
- Obtain 12-lead EKG with tachycardia.

AZOLES

Mechanism of Action

- Weaken structure of cell membrane by blocking the synthesis of cytochrome P450 enzyme lanosterol, preventing conversion to ergosterol

Indications

- Dermatophytosis, candidiasis, coccidioidomycosis, histoplasmosis/blastomycosis

Commonly Prescribed Medications

- Ketoconazole (oral and topical)
- Fluconazole, isavuconazonium, itraconazole, posaconazole, and voriconazole (oral and parenteral)
- Clotrimazole, econazole efinaconazole, ketoconazole, luliconazole, miconazole, sertaconazole, and sulconazole (topical)
- Butoconazole, clotrimazole, miconazole, terconazole, and tioconazole (intravaginal)

Diagnostic Testing

Baseline
- Fungal culture
- BMP and LFTs in suspected hepatorenal impairment
- CBC in suspected hemopoietic dysfunction
- 12-lead EKG to evaluate QT interval in patients at risk

Follow-Up
- Perform antifungal susceptibility testing if no response.
- Check BMP and LFTs in suspected hepatorenal impairment.
- Obtain CBC in suspected hemopoietic dysfunction.
- Obtain 12-lead EKG in suspected prolonged QT interval.
- Monitor BG more closely in diabetic patients.

POLYENES

Mechanism of Action

- Bind to ergosterol, creating pores in the cell membrane, leading to cell death

Indications

- *Superficial candidiasis (not systemic)*: Cutaneous, oropharyngeal, intestinal.
- Note: Life-threatening systemic candidiasis is treated with parenteral formulations.

Commonly Prescribed Medications

- Mycostatin (oral and topical)
- Amphotericin B, anidulafungin, caspofungin, micafungin (parenteral)

Diagnostic Testing

Baseline
- Obtain KOH smear.
- Check BMP, LFTs, and CBC before initiating parenteral formulations.

Follow-Up
- If no response, cultures or other diagnostic methods should be repeated.
- Check BMP and LFTs in suspected hepatorenal impairment.
- Obtain CBC in suspected hemopoietic dysfunction.

Table 2.5 Antifungals

Class	Contraindications/Precautions/Adverse Effects	Drug Interactions
Polyenes	• Hold for patients with allergy. • Do not use topical agents for treatment of systemic infections. • Monitor for local irritation, gastrointestinal upset. • Systemic polyenes can cause arrhythmias, hypotension/cardiogenic shock, anemia, nephropathy, ototoxicity, hypomagnesemia, hypokalemia, neuropathy. Parenteral formulations are associated with infusion reactions and phlebitis.	• None for oral suspension. • Parenteral infusions interact with blood products and antineoplastic therapy. There is synergistic hypokalemia with potassium-depleting diuretics, beta agonists, and insulin. • Increased risk of digoxin toxicity when taken with parenteral formulations.

Class	Contraindications/Precautions/Adverse Effects	Drug Interactions
Azoles	• Do not prescribe to patients with allergy to azoles, prolonged QT interval, myopathy, or liver disease. • Monitor for hepatotoxicity, adrenal insufficiency, testosterone insufficiency, hemolytic anemia, leukopenia, and thrombocytopenia. • Monitor for hypokalemia in patients taking azoles especially when combined with other agents that cause hypokalemia.	• Warfarin increases bleeding times. • QT-prolonging drugs are contraindicated. • Antacids, PPIs, and H2 antagonists may interfere with absorption of ketoconazole. • Azoles interact with medications that inhibit cytochrome P450 metabolism (benzodiazepines, immunosuppressants, anxiolytics, statins, celecoxib, some anticonvulsants). • Use caution when prescribing for patients taking digoxin, opioids, antiplatelets, anticoagulants, and urologic drugs.
Allylamine derivatives	• Hold in patients with allergy, liver disease, or SLE. • Monitor for infection, neutropenia, and hepatotoxicity. • Monitor liver enzymes and CBC. • Monitor for loss of taste and depression symptoms.	• CYP2D6 inhibitor increases drug effect of TCAs, MAOIs type B, and antiarrhythmics. • Terbinafine drug effect is increased by cimetidine.

ANTIVIRALS

Overview

- Antiviral therapy that is used to treat HIV and hepatitis B and C viruses is prescribed by HIV specialists and hepatologists, respectfully.
- HIV PrEP is prescribed at HIV clinics, Planned Parenthood, health centers, urgent care, and select primary care offices with specialized training.
- The most frequently treated viral infections in primary care are herpes viruses and influenza A and B viruses. Herpes virus medications reduce the severity of or suppress HSV 1, HSV 2, and varicella zoster.

General Guidelines

- PrEP health centers perform HIV and STI counseling and testing, assess renal function and prescribe daily dose combination antiretroviral therapy, and monitor patient every 3 months for tolerance, adherence, and outcomes.
- Gastroenterologist or hepatologist performs baseline testing for a tolerance of antiviral therapy for chronic hepatitis B, C infections. Periodic evaluation for a compilation of antivirals and interferons is performed. Screening for hepatitis C should be performed on all adults in primary care.
- Influenza antivirals are endonuclease or neuraminidase inhibitors that can be prescribed to reduce the severity of infection or prophylactically to prevent community spread. The CDC provides annual guidance with the specific agent and indications for use.
- Topical DNA polymerase inhibitors or prodrugs that inhibit DNA replication are prescribed to be taken close to the onset of presentation or continuously for 12 months for suppression.
- See Table 2.6 for contraindications, precautions, and adverse effects.

NEURAMINIDASE INHIBITORS

Mechanism of Action

- Inhibit viral neuraminidases to prevent the virus from crossing the mucous lining

Indications

- Influenza prophylaxis or to reduce the severity of the disease

Commonly Prescribed Medications

- Baloxavir marboxil, oseltamivir (oral)
- Peramivir (parenteral)
- Zanamivir (inhalation)

Diagnostic Testing

Baseline

- Nasal swab for influenza
- BMP and LFTs in suspected hepatorenal impairment
- CBC in suspected hemopoietic dysfunction

Follow-Up

- Check BMP and LFTs in suspected hepatorenal impairment.
- Obtain CBC in suspected bleeding.

NUCLEOSIDE ANALOGS

Mechanism of Action

- Inhibit viral DNA polymerase

Indications

- HSV 1, HSV 2, varicella zoster

Commonly Prescribed Medications

- Famciclovir, valacyclovir (oral)
- Acyclovir (oral and parenteral)
- Penciclovir (topical)

Diagnostic Testing

Baseline

- BMP and LFTs in suspected hepatorenal impairment
- CBC in suspected hemopoietic dysfunction

Follow-Up

- Check BMP and LFTs in suspected hepatorenal impairment.
- Obtain CBC in suspected hemopoietic dysfunction.

 POP QUIZ 2.2

A 15-year-old male presents to the primary care provider with an abscess to his left knee with localized erythema, edema, and tenderness. He states that it developed after he participated in a wrestling boot camp at school. What medications and monitoring should the nurse practitioner include in the plan?

Table 2.6 Antivirals

Class	Contraindications/Precautions/ Adverse Effects	Drug Interactions
Neuraminidase inhibitors	• Hold for patients with allergy. • Use caution in liver, renal, respiratory, or cardiac disease. • Monitor for delirium, seizure, rash, and GI bleeding.	• Clopidogrel decreases the drug level of medication. • Do not give within 2 weeks before or 48 hr after live virus influenza vaccination. • Probenecid increases the drug level.
Nucleoside analogs	• Hold for patients with allergy. • Monitor for CNS adverse events, hepatotoxicity, renal colic, nephropathy, thrombocytopenia, and GI symptoms. • Monitor for drug resistance.	• No significant drug interactions.

CARDIOVASCULAR MEDICATIONS

HEART FAILURE MEDICATIONS

Loop diuretics and digoxin will be discussed in this section. Refer to the Hypertension Medications section for other first-line heart failure medications, which are common to both hypertension and HF.

Overview

- Medications that are used in primary care to manage heart failure are ACEIs, ARBs, beta blockers, aldosterone antagonists, diuretics, vasodilators, neprilysin inhibitors/ARBs, digoxin, and ivabradine.
- Heart failure medications are prescribed by stage of disease.
  - *Stage A*: Risk factor modification of ASCVD, CKD, DM, HTN, and thromboembolic events. Use ACEIs, ARBs, or beta blockers in patients with HTN who are at risk for HF. Target SBP <130 mm.
  - *Stage B*: Use ACEIs, ARBs, or beta blocker in asymptomatic structural heart disease with EF ≤40%. Consider carvedilol to improve vascular outcomes.
  - *Stage C*: Titrate ACEIs, ARBs, and beta blocker with diuretics to reduce symptoms. Consider referral to cardiology.
  - *Stage D*: Refer to cardiology for ivabradine, sacubitril/valsartan, and chronic inotropes to restore organ perfusion and to enhance contractility in refractory HF.

General Guidelines

- Medications used in the management of comorbidities can cause exacerbations of HF.
- Check all medications for cardiotoxicity, nephrotoxicity, and altered fluid and electrolyte risks that can exacerbate hypertension and renal dysfunction.
- Target lower serum digoxin levels (0.5–0.9 ng/mL) in patients taking cardiac glycosides.
- Prescribe hydralazine and/or isosorbide dinitrate in African American patients or patients who cannot tolerate ACEIs or ARBs.
- See Table 2.7 at the end of this section for contraindications, precautions, and adverse effects.

LOOP DIURETICS

Mechanism of Action

- Inhibit sodium and chloride reabsorption at proximal and distal tubules and loop of Henle causing excretion of Na, K+, Mg, Ca, HCO_3 ion, and water.

Indications

- HF with fluid overload in stages 2 to 4

Commonly Prescribed Medications

- Torsemide (oral)
- Bumetanide, furosemide (oral and parenteral)

Diagnostic Testing

Baseline
- BMP and electrolytes for imbalance or renal impairment
- GFR and stage CKD
- CBC in suspected hemopoietic dysfunction
- Baseline uric acid in patients at risk for gout

Follow-Up
- Obtain BMP, Ca, Phos, Mg in suspected renal dysfunction or electrolyte anomalies.
- Monitor BG in patients with diabetes.
- Obtain CBC in suspected hematologic function.
- Obtain uric acid level in suspected gout or renal colic.

CARDIAC GLYCOSIDE

Mechanism of Action

- Slows down conduction through the AV node in atrial fibrillation and modestly improves cardiac contractility in SHF

Indications

- Symptomatic SHF stages 2 to 4, atrial fibrillation

Commonly Prescribed Medications

- Digoxin (oral and parenteral)

Diagnostic Testing

Baseline
- BMP, Mg, and Ca to evaluate electrolytes and renal function
- CBC in suspected hemopoietic dysfunction
- 12-lead EKG to evaluate for ventricular arrythmias, sick sinus syndrome, WPW syndrome, and bradycardia
- Echocardiogram to evaluate EF and the presence of idiopathic hypertrophic subaortic stenosis or pericarditis

Follow-Up
- Check BMP, LFTs, Mg, and Ca to evaluate electrolytes and hepatorenal function.
- Monitor BG in patients with diabetes.
- Obtain CBC in suspected hemopoietic dysfunction.
- Monitor serum digoxin level (0.5–0.9 ng/mL).
- Obtain 12-lead EKG, echocardiogram with suspected arrhythmia, decreased cardiac output, and periodic evaluation.

Table 2.7 Heart Failure Medications

Class	Contraindications/Precautions/Adverse Effects	Drug Interactions
Loop diuretics	• Hold with hypersensitivity to loop diuretics. Investigate allergies to sulfa and thiazide diuretics to identify the possibility of cross sensitivity. • Monitor for dehydration, AKI, GFR <30, and hypotension. • Monitor for pancreatitis, ototoxicity, and aplastic anemia. • Monitor for hypokalemia, hyponatremia, hypochloremia alkalosis, hyperglycemia, hyperuricemia, and hypocalcemia.	• Risk for digitalis toxicity increases with uncorrected hypokalemia from potassium-depleting diuretics. • *Monitor for addition of medications that potentiate hypokalemia*: Corticosteroids, insulin, beta agonists, and sympathomimetics and correct potassium to prevent adverse events. • Discontinue potassium supplementation when ACEIs, ARBs, or aldosterone antagonists are added to the medication profile.
Cardiac glycoside	• Hold for patients with digoxin toxicity, tachy/brady arrhythmias, bradycardia, and AV block. • Hypokalemia, hypomagnesemia, and hypercalcemia exacerbate digoxin toxicity. • Do not administer to patients with WPW syndrome or hypertrophic subaortic stenosis. • Use caution in patients with impaired renal function, thyroid disease, and MI.	• Potassium-depleting medications can increase the risk of digitalis toxicity. • Macrolide antibiotics, tetracyclines, quinidine, verapamil, amiodarone, propafenone, indomethacin, itraconazole, alprazolam, and spironolactone may raise the serum digoxin level. • Antacids, kaolin-pectin, sulfasalazine, neomycin, cholestyramine, certain anticancer drugs, metoclopramide, and rifampin may decrease serum digoxin level. • Concomitant use of digoxin and sympathomimetics or succinylcholine increases the risk of cardiac arrhythmias.

Note: All agents are contraindicated in the presence of hypersensitivity to the medication or one of its components.

HYPERLIPIDEMIA MEDICATIONS

Overview

• The ACC recommends statins as the primary medications for risk modification of lipids for ASCVD events. In this model of care, statins are prescribed based on personal risk for ASCVD, for patients age 40 to 75 years, or for patients in whom familial hypercholesterolemia is present.
• Medications are prescribed in patients in whom LDL ≥70 or ≤190, according to the percentile risk for an ASCVD event.
• Statin medications are prescribed according to their risk intensity—moderate or high based on the ASCVD risk calculator:
  • *No risk*: LDL level ≥190 mg/dL, prescribe high-intensity statin.
  • *Borderline risk*: 5% to 7.5%, prescribe moderate-intensity statin.
  • *Intermediate risk*: ≥7.6% to 20%, prescribe moderate- to high-intensity statin if risk enhancers present.
  • *High risk*: ≥20%, prescribe high-intensity statin to reduce LDL by ≥50%.

Mechanism of Action

- Prevent conversion of HMG-CoA to mevalonate, limiting the production of cholesterol
- Reduce LDL and raise HDL cholesterol

Indications

- Elevated LDL >190, diabetes mellitus, or risk for ASCVD event >5% with risk enhancers

Commonly Prescribed Medications

- *Low intensity*: Simvastatin 10 mg, lovastatin 20 mg (oral)
- *Moderate intensity*: Atorvastatin 10 to 20 mg, rosuvastatin 5 to 10 mg, lovastatin 40 to 80 mg, simvastatin 20 to 40 mg (oral)
- *High intensity*: Atorvastatin 40 to 80 mg, rosuvastatin 20 to 40 mg (oral)
- See Table 2.8 for contraindications, precautions, and adverse effects.

Diagnostic Testing

Baseline
- Check BMP and LFTs to evaluate for hepatorenal function.
- Check HbA1c to assess glycemic control.
- Evaluate CBC for hemopoietic function.
- Calculate ASCVD risk.

Follow-Up
- Check BMP and LFTs to evaluate for suspected hepatorenal dysfunction.
- Check HbA1c to assess glycemic control.
- Evaluate CBC in suspected pancytopenia.
- Evaluate CPK level with myalgia.
- Calculate ASCVD risk to evaluate effectiveness.

Table 2.8 Statin Medications

Contraindications/Precautions/Adverse Effects	Drug Interactions
<ul><li>Hold in rhabdomyolysis, active liver disease, pregnancy, nursing, coadministration with strong CYP3A4 inhibitors, gemfibrozil, cyclosporine, or danazol.</li><li>Monitor for myopathy seen with 3A4 medications, hepatotoxicity.</li><li>Monitor for increases in HbA1c, lupus-like syndromes, eosinophilia, rash, memory impairment, pancytopenia, with hemolytic anemia.</li></ul>	<ul><li>Do not give with strong CYP3A4 inhibitors, gemfibrozil, cyclosporine, azoles, macrolides, or danazol.</li><li>PPI, fluvoxamine, digoxin, amiodarone, diltiazem, verapamil, and cimetidine can increase the effect.</li><li>Niacin and grapefruit juice can increase myopathy.</li><li>St. John's wort, aluminum, and magnesium antacids decrease effect.</li></ul>

HYPERTENSION MEDICATIONS

Overview

- Antihypertensive medications (see Table 2.9 at the end of this section) reduce fluid volume, decrease arterial resistance, promote vasodilation, and optimize cardiac output. According to the ACC, the primary medications to treat hypertension are thiazide diuretics, ACEIs, ARBs, and calcium channel blockers. They are used in addition to lifestyle modifications to achieve desired outcomes.
- Goals for antihypertensive therapy are mutually agreed upon and consider the patients' percentile risk of ASCVD events and HF. The ACC's targets for blood pressure are based on risk and recommended therapy.
- NO RISK FOR ASCVD
  - Maintain SBP <120 and DBP <80.
  - Continue primary prevention and reassess in 1 year.
  - Target BP 120 to 129/80.
  - Use nonpharmacologic therapy and reassess in 3 to 6 months.
- *Stage 1 hypertension*: SBP 130 to 139, DBP 80 to 89
  - *ASCVD risk >10%*: Maintain SBP <130 or DBP <80.
  - Initiate BP medication and nonpharmacologic therapy.
  - Reevaluate in 1 month.
    - ○ *BP goal met*: Reassess in 3 to 6 months.
    - ○ *BP goal not met*: Optimize adherence and consider intensification of therapy.
  - *ASCVD risk <10%*: Maintain SBP <140 or DBP <90.
  - Reassess BP every 3 to 6 months if ASCVD risk is <10%; provide nonpharmacologic therapy; monitor for progression.
- *Stage 2 hypertension*: SBP ≥140/90
  - Initiate BP medication and nonpharmacologic therapy.
  - Reevaluate in 1 month.
    - ○ *BP goal met*: Reassess in 3 to 6 months.
    - ○ *BP goal not met*: Optimize adherence and consider intensification of therapy.

General Guidelines

- Prescribe thiazide diuretic as the initial medication if there is no compelling indication for alternative agents.
  - HCTZ is recommended for African American or Black patients of Caribbean descent, patients with edema, and geriatric and pediatric patients.
  - HCTZ can exacerbate hypokalemia when prescribed with loop diuretics in HF.
- Prescribe ACEI or ARB to patients with a higher risk of HF.
  - Do not prescribe to women who are pregnant or women who are trying to conceive.
  - Do not prescribe ACEIs and ARBs together with or without aldosterone antagonists or renin inhibitors.
  - Do not prescribe with potassium supplements or hyperkalemia in CKD. May be prescribed to patients with CKD who have normokalemia or are on dialysis.
- Prescribe CCB in patients who are older adults, are African American, are diagnosed with Prinzmetal angina, have Raynaud's syndrome, or are renal colic.
  - Do not prescribe to patients with HF.
  - Do not prescribe nondihydropyridine CCB to patients with bradycardia, heart block, or sick sinus syndrome.
- Prescribe cardioselective beta blockers as an adjunct to ACEI or ARB in patients with HF or myocardial infarction.
  - To avoid rebound hypertension, do not stop beta blocker abruptly.
- Prescribe hydralazine to African American patients with HF.
- Prescribe loop diuretics, aldosterone antagonists, hydralazine, beta blockers, central acting agents, and direct vasodilators as second-line therapy or if there is a compelling reason to prescribe.

General Precautions

- Conduct fall risk assessment and provide instruction to protect from fall injury due to orthostatic changes.
- Never prescribe two medications of the same class or target the same action except for opposing diuretics and CCB.
- Never prescribe ACEIs, ARBs, or aldosterone antagonist together, nor to a woman who is pregnant or trying to conceive.
- Prescribe centrally acting agents as a last-line therapy.
  - Note that hypertensive crisis in the abrupt withdrawal of clonidine precludes their use where there is no compelling indication.
- Prescribe alpha-1 blockers (terazosin, prazosin) as second-line therapy in BPH. There is a greater risk of orthostatic hypotension and falls in older adults.
- Do not prescribe nonselective beta blockers to patients with asthma/COPD or depression.

Patient Population Considerations

Women (conception/pregnancy/lactation)

- Screen pregnant women at each visit. Criteria for the diagnosis of preeclampsia include elevated blood pressure ($\geq140/90$) on two occasions 4 hr apart, after 20 weeks.
- Target BP <160/110 in pregnant women with chronic hypertension. Prescribe labetalol (alpha–beta blocker) or extended-release nifedipine. Consider its use in women of reproductive age.

Geriatrics

- Consider target BP <150/90 in patients age 65 or older.
- Weigh the risk of orthostatic hypotension, adverse effects, and falls against polypharmacology.

Pediatrics

- Pediatric hypertension is diagnosed in children age <13 years by averaging BP over three visits and excluding secondary causes. Children and adolescents who have failed lifestyle modifications or who have stage 2 HTN with no modifiable risk factors (i.e., obesity) should be started on an ACEI, ARB, CCB, or thiazide diuretic.

THIAZIDE DIURETICS

Mechanism of Action

- Inhibit sodium reabsorption at distal tubules causing excretion of Na, K+, HCO_3 ion, and water

Indications

- First-line HTN therapy for patients of African or Caribbean descent, patients with HF or edema, and geriatric and pediatric patients

Commonly Prescribed Medications

- Chlorthalidone, chlorothiazide, hydrochlorothiazide, indapamide, methyclothiazide, metolazone (oral)

Diagnostic Testing

Baseline

- Check BMP and electrolytes for imbalance or renal impairment.
- Calculate GFR and stage CKD.
- Obtain CBC in suspected hemopoietic dysfunction.
- Obtain baseline lipid levels.
- Obtain baseline uric acid in patients at risk for gout.

Follow-Up
- Obtain BMP, Ca, Phos, Mg in suspected renal dysfunction or electrolyte anomalies.
- Monitor BG in patients with diabetes.
- Monitor for elevated lipid levels.
- Obtain CBC in suspected hematologic function.
- Obtain uric acid level in suspected gout or renal colic.

ANGIOTENSIN CONVERTING ENZYME INHIBITORS

Mechanism of Action

- Inhibit the conversion of angiotensin I to angiotensin II to dilate arteries and veins, inhibit aldosterone promoting diuresis, are nephroprotective due to renal arteriole vasodilation, limit cardiac and vascular remodeling, and inhibit bradykinin

Indications

- First-line agent for HTN in patients experiencing or at risk for HF, LVH, CVHD, DM, or CKD on dialysis
- For patients with CKD without hyperkalemia who can tolerate the medication with close monitoring of GFR
- Fewer benefits realized in African American patients

Commonly Prescribed Medications

- Benazepril, captopril, fosinopril, lisinopril, moexipril, perindopril, quinapril, ramipril, trandolapril (oral)
- Enalapril (oral and parenteral)

Diagnostic Testing

Baseline
- Check BMP and electrolytes for imbalance or renal impairment.
- Calculate GFR and stage CKD.
- Obtain CBC in suspected hemopoietic dysfunction.

Follow-Up
- Obtain BMP in suspected renal dysfunction or hyperkalemia and hyponatremia.
- Obtain CBC in suspected pancytopenia.

ANGIOTENSIN RECEPTOR BLOCKERS

Mechanism of Action

- Block vasoconstriction and aldosterone-secreting effects of angiotensin II to promote natriuresis and vasodilation

Indications

- First-line agent for patients at risk for or experiencing HF, LVH, nephropathy, DM
- Fewer benefits realized in African American patients

Commonly Prescribed Medications

- Azilsartan, candesartan, eprosartan, irbesartan, losartan, olmesartan, telmisartan, valsartan (oral)

Diagnostic Testing

Baseline
- Check BMP and electrolytes for imbalance or renal impairment.
- Calculate GFR and stage CKD.
- Obtain CBC in suspected hemopoietic dysfunction.

Follow-Up
- Obtain BMP in suspected renal dysfunction or hyperkalemia and hyponatremia.
- Obtain CBC in suspected pancytopenia.

CALCIUM CHANNEL BLOCKERS

Mechanism of Action

- Reduce peripheral resistance by inhibiting calcium ion influx in the arterial vascular smooth muscle of peripheral circulation.
- Reduce stroke volume through their effect on the cardiac muscle.

Indications

- First-line agent in hypertension.
- Can be considered in older adults and African American patients who do not respond to thiazide diuretics.
- Parenteral formulations can be used in hypertensive emergencies without acute MI or HF.
- For HTN in pregnant patients with chronic hypertension.
- Dihydropyridine causes dose-related peripheral edema.
- Nondihydropyridine lowers heart rate and can be used in atrial fibrillation and supraventricular tachycardias without heart failure but should not be used in ventricular dysrhythmia, in acute MI, or in combination with beta blockers.

Commonly Prescribed Medications

- *Dihydropyridine*: Amlodipine, felodipine, isradipine, nisoldipine (oral)
- Clevidipine (parenteral)
- Nicardipine (oral and parenteral)
- Nifedipine (oral and sublingual)
- *Nondihydropyridine*: Diltiazem, verapamil (oral and parenteral)

Diagnostic Testing

Baseline
- Check BMP and LFTs to evaluate hepatorenal function.
- Monitor BG in patients with diabetes.
- Obtain 12-lead EKG to exclude bradycardia and heart block with non-dihydropyridines.
- Obtain echocardiogram to exclude heart failure.

Follow-Up
- Check BMP and LFTs in suspected hepatorenal dysfunction.
- Monitor BG in patients with diabetes.
- Obtain 12-lead EKG to evaluate for bradycardia and heart block with non-dihydropyridines.
- Obtain echocardiogram in suspected heart failure.

CARDIOSELECTIVE BETA BLOCKERS

Mechanism of Action

- Antagonism of catecholamines at beta receptors reduces stroke volume and heart rate; central effect leading to reduced sympathetic peripheral outflow
- Suppression of renin supports vasodilation (metoprolol)

Indications

- For HTN in patients at risk for or experiencing ACS, HF, or tachyarrhythmias.
  - Metoprolol is cardioselective and decreases mortality in MI.
- Propranolol is a *nonselective beta blocker* used in thyrotoxicosis, panic disorder, and tremor.

Commonly Prescribed Medications

- Nonselective
  - Nadolol (oral)
  - Propranolol, sotalol (oral and parenteral formulations)
- Cardioselective
  - Acebutolol, atenolol, betaxolol, bisoprolol (oral)
  - Metoprolol (oral and parenteral)
  - Esmolol (parenteral)

Diagnostic Testing

Baseline
- Check BMP and LFTs to evaluate hepatorenal function.
- Obtain baseline lipid levels.
- Monitor BG in patients with diabetes.
- Obtain 12-lead EKG to exclude bradycardia and heart block.
- Obtain echocardiogram to evaluate for the presence of heart failure.

Follow-Up
- Check BMP and LFTs in suspected hepatorenal dysfunction.
- Monitor for hypoglycemia and hypoglycemia unawareness in patients with diabetes.
- Monitor for hyperlipidemia.
- Obtain 12-lead EKG to evaluate for bradycardia and heart block.
- Obtain echocardiogram in suspected heart failure.

ALPHA–BETA BLOCKERS

Mechanism of Action

- Antagonism of catecholamines at beta receptors reduces stroke volume and heart rate and enhances vasodilation and reduces peripheral resistance due to alpha blockade.

Indications

- For HTN in patients at risk for or experiencing HF

Commonly Prescribed Medications

- Alpha–beta selective:
  - Carvedilol (oral)
  - Labetalol (oral and parenteral)

Diagnostic Testing

Baseline
- Check BMP and LFTs to evaluate hepatorenal function.
- Obtain baseline lipid levels.
- Monitor BG in patients with diabetes.
- Obtain 12-lead EKG to exclude bradycardia and heart block.
- Obtain echocardiogram to evaluate ejection fraction and wall motion.

Follow-Up
- Check BMP and LFTs in suspected hepatorenal dysfunction.
- Monitor for hypoglycemia and hypoglycemia unawareness in patients with diabetes.
- Monitor for hyperlipidemia.
- Obtain 12-lead EKG to evaluate for bradycardia and heart block.
- Obtain echocardiogram in worsening heart failure.

ALDOSTERONE RECEPTOR ANTAGONISTS

Mechanism of Action

- Aldosterone antagonist binds at the Na–K exchange site in distal tubules, causing Na, Cl^-, and water excretion.

Indications

- Second-line agent in hypertension with hypokalemia secondary to potassium-depleting diuretic; adjunct to potassium-depleting diuretics in patients who cannot tolerate ACEI or angiotensin II blockade
- Primary hyperaldosteronism, edema in cirrhosis, nephrotic syndrome

Commonly Prescribed Medications

- Spironolactone, eplerenone (oral)

Diagnostic Testing

Baseline
- Obtain BMP and LFTs to evaluate electrolytes and hepatorenal function.
- Calculate GFR and stage CKD.
- Obtain baseline serum Ca, Mg, uric acid, and BG.
- Check CBC for agranulocytosis and thrombocytopenia.

Follow-Up
- Monitor BMP and LFTs for hepatorenal dysfunction.
- Monitor serum Ca, Mg, potassium, uric acid, and BG periodically.
- Monitor CBC for agranulocytosis and thrombocytopenia.

 POP QUIZ 2.3

A 55-year-old female presents to the primary care provider with a blood pressure of 210/108 mm-Hg. She denies symptoms of stroke, heart failure, and MI. She reports that she has gained 25 lbs over the past 2 years and her BMI is now 29. She has a prior history of gestational diabetes. What medications and monitoring should be included in the plan?

Table 2.9 Antihypertensive Medications

Class	Contraindications/Precautions/ Adverse Effects	Drug Interactions
Thiazide diuretics	• Hold with known allergy to sulfonamide-derived drugs. • Monitor for AKI, dehydration, and hypotension. • Monitor for hypokalemia, hyponatremia, hypochloremia, alkalosis, and hyperglycemia. • Monitor for worsened hypokalemia in patients with history of bronchial asthma using beta agonists or patients with diabetes using insulin. • Monitor for hyperuricemia, hypercalcemia, hyperlipidemia, and aplastic anemia.	• Digitalis toxicity may occur with hypokalemia. • Potentiates hypokalemia with an agent that decreases potassium such as loop diuretics, corticosteroids, insulin, beta agonists, and sympathomimetics. • Discontinue potassium supplementation when ACEIs, ARBs, or aldosterone antagonist are added to medication profile.
ACEIs	• Hold in the presence of bradykinin cough, angioedema, pregnancy, AKI. • Monitor for hyperkalemia, hyponatremia, hypotension, agranulocytosis. • Monitor for acute renal failure and hepatic dysfunction.	• *Potentiates hyperkalemia with any agent that can increase potassium or dual blockade of RAS*: Aliskiren, spironolactone, ARBs, NSAIDs, potassium supplements, heparin, trimethoprim, triamterene, amiloride. • Increased risk of lithium toxicity. • ASA, NSAIDs, and COX-2 inhibitors decrease the efficacy of drug and may decrease renal function.
ARBs	• Hold in the presence of bradykinin cough, angioedema, pregnancy, AKI. • Monitor for hyperkalemia, hyponatremia, hypotension, agranulocytosis, and anemia. • Monitor for acute renal failure and hepatic dysfunction.	• *Potentiates hyperkalemia with any agent that can increase potassium or dual blockade of RAS*: Aliskiren, spironolactone, ACEIs, NSAIDs, COX-2 inhibitors, potassium supplements, heparin, trimethoprim, triamterene, and amiloride. • Increased risk of lithium toxicity. • ASA, NSAIDs, and COX-2 inhibitors decrease the efficacy of drug and may decrease renal function.

(continued)

Table 2.9 Antihypertensive Medications (*continued*)

Class	Contraindications/Precautions/ Adverse Effects	Drug Interactions
CCBs: Nifedipines	• Hold in patients with worsening HF/ cardiogenic shock and acute myocardial infarction ≤4weeks. • Monitor for HF, peripheral edema, reflex tachycardia, hypotension, and hyperglycemia. • Use cautiously in the presence of depression, aortic stenosis, GI stenosis/ constipation, cirrhosis, and dizziness. • Monitor for agranulocytosis and thrombocytopenia. • Monitor hepatic, renal, and cardiac function closely in older patients. • Use caution with concurrent use of beta blockers due to increased risk of HF.	• Concomitant administration with strong CYP3A4 inducers (i.e., rifampin, rifabutin, phenobarbital, phenytoin, carbamazepine, St. John's wort) significantly reduces the nifedipine effect. • CYP3A inhibitors (i.e., fluoxetine, phenytoin, valproic acid, ketoconazole, fluconazole, itraconazole clarithromycin, erythromycin, grapefruit, nefazodone, saquinavir, indinavir, nelfinavir, ritonavir, quinidine), and substrates (tacrolimus) may increase nifedipine effect. • Increased hypotension with timolol, central-acting alpha-1 blockers, diuretics, and PDE5 inhibitors. • Digoxin toxicity when added to digoxin. • Increased PT/INR with warfarin.
CCBs: Diltiazem	• Hold in patients with HF, bradycardia, acute MI, heart block, and hypotension. • Monitor for hepatotoxicity, severe skin reactions, and worsening HF. • Monitor for agranulocytosis, thrombocytopenia, and hyperglycemia.	• Diltiazem is a substrate and inhibitor of P450 3A4. • Limit doses of statins and avoid coadministration with rifampin. • Do not coadminister with beta blocker to avoid bradycardia.
Cardioselective beta blockers	• Hold in bradycardia and second- or third-degree heart block, decompensated HF/cardiogenic shock, bronchospastic disease, and hypotension. • Use caution in patients with diabetes, depression, HF, COPD, Raynaud's syndrome, and liver impairment. • Monitor for liver impairment, agranulocytosis, thrombocytopenia, hypoglycemia, and hyperkalemia.	• Catecholamine-depleting drugs (reserpine, MAOIs) may have an additive effect. • CYP2D6 inhibitors such as quinidine, fluoxetine, paroxetine, and propafenone are likely to increase metoprolol concentration. • Digoxin, verapamil, and diltiazem can increase the risk of bradycardia. • Hyperkalemia can occur with some beta blockers, especially when combined with agents that increase potassium.

Class	Contraindications/Precautions/ Adverse Effects	Drug Interactions
Alpha–beta blockers	• Hold in bradycardia, second- or third-degree heart block, decompensated HF/cardiogenic shock, bronchospastic disease, hypotension. • Use caution in diabetes, depression, worsening HF, Raynaud's, liver impairment. • Monitor for liver impairment, agranulocytosis and thrombocytopenia, hypoglycemia, and hyperkalemia.	• Contraindicated in iobenguane I 123 used in diagnostic testing. • Catecholamine-depleting drugs (reserpine, MAOIs) may have an additive effect. • Quinidine, amiodarone, SSRIs, SNRIs, cimetidine, omeprazole, dabigatran, azoles, and chlorpromazine are likely to increase drug concentration. • Digoxin, clonidine, timolol, verapamil, and diltiazem can increase the risk of bradycardia. Increased serum potassium when prescribed with ASA, NSAIDs, RAAS inhibitors, potassium supplements, and agents that can precipitate hyperkalemia.
Aldosterone receptor antagonists	• Hold with hyperkalemia, dehydration and AKI, Addison's disease/adrenal insufficiency, hypotension, hyponatremia, hypocalcemia, hypomagnesemia, hyperchloremic alkalosis, hyperglycemia, and hyperuricemia. • Hold in patients who are pregnant. • Use caution with patients who have renal/hepatic impairment.	• Do not prescribe with ACEIs, ARBs, renin inhibitors, NSAIDs, heparin, or trimethoprim. • Interfere with some digoxin assays. • Combined with cholestyramine can cause hyperkalemic acidosis. • Increased risk of lithium toxicity. • ASA, NSAIDs, and COX-2 inhibitors decrease the efficacy of drug and renal function.

Note: All agents would be contraindicated in the presence of hypersensitivity to the medication or one of its components. All antihypertensives potentiate hypotension when combined with other antihypertensives.

Erectile dysfunction has been reported with use of thiazide diuretics, aldosterone receptor blockers, centrally acting agents, alpha blockers, and beta blockers.

ANTITHROMBOTIC MEDICATIONS

Overview

- Common antithrombotic agents are heparin, vitamin K antagonists, antiplatelets, and direct thrombin inhibitors that are prescribed to prevent thromboembolic complications.
- Types of medications prescribed include ASA, antiplatelets, heparins, vitamin K antagonists, and direct thrombin inhibitors.
- See Table 2.10 at the end of this section for complications, precautions, and interactions.

General Guidelines

- There is an increased risk of bleeding with other antiplatelets, antithrombotics, thrombolytics, anticoagulants, fish oil, and garlic.
- Instruct in safety protocols to prevent bleeding injury that is appropriate for age and condition.
  - *Adolescents and young adults*: No contact sports.
  - *Older adults*: Fall precautions; direct thrombin inhibitors may offer a safer alternative to warfarin in older patients requiring anticoagulation for atrial fibrillation.

(continued)

General Guidelines (*continued*)

- In suspected occult bleeding, perform point-of-care occult blood testing.
- Refer patients who have uncontrolled bleeding or symptoms of ICH to the ED.
- Be aware of antidotes in the presence of excessive bleeding. They include the following:
  - *Antiplatelets*: Platelet transfusions
  - *Heparin*: Protamine sulfate for reversal of prolonged PTT
  - *Warfarin*: Vitamin K oral or injection with or without fresh frozen plasma according to INR
  - *Direct thrombin inhibitor (dabigatran)*: Idarucizumab, a reversal of prolonged TT
  - *Direct thrombin Xa inhibitor (rivaroxaban, apixaban, edoxaban)*: Andexanet alfa, a reversal of prolonged PT, PTT
- Monitor therapeutic levels for warfarin according to condition.
  - Low molecular weight heparin does not require titration according to PTT.
- Prescribe agents according to conditions for the recommended time frame.
- Provide education for bleeding precautions and injury prevention based on age/lifestyle.

General Precautions

- Active bleeding, bleeding diathesis, head trauma, and bleeding strokes are absolute contraindications.
- Use caution in patients with GERD, PUD, liver disease, inflammatory bowel disease.
- Refer to current surgical or procedure guidelines for the management of antithrombotic medication according to condition.

SALICYLATE (ASPIRIN)

Mechanism of Action

- Inhibits platelet aggregation

Indications

- ACS, recent MI, stroke, PAD, CABG, and as part of dual antiplatelet therapy in PCI
- Kawasaki disease in pediatrics

Commonly Prescribed Medications

- Aspirin, enteric coated aspirin (oral)

Diagnostic Testing

Baseline
- Check BMP and LFTs to evaluate hepatorenal function.
- Obtain CBC to evaluate hemopoietic function.

Follow-Up
- Check BMP and LFTs in suspected hepatorenal dysfunction.
- Obtain CBC in suspected hemopoietic dysfunction.

ANTIPLATELETS

Mechanism of Action

- Inhibit platelet coagulation at ADP-induced pathway

Indications

- ACS, recent MI, stroke, PAD, CABG, and as part of dual antiplatelet therapy in PCI

Commonly Prescribed Medications

- Clopidogrel, prasugrel, ticagrelor (oral)

Diagnostic Testing

Baseline
- BMP and LFTs to evaluate hepatorenal function
- CBC to evaluate hemopoietic function

Follow-Up
- Check BMP and LFTs in suspected hepatorenal dysfunction.
- Obtain CBC, bleeding times in suspected hemopoietic dysfunction.

HEPARINS

Mechanism of Action

- *UFH*: Anticoagulation through activated coagulation factors involved in the clotting sequence; prolong aPTT
- *LMWH*: Anticoagulation through inhibition of factor Xa; do not increase PT/PTT

Indications

- *UFH*: Acute MI, PE, DVT
- *LMWH*: DVT, ACS, NSTEMI prophylaxis, STEMI, DVT/PE treatment

Commonly Prescribed Medications

- Unfractionated heparin, enoxaparin (parenteral)

Diagnostic Testing

Baseline
- BMP and LFTs to evaluate hepatorenal function
- CBC, PTT, and PT/INR to evaluate hemopoietic function and bleeding times

Follow-Up
- Check BMP and LFTs in suspected hepatorenal dysfunction.
- Obtain CBC and bleeding times in suspected hemopoietic dysfunction.
- Monitor PTT in unfractionated heparin and titrate medication to achieve target therapeutic bleeding times according to condition.

COUMARINS

Mechanism of Action

- *Inhibit synthesis of vitamin K-dependent clotting factors*: Factors 2, 7, 9, and 10, and anticoagulant proteins C and S

Indications

- DVT/PE, atrial fibrillation, and prosthetic valve replacement prophylaxis to prevent prosthetic valve thrombosis
- For prophylactic use against systemic embolization and stroke in patients who have had recurrent MI, structural defects of the heart, and heart failure

Commonly Prescribed Medications

- Warfarin (oral)

Diagnostic Testing

Baseline
- BMP, CBC, LFTs, PT/INR

Follow-Up
- Monitor CMP, CBC, LFTs INR for the following conditions:
  - DVT, PE, MI, atrial fibrillation, some mechanical valves (INR range 2–3)
  - Caged ball or caged disk valves (INR range 2.5–3.5)

DIRECT THROMBIN INHIBITORS

Mechanism of Action

- Inhibit thrombin or Factor Xa and conversion of fibrinogen to fibrin in the coagulation cascade

Indications

- DVT/PE, nonvalvular atrial fibrillation prophylaxis and treatment
- Procedures and conditions treatable by heparin where the patient is at risk for heparin-induced thrombocytopenia

Commonly Prescribed Medications

- Dabigatran, rivaroxaban, apixaban, edoxaban, betrixaban (oral)
- Argatroban, bivalirudin, desirudin, and lepirudin (parenteral)

Diagnostic Testing

Baseline
- Check BMP and LFTs to evaluate electrolytes and hepatorenal function.
- Obtain CBC, aPPT, and PT/INR as baseline.
- Obtain factor Xa before administration of rivaroxaban.

Follow-Up
- Check electrolytes and hepatorenal function in suspected dysfunction.
- Obtain CBC, aPPT, and PT/INR in suspected bleeding.

Table 2.10 Antithrombotic Medications

Class	Contraindications/Precautions/ Adverse Effects	Drug Interactions

Salicylate	• Hold in patients with allergy to ASA and NSAIDs, with active bleeding, and with aspirin-intolerant asthma.
	• Use caution in patients with renal impairment, peptic ulcer disease, and esophagitis.
	• Contraindicated in
	  • Inflammatory bowel disease
	  • Decompensated heart failure
	  • Tinnitus
	  • Viral syndrome in children
	  • Pregnancy (except preeclampsia)
		• Decreased effect of ASA with NSAIDs.
		• Decreased effect of chloramphenicol, probenecid, aliskiren, alpha antagonist.
		• Decreased renal function when coadministered with ACEIs or ARBs.
		• Increased toxicity with ARBs, ketorolac, and green tea.
		• Increased potassium with atenolol, acebutolol, digoxin.
		• Increased risk of other drug concentrations with methotrexate, SNRIs, SSRIs, sulfa agent, insulin, and cortisone.

Antiplatelets	• Hold in patients with neuraxial blockade, intracranial hemorrhage, or liver failure.
	• Use caution in patients with renal impairment.
	• Contraindicated in the following conditions:
	  • Active bleeding
	  • Inflammatory bowel disease
	  • Hemodialysis
	  • Aplastic anemia
	  • TTP
	  • Vasculitis
	  • Abdominal hemorrhage with colitis, appendicitis, and pancreatitis
		• *CYP2C19 inhibitors*: Avoid concomitant use of omeprazole or esomeprazole.
		• CYP3A4 inhibitors decrease the effects of clopidogrel (grapefruit, azoles, diltiazem, nifedipine, ritonavir, INH).
		• Increased risk of bleeding with SSRIs, SNRIs, barbiturates, phenytoin, corticosteroids, rifapentine, topiramate, and green tea.

Heparins	• Hold in patients with pork allergy, active bleeding, bleeding diathesis, neuraxial blockade, hemorrhagic stroke, head trauma, heparin-induced thrombocytopenia, and thrombocytopenia of alternative cause. • Obtain informed consent from patients with religious objections to pork products. • Use caution with patients who have peptic ulcer disease, uncontrolled HTN, or renal impairment. • Monitor for hyperkalemia and anemia.	• Increased risk of hyperkalemia with ACEIs, ARBs, aldosterone antagonists, and potassium supplements. • Barbiturates and prednisone decrease the effects of LMWH. • Increased risk of bleeding with macrolides, PCNs, cephalosporins, quinine, sulfasalazine, sulfamethoxazole, ARBs, SNRIs, phenytoin, and saw palmetto.

(*continued*)

Table 2.10 Antithrombotic Medications (*continued*)

Class	Contraindications/Precautions/ Adverse Effects	Drug Interactions
Coumarins	• Hold in patients with INR >3.5–4, active bleeding, uncontrolled hypertension, preeclampsia, pregnancy, neuraxial blockade. • Monitor for skin necrosis and purple toe syndrome.	• Medications that decrease the effects of warfarin include barbiturates, prednisone, estrogen, carbamazepine, phenytoin, pentoxifylline, rifampin, spironolactone, and smoking. • Increased risk of bleeding with allopurinol, amiodarone, propranolol, macrolides, PCNs, cephalosporins, azoles, alpha antagonists, quinine, ritonavir, sulfasalazine, sulfamethoxazole , ARBs, SNRIs, SSRIs, phenytoin, saw palmetto, glyburide, and omeprazole. • Simvastatin increases availability of coumarins.
Direct thrombin inhibitors	• Hold in patients with neuraxial blockade and active bleeding. • Hold with mechanical heart valve when prescribing dabigatran. • Adjust dose according to renal function. Hold for CrCl <15 mL/min. • Use caution in patients with uncontrolled hypertension. • Monitor for agranulocytosis. • Increased risk of thrombosis if stopped prematurely.	• St. John's wort, phenytoin, rifampin, barbiturates, and carbamazepine decrease the effect of dabigatran. • Increased risk of bleeding with strong CYP3A inhibitors.

Note: All agents would be contraindicated in the presence of hypersensitivity to the medication or one of its components.

ENDOCRINE MEDICATIONS

DIABETES MEDICATIONS

TYPE 2 DIABETES POLYPHARMACOLOGY REVIEW

Drug Selection

- *First-line therapy:* Metformin is the initial agent for type 2 DM and in certain cases of prediabetes.
- *Second-line therapy:* If the patient is not at target HbA1c after metformin, select an additional agent based on compelling indications, disease states, hypoglycemia risk, weight control, and cost. Combination pills may enhance compliance when available. Second-line therapy for the following indications are as follows:
  - *ASCVD:* GLP-1 RA or SGLT2I
  - *HF or risk of CKD progression:* SGLT2I or GLP-1 RA
  - *Hypoglycemia risk:* DPP-4I, GLP-1 RA, SGLT2I, or TZD
  - *Weight loss/minimize gain:* GLP-1 RA or SGLT2I
  - *Cost is a major issue:* SU or TZD
- *Third-line therapy:* Add alternative from second-line therapy options for compelling indication, based on compelling indication if the patient is still not at target. Note that there is no additional benefit combining DDP-4I and GLP-1 RA.

- *Quadruple therapy:* If the patient's response is inadequate, a fourth agent may be considered as follows:
  - *ASCVD:* Basal insulin, TZD, or SU
  - *HF:* Basal insulin, SU, may consider DDP-4I if not on GLP-1 RA
  - *Risk of CKD progression:* Same as HF; may also consider TZD or SU
  - *Hypoglycemia risk:* Later-generation SU or basal insulin
  - *Weight loss/minimize gain:* DDP-4I if not on GLP-1 RA
  - *Cost is a major issue:* Least expensive basal insulin, DPP-4, or SGLT2I
- See Table 2.11 at the end of this section for contraindications, precautions, and interactions.

General Guidelines

- *General contraindications:* Allergy to medication, type 1 DM, diabetic ketoacidosis.
- *General drug interaction:* Agents that minimize the risk of hypoglycemia (metformin, DPP-4I, GLP-1 RA, SGLT2I, TZD) increase the risk for hypoglycemia when insulin secretagogues or insulin is added.

Patient Population Considerations

Women (conception/pregnancy/lactation)
- Discontinue oral agents in patients with type 2 DM seeking to conceive or those who are pregnant or breastfeeding and prescribe insulin in their place.

Geriatrics
- Avoid overtreatment and simplify complex regimens to avoid hypoglycemia to target HbA1c of <8.5%. Evaluate for the development of chronic diseases and cognitive impairment that could impede medication compliance and increase the risk for drug–drug interactions. Monitor for events that could exacerbate renal injury and affect GFR.

Pediatrics
- *Age 10 and older:* Start on metformin and add basal insulin if not at target HbA1c. If glycemic targets are no longer met with metformin (with or without basal insulin), add GLP-1 RA (liraglutide) if the patient has no past medical history or family history of medullary thyroid carcinoma or multiple endocrine neoplasia type 2.

Patients With Renal Dysfunction: GFR <30 mL/min
- Metformin is contraindicated. Consider DPP-4I, GLP-1 RA, or TZDs.

Patients Undergoing Surgery
- Withhold metformin on day of surgery and use insulin to target BG 80 to 180 mg/dL. If the patient is receiving oral hypoglycemics, withhold on the morning of surgery/procedure. If prescribed insulin therapy, order half of the NPH dose or 60% to 80% doses of basal insulin and increase the frequency of SMBG. Use short- or rapid-acting insulin for correction.

  BIGUANIDES

Mechanism of Action

- Decrease hepatic glucose production and intestinal absorption of glucose.
- Improve insulin sensitivity by increasing peripheral glucose uptake.
- Produce modest weight loss; do not cause hypoglycemia alone.

Indications

- First-line antidiabetic agent for patients with type 2 DM
- Consider for the patient with prediabetes under age 60 (confirmed HbA1c 5.7%–6.4% or BG 100–125 mg/dL), with BMI ≥35, or in women with a history of gestational diabetes
- For ages 10 and over

Commonly Prescribed Medications

- Metformin (oral) is the only biguanide.

Diagnostic Testing

Baseline
- HbA1c, BMP, CBC, serum B_{12} level, LFTs; calculate GFR

Follow-Up
- HbA1c every 3 to 4 months
- BMP, vitamin B_{12} level; calculate GFR; hold drug and check for elevated serum lactate >5 mmol/L with symptoms of lactic acidosis

DIPEPTIDYL PEPTIDASE IV

Mechanism of Action

- Decreases glucagon, increases insulin synthesis, and decreases gastric emptying
- Does not promote weight loss or gain; does not produce hypoglycemia

Indications

- Added to metformin as a second-line agent for patients with type 2 DM and without ASCVD, HF, or CKD
- Reduces the risk for hypoglycemia when added to metformin in cases where HbA1c is above target

Commonly Prescribed Medications

- Alogliptin, linagliptin, saxagliptin, sitagliptin, vildagliptin (oral)

Diagnostic Testing

Baseline
- Obtain HbA1c, BMP; calculate GFR, amylase, lipase level, triglyceride level

Follow-Up
- HbA1c every 3 to 4 months
- BMP, calculate GFR
- Monitor for amylase, lipase, and triglycerides level with abdominal pain
- Check BMP with acute renal failure

GLP-1 RECEPTOR ANTAGONISTS

Mechanism of Action

- Stimulate insulin release in the presence of increased glucose
- Decrease glucagon secretion and delay gastric emptying
- Promote weight loss; do not produce hypoglycemia on their own
- Decrease the risk of ASCVD death

Indications

- Reduce the risk of ASCVD, weight gain, or hypoglycemia
- Added to metformin as second-line therapy in cases where HF or CKD predominates and SLGT2 inhibition is contraindicated
- Cannot be prescribed with DPP4I

Commonly Prescribed Medications

- Albiglutide, dulaglutide, exenatide (IR and ER), liraglutide, lixisenatide (injectable)
- Semaglutide (oral and injectable)

Diagnostic Testing

Baseline
- HbA1c, BMP; LFTs, amylase, lipase, triglyceride level, and bilirubin
- Calculate GFR

Follow-Up
- HbA1c every 3 to 4 months
- BMP; calculate GFR
- LFTs, amylase, and lipase in the presence of jaundice, and s/s of pancreatitis
- Serum calcitonin level and thyroid ultrasound in the presence of thyroid symptoms; values >50 ng/L are significant

METGLITINIDES

Mechanism of Action
- Stimulate insulin secretion from the pancreas to reduce postprandial glucose
- Contribute to weight gain and hypoglycemia

Indications
- Adjuvant to SU in cases where added effect to reduce postprandial BG is required

Commonly Prescribed Medications
- Nateglinide, repaglinide (oral)

Diagnostic Testing

Baseline
- HbA1c, BMP, LFTs, bilirubin
- GFR

Follow-Up
- HbA1c every 3 to 4 months
- BMP, LFTs, bilirubin
- GFR
- Serum uric acid with renal colic symptoms or gouty arthritis

SODIUM-GLUCOSE COTRANSPORTER 2 INHIBITORS

Mechanism of Action
- Reduce renal glucose reabsorption, lower the renal threshold for glucose, and increase urinary glucose excretion

Indications
- Added as second-line therapy to metformin in type 2 DM to reduce the risk of HF or CKD, weight gain, or hypoglycemia
- Added to metformin in cases where ASCVD predominates and GLP-1 RA is contraindicated

Commonly Prescribed Medications
- Canagliflozin, dapagliflozin, empagliflozin (oral)

Diagnostic Testing

Baseline
- HbA1c, BMP
- GFR

Follow-Up
- HbA1c every 3 to 4 months
- BMP, urinalysis, LDL
- GFR
- Hold drug and check for BMP in NPO states
- ABGs if DKA suspected

SULFONYLUREAS

Mechanism of Action

- Stimulate insulin secretion from the beta cells
- Promote weight gain and cause hypoglycemia

Indications

- Second-line agent when there is no ASCVD, HF, CKD, or competing need to minimize hypoglycemia or weight gain

Commonly Prescribed Medications

- *First generation*: Chlorpropamide, tolbutamide, tolazamide (oral)
- *Second generation*: Glimepiride, glipizide, glyburide (oral)

Diagnostic Testing

Baseline
- HbA1c, CBC, BMP, LFTs, bilirubin
- GFR

Follow-Up
- HbA1c every 3 to 4 months
- BMP, CBC, LFTs, bilirubin
- GFR

THIAZOLIDINEDIONES

Mechanism of Action

- Increase insulin sensitivity, decrease insulin resistance, and reduce hepatic glucose output
- Can promote weight gain but does not cause hypoglycemia

Indications

- Added to metformin as a second-line therapy when there is a compelling need to minimize hypoglycemia

Commonly Prescribed Medications

- Pioglitazone, rosiglitazone (oral)

Diagnostic Testing

Baseline
- HbA1c, CBC, BMP, lipid panel, LFTs, bilirubin
- GFR
- Bone density testing

Follow-Up
- HbA1c every 3 to 4 months
- BMP, lipid panel
- Calculate GFR
- Hold drug and check for LFTs and bilirubin in the presence of jaundice

INSULIN—TYPE 1 AND TYPE 2 DIABETES

Drug Selection

- In selecting insulin, it is critical to consider patient preferences, ability to perform injections and adhere to plan, affordability, and risk for hypoglycemia.
- *Type 1 DM:* Basal/bolus insulin according to SMBG and patient preferences.
  - Insulin glargine at bedtime with premeal short- or rapid-acting insulin injections
  - NPH twice daily with premeal short- or rapid-acting insulin injections
  - Insulin pump using short-acting or rapid-acting insulin
- *Type 2 DM:* Introduce insulin when not meeting target A1c on oral agents and patient states preference for injectable therapy.
  - *Step 1:* Insulin glargine at bedtime or NPH.
  - *Step 2:* Not at target HbA1c—consider titration, NPH twice daily, and/or prandial insulin.
  - *Step 3:* Not at target HbA1c—consider titration, consider full basal/bolus regimen versus mixed NPH/regular insulin or premixed NPH/regular insulin twice daily.
  - See Table 2.12 for a review of insulin.

General Guidelines

- Counsel patient in s/s of heart failure, hypokalemia, and infection to report immediately.
- Ensure the patient is performing SMBG according to preference and refrigerates unused insulin.
- Refer all patients to a diabetes educator. Education includes the following:
  - SMBG, injection technique, site selection (rotating sites within a region), mixing insulin (if applicable), insulin storage and inspection, hypoglycemia management and sick day rules, infection protection, and sharps management in the community

General Precautions

- *Contraindications:*
  - Hypersensitivity to insulin glargine or its components
  - Not to be used during hypoglycemia episode
- *Warnings/precautions:*
  - Bloodborne pathogen/infection transmission, medication errors, lipodystrophy, and injection site reactions
  - Hyperglycemia/hypoglycemia, hypokalemia
  - Fluid retention and HF with TZDs
  - Weight gain
- *Drug–drug interactions with all insulins:*
  - *Decreased BG/awareness:*
    - Antidiabetic agents, ACEIs, angiotensin II receptor blocking agents, disopyramide, fibrates, fluoxetine, MAOIs, pentoxifylline, pramlintide, salicylates, somatostatin analogs (e.g., octreotide), and sulfonamide antibiotics **decrease BG**. Beta blockers, clonidine, guanethidine, and reserpine may blunt awareness.

(continued)

General Precautions (*continued*)

- *Increase BG*:
  - ○ Atypical antipsychotics (e.g., olanzapine and clozapine), corticosteroids, danazol, diuretics, estrogens, glucagon, isoniazid, niacin, oral contraceptives, phenothiazines, progestogens (e.g., in oral contraceptives), protease inhibitors, somatropin, sympathomimetic agents (e.g., albuterol, epinephrine, terbutaline), and thyroid hormones.
  - ○ Alcohol, beta blockers, clonidine, and lithium salts. Pentamidine may cause hypoglycemia, which may sometimes be followed by hyperglycemia.

Patient Population Considerations

Women (conception/pregnancy/lactation)
- Start reproductive counseling, beginning in puberty. Discuss family planning and contraceptives when oral agents are in use and the importance of maintaining an optimal A1c < 6.5% to reduce risks to the fetus. Women are switched from oral agents to insulin when attempting to conceive through pregnancy and breastfeeding.

Geriatrics
- Simplification of complex regimens are considered in older adults with chronic medical conditions, and A1c targets may be increased to prevent hypoglycemia. Caregivers in assisted living or nursing homes may need additional staff development.

Hospitalized Patients
- All patients with diabetes get an A1c level if not done in the past 3 months. Prescribe insulin administration using standardized protocols.

NPO Status
- Procedures/tests and surgery increase the risk of hypoglycemia in patients with diabetes. Reduce insulin dose, increase BG testing, and correct BG values using short-acting insulin. Target BG at 140 to 180 mg/dL perioperatively.

Table 2.11 Antidiabetic Agents for Type 2 Diabetes

Class	Contraindications/Precautions/Adverse Effects	Drug Interactions
Biguanides	• Hold in patients with renal failure, acute/chronic acidosis, or evidence of hepatic disease. • Hold on day of contrast dye procedures and restart after 48 hr if repeat BMP reveals normal renal function. • Hold in nursing women to prevent infant hypoglycemia. • Monitor for conditions that increase the risk of renal failure (NPO status, dehydration, hypotension, nephropathy secondary to HF) or hepatic impairment (binge drinking, hepatotoxins) to avoid acidosis. • Start with a low dose, titrate slowly, and take with meals to manage GI upset. • Not for use in children under age 10.	Do not prescribe with medications that increase the risk for lactic acidosis (especially nephrotoxins or hepatotoxins): Topiramate, zonisamide, acetazolamide, dichlorphenamide, ranolazine, vandetanib, dolutegravir, and cimetidine, alcohol.
DPP4I	• Hold with s/s of pancreatitis. • Monitor for elevations in LFTs and rising azotemia. • Adjust dosing with renal insufficiency and monitor for conditions that increase the risk of its development. • Not for use in children under age 18.	Digoxin levels increase slightly when medication is added.

Class	Contraindications/Precautions/Adverse Effects	Drug Interactions
GLP-1 RA	• Hold with personal or family history of MTC, MEN2, gastroparesis. • Monitor for s/s of pancreatitis and gallbladder disease and worsening renal or hepatic function. • Monitor injection site for infections or behaviors that increase the risk of infection transmission with injectables. • Not for use in children under age 10.	GLP-1 RA can delay the absorption of concomitantly administered oral medications.
Meglitinides	• Hold with hypoglycemia or skipped meals. • Increased risk of hypoglycemia with hepatic impairment. • Monitor for gout, arthropathy, elevation in uric acid. • Can cause weight gain.	• Triazole antifungals, amiodarone, alcohol, NSAIDs, salicylates, MAOIs, beta-blocking agents, and anabolic steroids **decrease BG.** • Thiazides, corticosteroids, thyroid products, sympathomimetics, somatropin, somatostatin analogs, rifampin, phenytoin, and St. John's wort **increase BG.**
SGLT2I	• Hold in severe renal failure, ESRD, and dialysis. • Monitor for hypotension, ketoacidosis, hyperlipidemia, signs of UTI, or fungal infections. • Monitor for risk of decreased renal function in hypotension, decreased cardiac output, volume depletion, and AKI. • Not for use in children under age 18.	Diuretics, ACEIs, ARBs, and NSAIDs may increase the risk for acute kidney injury.
SU	• Hold with hypersensitivity to sulfa agents or G6PD deficiency. • Hold with hypoglycemia and anorexia. Reduce dose before surgery. • Monitor for pancytopenia. • Monitor for increased risk of cardiovascular mortality. • Use cautiously with renal and liver dysfunction. • Use extended-release agents cautiously in geriatric patients. • Can cause weight gain.	• Triazole antifungals, salicylates, sulfonamides, chloramphenicol, probenecid, coumarins, MAOIs, quinolones, and beta-blocking agents **decrease BG.** • Diuretics, corticosteroids, phenothiazines, thyroid products, estrogens, oral contraceptives, phenytoin, nicotinic acid, sympathomimetics, CCB drugs, and isoniazid **increase BG.**
TZD	• Hold in symptomatic HF (NYHA Class III/IV) and monitor for its development in a patient at risk. • Hold in patients with hepatotoxicity or bladder cancer. • Monitor BMD, lipid panel, renal, and liver function. • Weight gain and peripheral edema may occur. If present, evaluate for progression of HF.	• CYP2C8 inhibitors (rifampin) increase drug levels. • CYP2C8 inducers (gemfibrozil) decrease drug levels. • Topiramate decreases drug levels.

Table 2.12 Insulin Review

Type of Insulin	Onset	Peak	Duration	Considerations
Basal insulin	1–4 hr	Minimal	24 hr	• Take at bedtime. • Do not mix with other insulins in syringe.
Insulin NPH	2–4 hr	4–10 hr	14–18 hr	• May be divided into two doses.
Insulin human recombinant	30–60 min	2–3 hr	4–6 hr	• Take BG test 30 min before eating and administer at that time.
Insulin lispro	<15 min	30–90 min	<5 hr	• Take BG test immediately before eating and administer with food.

THYROID MEDICATIONS

Drug Selection

- *Hypothyroidism:* Levothyroxine (T4) is the initial agent prescribed for primary or secondary hypothyroidism. Titrate every 4 to 8 weeks to achieve a serum TSH level of 0.5 to 4 mIU/mL.
- *Hyperthyroidism:* Prescribe antithyroid agents to inhibit thyroid hormone synthesis, decrease vascularity, or manage symptoms in hyperthyroidism. These medications may be prescribed in preparation for, or in place of, procedures to manage hyperthyroidism. Expect patients who have been treated with antithyroid treatment to require lifelong thyroid replacement hormone.
  - *Refer to endocrinology for acute management*
  - Prescribe methimazole as the first-choice agent. Reserve propylthiouracil for patients who cannot tolerate methimazole. It may take 1 to 2 years to achieve effectiveness.
  - Order beta blocker propranolol to minimize symptoms of tachycardia, hypertension, and tremor.
  - Consult endocrinology and surgery to prescribe SSKI solution to reduce thyroid vascularity before surgery or manage critical patients in thyroid storm.
  - Manage exophthalmos of Graves' disease with artificial tears.
- See Table 2.13 at end of section for contraindications, precautions, and interactions.

General Guidelines

- *General contraindication:* Allergy to the medication.
- *General drug interaction:* Many agents can impede the absorption of levothyroxine, especially MVI with iron and cholestyramine, sucralfate, antacids, and calcium carbonate. Therefore, this medication should be taken on an empty stomach, 30 min before eating with a full glass of water.
- *General precautions:*
  - *Hyperthyroidism:* Patients are not euthyroid following completion of antithyroid therapy. Discuss the need for management of hypothyroidism at its conclusion.
  - *Hypothyroidism:* Advise patients to use the same brand of levothyroxine, taken by itself at the same time daily for the best effect. If a substitution is likely, titrate the patient on a single brand and prescribe the drug to be dispensed as written. Remind patients that thyroid replacement hormone therapy is lifelong.

Patient Population Considerations

Women (conception/pregnancy/lactation)

- *Hypothyroidism:* Evaluate serum TSH levels each trimester during pregnancy. Pregnant women with preexisting hypothyroidism by history may have increased requirements during pregnancy and the postpartum period.
- *Hyperthyroidism:* PTU is prescribed instead of methimazole in women of childbearing age, pregnancy, and lactation.

Geriatrics
- *Hypothyroidism:* Use a lower starting dose and titrate levothyroxine slowly to avoid cardiac side effects of hyperthyroidism. Avoid overtreatment with levothyroxine in geriatric patients to trigger secondary hyperthyroidism that can cause MI and HF.
- *Hyperthyroidism:* Manage symptoms of tachycardia and hypertension with propranolol in the older adult.

Pediatrics
- *Hypothyroidism:* Congenital hypothyroidism requires referral to a pediatric endocrinologist. Most cases are a result of irradiation or Hashimoto's thyroiditis. Doses as high as 4 to 10 mcg/kg/day may be necessary due to faster metabolism.
- *Hyperthyroidism:* Prescribe methimazole in consultation with endocrinology for children with Graves' disease.

THYROID REPLACEMENT HORMONE

Mechanism of Action
- Replaces circulating thyroxine

Indications
- Primary or secondary hypothyroidism

Commonly Prescribed Medications
- Liothyronine, liotrix, thyroid desiccated (oral)
- Levothyroxine (oral and parenteral formulation)

Diagnostic Testing

Baseline
- TSH (repeat abnormal results and add free T4 to a second blood test)

Follow-Up
- TSH, bone density, lipid panel

ANTITHYROID SYNTHESIS AGENTS

Mechanism of Action
- Inhibit thyroid hormone synthesis by blocking the oxidation of iodine

Indications
- Hyperthyroidism, Graves' disease

Commonly Prescribed Medications
- Methimazole, propylthiouracil (oral)

Diagnostic Testing

Baseline
- TSH, T3, T4, CBC, LFTs, beta hCG
- 12-lead EKG, baseline DEXA scan in the geriatric patient

Follow-Up
- TSH, T3, T4, BMP. CBC, LFTs, ANCA panel in the presence of vasculitis

POP QUIZ 2.4

A 25-year-old male presents to the primary care provider for evaluation of type 2 DM with a HbA1c of 8%. He is taking metformin 100 mg BID. He has no signs of microvascular or macrovascular disease. His BMI is 32. What medications should be included in the plan?

Table 2.13 Medications for Thyroid Disorders

Class	Contraindications/Precautions/ Adverse Effects	Drug Interactions
Levothyroxine	• Hold with s/s of hyperthyroidism or adrenal insufficiency. • Monitor weight loss and explain that medication is not a substitute for obesity management. • Monitor for tachycardia, hypertension, and ischemic symptoms. • Monitor for hyperglycemia in diabetic patients. • A change in brands may manifest with signs of under/overmedication.	• Do not prescribe with sympathomimetics or stimulants. Concurrent use with ketamine can cause hypertension. • TCAs can cause toxicity of both agents. • Tyrosine-kinase inhibitors can reduce the effect of medication. Amiodarone inhibits the peripheral conversion of T4. • Levothyroxine can decrease the effect of digitalis.
Methimazole	• Hold for s/s hypothyroidism. • Not for use in the first trimester of pregnancy. • Monitor for agranulocytosis, liver toxicity, and vasculitis.	• This medication blocks vitamin K activity. Monitor PT/PTT in inpatients on anticoagulants. • May require higher doses of beta blockers, digoxin, and theophylline during therapy and reduced amounts when the patient is euthyroid.
Propylthiouracil	• Hold for s/s hypothyroidism. • Hold if the patient can tolerate methimazole. • Monitor for liver failure, glomerulonephritis, agranulocytosis, bleeding, and vasculitis. • Avoid administration after the first trimester of pregnancy. • Monitor for exfoliating skin rash. • Monitor for overdose.	• May require higher doses of beta blockers, digoxin, theophylline during therapy, and reduced amounts when euthyroid. • The medication blocks vitamin K activity. Monitor PT/PTT in inpatients on anticoagulants.

GERD MEDICATIONS

ANTACIDS

Mechanism of Action

- These are compounds using calcium, aluminum, and magnesium to neutralize acid in the stomach. Inhibition of peptic activity may suppress *Helicobacter pylori* growth.
- May be combined with simethicone to reduce gas.
- See contraindications, precautions, and interactions for this and other GERD medications in Table 2.14.

Indications

- Prescribed with *Helicobacter pylori* eradication drug therapy or for symptomatic relief of dyspepsia. Binds phosphate

Commonly Prescribed Medications

- Aluminum/magnesium, magnesium hydroxide, calcium carbonate (oral)

Diagnostic Testing

Baseline
- None

Follow-Up
- None

H2 ANTAGONIST

Mechanism of Action
- H2 inhibition of gastric secretions

Indications
- GERD, erosive esophagitis, duodenal and gastric ulcer
- Hypersecretory conditions Zollinger–Ellison, MEN

Commonly Prescribed Medications
- Cimetidine, nizatidine
- Famotidine (oral and parenteral formulations)

Diagnostic Testing

Baseline
- None in OTC use

Follow-Up
- CBC, BMP in refractory dyspepsia, endoscopy

PROTON PUMP INHIBITOR

Mechanism of Action
- Suppresses binding to gastric parietal cells inhibiting basal and stimulated gastric acid secretion to promote healing of erosions

Indications
- Erosive esophagitis, GERD, hypersecretory conditions Zollinger–Ellison, MEN

Commonly Prescribed Medications
- Omeprazole, rabeprazole (oral)
- Pantoprazole, esomeprazole, lansoprazole (oral and parenteral)

Diagnostic Testing

Baseline
- None in OTC use

Follow-Up
- CBC, BMP, endoscopy in refractory dyspepsia

 POP QUIZ 2.5

A 78-year-old male presents to the primary care provider for evaluation of dyspepsia associated with dysphagia that no longer responds to over-the-counter famotidine that he has taken for the past 2 years with positive effect. He reports increased pallor, fatigue, and unintentional weight loss. What is the most appropriate next step?

Table 2.14 GERD Medications

Drug	Contraindications/Precautions/Adverse Effects	Drug Interactions
Antacids	• Hold in CKD or AKI with reduced renal clearance. • Avoid calcium salts with hyperparathyroidism. • Monitor for hypophosphatemia, constipation, and bowel obstruction with excess calcium. • Monitor for hypermagnesemia, diarrhea with excess magnesium especially in concurrent bowel disease, and renal failure. • Monitor for aluminum toxicity with overuse and renal insufficiency.	• Taking medications with antacids may decrease absorption and effect.
H2 antagonists	• Use caution in renal and liver impairment. • Advise patients that this medication can mask the symptoms of malignancy. • Monitor for arrhythmia and QT prolongation. • Monitor for CNS toxicity, anxiety, and depression especially in the older adults. • Monitor for pancytopenia.	• Cimetidine is a P450 inhibitor. Monitor when administered with substrates, inhibitor, or inducers for alteration in effect.
PPIs	• Advise patients that this medication can mask the symptoms of malignancy. • Monitor for *Clostridium difficile* infections and pneumonia. • Monitor for nephritis, osteoporosis, SLE reactions, and pancytopenia. • Monitor for hypocalcemia, hypomagnesemia, arrhythmia, seizures, *Helicobacter pylori*, gastric cancer, and increased infections with long-term use. • Monitor for rebound hypergastrinemia after withdrawal.	• Medications are metabolized by CYP2C19, CYP3A4, or both causing a risk drug effect. Monitor when administered with substrates, inhibitor, or inducers for alteration in effect. • Increased risk of bleeding with warfarin; increased drug effect of methotrexate.

Note: All agents would be contraindicated in the presence of hypersensitivity to the medication or one of its components.

RESPIRATORY MEDICATIONS

INHALED CORTICOSTEROIDS

Mechanism of Action

- Antiinflammatory agent that may decrease the number and activity of inflammatory cells, cytokine, and inflammatory mediators.
- A decrease in inflammation reduces airway hyperresponsiveness and bronchoconstriction.
- See Table 2.15 at the end of this section for contraindications, precautions, and interactions for respiratory medications.

Indications

- As an adjunct to LABA/LAMA in COPD to reduce the number of exacerbations
- As a daily maintenance dose in step 2 asthma
- As an adjunct to SABA in adults and adolescents in step 1 asthma who are not taking maintenance therapy

Commonly Prescribed Medications

- Fluticasone, budesonide, mometasone, flunisolide, ciclesonide (oral)

Diagnostic Testing

Baseline
- Pulmonary function testing

Follow-Up
- Daily peak flow and periodic pulmonary function testing

LONG-ACTING BETA AGONISTS

Mechanism of Action

- Relax bronchiole smooth muscle at beta-2 receptor; long-acting effect
- Not for acute respiratory events

Indications

- Maintenance therapy for asthma and COPD in conjunction with an inhaled corticosteroid

Commonly Prescribed Medications

- Formoterol (in budesonide–formoterol inhaler)
- Salmeterol (inhaler)

Diagnostic Testing

Baseline
- Pulmonary function testing
- 12-lead EKG

Follow-Up
- Daily peak flow and periodic pulmonary function testing, 12-lead EKG with palpitations

LONG-ACTING MUSCARINIC AGONISTS

Mechanism of Action

- Anticholinergic that relaxes bronchiole smooth muscle at the muscarinic receptor; long-acting effect
- Not for acute respiratory events

Indications

- Maintenance therapy for asthma and COPD

Commonly Prescribed Medications

- Tiotropium bromide (inhaler)

Diagnostic Testing

Baseline
- Pulmonary function testing
- 12-lead EKG

Follow-Up
- Daily peak flow and periodic pulmonary function testing, 12-lead EKG with palpitations

SHORT-ACTING BETA AGONISTS

Mechanism of Action

- Relax bronchiole smooth muscle at beta-2 receptor

Indications

- Short-acting rescue agent for asthma and COPD
- In asthma, may be combined with ICS to improve the course of the disease

Commonly Prescribed Medications

- Albuterol, levalbuterol (inhaler)

Diagnostic Testing

Baseline
- Pulmonary function testing

Follow-Up
- Daily peak flow and as needed before SABA and periodic pulmonary function testing

POP QUIZ 2.6

A 35-year-old female with a history of asthma and GERD presents to the primary care provider for frequent episodes of wheezing that wakes her up from sleep on most nights of the week. She is prescribed a rescue albuterol inhaler that she uses for wheezing, and omeprazole, which she takes each morning. What are the next steps in managing this patient?

Table 2.15 Respiratory Medications

Class	Contraindications/Precautions/Adverse Effects	Drug Interactions
ICS	• Hold in allergy, status asthmaticus. • Monitor for thrush, secondary infection, cough. • Use with caution in immunosuppressed. • Excessive use can suppress the HPA axis, causing adrenal insufficiency with abrupt withdrawal.	• ICS are inhibitors of cytochrome P450 3A4. There may be an increased incidence of adrenal insufficiency and Cushing's due to coadministration of cytochrome P450 3A4 substrates and inducers, and inhibitors.
LABA	• Contraindicated in monotherapy (increased risk of fatality in asthma). • Use caution in patients at risk for tachyarrhythmias, HTN, CVHD, ASCVD, aneurysm, and severe asthma. • Monitor for elevated HR, BP, chest pain, tremor, paradoxical bronchospasm. • Monitor for hypokalemia, hyperglycemia, and atrial fibrillation.	• Salmeterol is metabolized by CYP 3A4. Prolonged QT interval has been observed with coadministration with strong CYP3A4 inhibitor (ketoconazole) and increased drug levels with moderate inhibitor (erythromycin). • Formoterol is not a CYP 3A4 substrate but when combined with budesonide is metabolized by it. Use caution when prescribing budesonide-formoterol with CYP 3A4 inhibitors or inducers.

Class	Contraindications/Precautions/ Adverse Effects	Drug Interactions
LAMA	• Contraindicated in patients with milk allergy. • Use caution in patients at risk for urinary retention, glaucoma, and sinus infections • Monitor for anticholinergic side effects and paradoxical bronchospasm. • Monitor for renal impairment.	• Metabolized by enzymatic pathway and can be inhibited by CYP450 2D6 and 3A4 inhibitors, such as quinidine, ketoconazole, and gestodene.
SABA	• Contraindicated in allergy. • Monitor for paradoxical bronchospasm, worsening asthma, and ineffective monotherapy. • Monitor for chest pain, HTN, tachycardia, tremor, hypokalemia, and hyperglycemia. • Monitor for anxiety.	• Increase in hypokalemia with insulin and loop and thiazide diuretics. • Increase in digoxin level. • Increase CV symptoms with MAOIs or TCAs.

RESOURCES

ADAA. (2015). *Clinical practice review for GAD.* https://adaa.org/resources-professionals/practice-guidelines-gad

Alexander, M. (2020). *Hypertension.* https://emedicine.medscape.com/article/241381-overview

Alidoost, M., Conte, G. A., Agarwal, K., Carson, M. P., Lann, D., & Marchesani, D. (2020). Iatrogenic Cushing's syndrome following intra-articular triamcinolone injection in an HIV-infected patient on cobicistat presenting as a pulmonary embolism: Case report and literature review. *International Medical Case Reports Journal, 13,* 229–235. https://doi.org/10.2147/IMCRJ.S254461

American College of Cardiology. (2018). *Diabetes management in older adults with cardiovascular disease.* https://www.acc.org/latest-in-cardiology/articles/2018/02/28/12/19/diabetes-management-in-older-adults-with-cvd

American College of Cardiology. (2019). *AHA/ACC/HRS Focused update of the 2014 guideline for management of patients with atrial fibrillation.* https://www.ahajournals.org/doi/full/10.1161/CIR.0000000000000665

American Psychological Association. (2019). *Clinical practice guideline for the treatment of depression across three age cohorts.* https://www.apa.org/depression-guideline/guideline.pdf

Arnett, D. K., Blumenthal, R. S., Albert, M. A., Buroker, A. B., Goldberger, Z. D., Hahn, E. J., Himmelfarb, C. D., Khera, A., Lloyd-Jones, D., William McEvoy, J., Michos, E. D., Muñoz, D., Smith, S. C., Virani, S. S., Williams, K. K., Yeboah, J., & Ziaeian, B. (2019). 2019 ACC/AHA guideline on the primary prevention of cardiovascular disease: A report of the American College of Cardiology/American Heart Association task force on clinical practice guidelines. *Journal of the American College of Cardiology, 74*(10), e177–e232. https://doi.org/10.1161/CIR.0000000000000678

Averitas Pharma. (2020). *Qutenza 8% patch administration.* https://www.qutenza.com/hcp/dpn/administration/

Ayoade, F. (2018). *Medscape: Herpes simplex medications.* https://emedicine.medscape.com/article/218580-medication#2

Banach, M., Patti, A. M., Giglio, R. V., Cicero, A. F., Atanasov, A. G., Bajraktari, G., Bruckert, E., Descamps, O., Djuric, D. M., Ezhov, M., Fras, Z., von Haehling, S., Katsiki, N., Langlois, M., Latkovskis, G., Mancini, G. B. J., Mikhailidis, D. P., Mitchenko, O., Moriarty, P. M., . . . Muntner, P. (2018). The role of nutraceuticals in statin intolerant patients. *Journal of the American College of Cardiology, 72*(1), 96–118. https://doi.org/10.1016/j.jacc.2018.04.040

Baniasadi, S. (2020). Metabolism-based drug-drug interactions in patients with chronic respiratory diseases: A review focusing on drugs affecting the respiratory system. *Current Drug Metabolism, 21*(9), 704–713. https://doi.org/10.2174/1389200221999200820164038

Bates, D., Schultheis, B. C., Hanes, M. C., Jolly, S. M., Chakravarthy, K. V., Deer, T. R., Levy, R. M., & Hunter, C. W. (2019). A comprehensive algorithm for management of neuropathic pain. *Pain Medicine, 20*(Suppl. 1), S2–S12.

Bernardo, J. (2017). *Medscape: Aluminum toxicity.* https://emedicine.medscape.com/article/165315-overview#a4

Bhatt, N. (2019). *Medscape: Anxiety.* https://emedicine.medscape.com/article/286227-overview

Cash, J. C., & Glass, C. A. (Eds.). (2019). *Adult-gerontology practice guidelines* (2nd ed.). Springer Publishing Company.

Cattaneo, D., Giacomelli, A., Pagani, G., Filice, C., & Gervasoni, C. (2021). Ritonavir/cobicistat-induced Cushing syndrome in HIV patients treated with non-oral corticosteroids: A call for action? *The American Journal of the Medical Sciences, 361*(1), 137–139. https://doi.org/ 10.1016/j.amjms.2020.08.013

CDC. (2017). *Antibiotic prescribing and user in doctor's office: Adult treatment recommendation.* https://www.cdc.gov/antibiotic-use/community/for-hcp/outpatient-hcp/adult-treatment-rec.html

CDC. (2019). *Antibiotic use in the United States, 2018 update: Progress and opportunities.* US Department of Health and Human Services.

CDC. (2020a). *Antibiotic/antimicrobial resistance.* https://www.cdc.gov/drugresistance/protecting_patients.html

CDC. (2020b). *Fungal disease: Antifungal resistance.* https://www.cdc.gov/fungal/antifungal-resistance.html

CDC. (2020c). *Hepatitis: Health professional tools.* https://www.cdc.gov/hepatitis/resources/healthprofessionaltools.htm

CDC. (2020d). *HIV PrEP.* https://www.cdc.gov/hiv/basics/prep.html

CDC. (2020e). *Influenza health care providers.* https://www.cdc.gov/flu/season/health-care-professionals.htm

Codina Leik, M. T. (2018). *Family nurse practitioner certification: Intensive review.* Springer Publishing Company.

DailyMed. (2016a). *Buspirone hydrochloride tablet.* https://dailymed.nlm.nih.gov/dailymed/drugInfo.cfm?setid=33accd6b-10a6-5bd3-e054-00144ff88e88

DailyMed. (2016b). *TUMS-calcium carbonate tablet.* https://dailymed.nlm.nih.gov/dailymed/drugInfo.cfm?setid=35f79dcf-1743-4d9f-aba5-5ead6b056309

DailyMed. (2018a). *Carvedilol tablet.* https://dailymed.nlm.nih.gov/dailymed/drugInfo.cfm?setid=a9314bc0-fd5d-477b-bef5-3bee532774c0

DailyMed. (2018b). *Omeprazole capsule.* https://dailymed.nlm.nih.gov/dailymed/lookup.cfm?setid=c63b2dd4-ac8a-47a1-889b-94d68137bd01

DailyMed. (2018c). *Pregabalin capsule.* https://dailymed.nlm.nih.gov/dailymed/drugInfo.cfm?setid=cf7b4b67-b017-47ac-af3f-bde5bd07bb0c

DailyMed. (2018d). *Spironolactone tablet.* https://dailymed.nlm.nih.gov/dailymed/drugInfo.cfm?setid=a7510768-8a52-4230-6aa0-b0d92d82588f

DailyMed. (2018e). *Tizanidine.* https://dailymed.nlm.nih.gov/dailymed/drugInfo.cfm?setid=413ee468-c7e8-4283-8e2b-b573dcc1f607

DailyMed. (2019a). *Amoxicillin and clavulanate potassium tablet.* https://dailymed.nlm.nih.gov/dailymed/lookup.cfm?setid=d75b0a7e-cb9b-4102-bcac-097403b25129

DailyMed. (2019b). *Digoxin tablet.* https://dailymed.nlm.nih.gov/dailymed/drugInfo.cfm?setid=f3d29508-e7cc-47ff-845d-b5375ee30407

DailyMed. (2019c). *Erythromycin tablet.* https://dailymed.nlm.nih.gov/dailymed/drugInfo.cfm?setid=e9b5abbb-2952-44ce-8cbb-415d9be23df4

DailyMed. (2019d). *Oxycodone.* https://dailymed.nlm.nih.gov/dailymed/drugInfo.cfm?setid=094b64b3-cd32-4de5-afb6-ea00d9caad74

DailyMed. (2019e). *Symbicort-budesonide and formoterol dihydrate aerosol.* https://dailymed.nlm.nih.gov/dailymed/drugInfo.cfm?setid=fafa4cf1-99c2-43d5-73ad-51f256de3be0

DailyMed. (2020a). *Acyclovir.* https://dailymed.nlm.nih.gov/dailymed/drugInfo.cfm?setid=5f95a4f4-4822-4502-afbf-b592cafc1ae9

DailyMed. (2020b). *Albuterol sulfate inhalant.* https://dailymed.nlm.nih.gov/dailymed/drugInfo.cfm?setid=c4d6d76a-14b8-411a-8019-e2c923c2c532

DailyMed. (2020c). *Ciprofloxacin tablet.* https://dailymed.nlm.nih.gov/dailymed/drugInfo.cfm?setid=888dc7f9-ad9c-4c00-8d50-8ddfd9bd27c0

DailyMed. (2020d). *Clonazepam tablet.* https://dailymed.nlm.nih.gov/dailymed/lookup.cfm?setid=c707caa1-d6fd-4790-9a64-f749bf93ef18&version=11

DailyMed. (2020e). *Doxycycline.* https://dailymed.nlm.nih.gov/dailymed/drugInfo.cfm?setid=9b52e0a7-f024-4d8a-a59e-374946e60b44

DailyMed. (2020f). *Enalapril tablet.* https://dailymed.nlm.nih.gov/dailymed/drugInfo.cfm?setid=a839e6df-7003-8e6a-e053-2995a90a7536

DailyMed. (2020g). *Famotidine tablet.* https://dailymed.nlm.nih.gov/dailymed/drugInfo.cfm?setid=f149eccl-d66c-42f9-a3f4-2ab6a522942b#:~:text=Take%20famotidine%20tablets%20once%20daily%20before%20bedtime%20or,may%20report%20side%20effects%20to%20FDA%20at%201-800-FDA-1088

DailyMed. (2020h). *Fluconazole.* https://dailymed.nlm.nih.gov/dailymed/drugInfo.cfm?setid=737e0fac-a2d2-4053-a0d7-edbfb6248f69

DailyMed. (2020i). *Furosemide tablet*. https://dailymed.nlm.nih.gov/dailymed/drugInfo. cfm?setid=b5c6fcf4-fd37-4fee-8dac-1a3273d95ffe

DailyMed. (2020j). *Hydroxyzine hydrochloride tablet*. https://dailymed.nlm.nih.gov/dailymed/drugInfo. cfm?setid=adc4cb73-77c6-48ff-aaf2-b3568d53de1f

DailyMed. (2020k). *Losartan tablet*. https://dailymed.nlm.nih.gov/dailymed/drugInfo.cfm?setid=cafd54e8-42a8-474c-8ea8-49ec74c2b0d3#:~:text=1.1%20Hypertension%20-%20Losartan%20potassium%20tablets%20are%20 indicated,of%20age%20and%20older%2C%20to%20lower%20blood%20pressure

DailyMed. (2020l). *Nystatin*. https://dailymed.nlm.nih.gov/dailymed/drugInfo. cfm?setid=28b4e26e-206a-4e8a-abfe-774b780e91c3

DailyMed. (2020m). *Oseltamivir phosphate capsule*. https://dailymed.nlm.nih.gov/dailymed/drugInfo. cfm?setid=e5cd4c23-7edb-42df-a96b-860841322efb

DailyMed. (2020n). *Pantoprazole*. https://dailymed.nlm.nih.gov/dailymed/drugInfo. cfm?setid=eda64039-771b-41d7-b9c4-970cfbf5fbb9

DailyMed. (2020o). *Serevent Diskus-salmeterol xinafoate powder metered*. https://dailymed.nlm.nih.gov/dailymed/ drugInfo.cfm?setid=12d9728e-6b5c-4aee-bfb0-745e542ed2e4

DailyMed. (2020p). *Simvastatin tablet*. https://dailymed.nlm.nih.gov/dailymed/drugInfo. cfm?setid=fdbfe194-b845-42c5-bb87-a48118bc72e7

DailyMed. (2020q). *Sulfamethoxazole and trimethoprim*. https://dailymed.nlm.nih.gov/dailymed/drugInfo. cfm?setid=a6182855-6287-45e9-b6b4-7b57efc9c76e

DailyMed. (2020r). *Tebifinafine*. https://dailymed.nlm.nih.gov/dailymed/lookup. cfm?setid=ae523286-64e7-4632-866b-ccdee2523eb2&version=3

DailyMed. (2020s). *Tramadol*. https://dailymed.nlm.nih.gov/dailymed/lookup. cfm?setid=5babcfcf-331b-5db9-e053-2a91aa0aaf89&version=2

Department of Veterans Affairs. (2019). *Managing heart failure in primary care: Improving outcomes through the use of evidence -based medicine*. https://www.pbm.va.gov/PBM/AcademicDetailingService/Documents/Academic_ Detailing_Educational_Material_Catalog/HeartFailure_Provider_ProviderGuide_IB101161.pdf

Dowell, D., Haegerich, T. M., & Chou, R. (2016). CDC guideline for prescribing opioids for chronic pain—United States, 2016. *JAMA, 315*(15), 1624–1645.

Duma, S. R., & Fung, V. S. (2019). Drug-induced movement disorders. *Australian Prescriber, 42*(2), 56–61. https:// doi.org/10.18773/austprescr.2019.014

Fulop, T. (2020). *Medscape: Hypermagnesemia*. https://emedicine.medscape.com/article/246489-overview#a1

Galdo, J. A. (2013). Long-term consequences of chronic proton pump inhibitor use. *US Pharm, 38*(12), 38–42.

Haastrup, P. F., Thompson, W., Søndergaard, J., & Jarbøl, D. E. (2018). Side effects of long-term proton pump inhibitor use: A review. *Basic & Clinical Pharmacology & Toxicology, 123*(2), 114–121. https://doi.org/10.1111/ bcpt.13023

Halverson, J. (2019). *Medscape: Depression*. https://emedicine.medscape.com/article/286759-overview

Hornor, M. A., Duane, T. M., Ehlers, A. P., Jensen, E. H., Brown, P. S., Jr., Pohl, D., da Costa, P. M., Ko, C. Y., & Laronga, C. (2018). American College of Surgeons' guidelines for the perioperative management of antithrombotic medication. *Journal of the American College of Surgeons, 227*(5), 521–536.e1. https://doi. org/10.1016/j.jamcollsurg.2018.08.183

IU Department of Medicine. (n.d.). *Flockhart table: Drug interactions table*. https://drug-interactions.medicine. iu.edu/MainTable.aspx

Jordan, S., Davies, G. I., Thayer, D. S., Tucker, D., & Humphreys, I. (2019). Antidepressant prescriptions, discontinuation, depression and perinatal outcomes, including breastfeeding: A population cohort analysis. *PLoS ONE, 14*(11), e0225133. https://doi.org/10.1371/journal.pone.0225133

Katholi, R. E., Stormer, E. A., Castro-Torres, Y., & Ervin, M. R. (2020). Is real world use of carvedilol in patients with HFrEF consistent with clinical trial data? A 21-year experience in a private cardiologist's practice. *Journal of Cardiology Research, 3*(1), 30. https://doi.org/gsl.jcr.2020.000030

Kolasinski, S. L., Neogi, T., Hochberg, M. C., Oatis, C., Guyatt, G., Block, J., Callahan, L., Copenhaver, C., Dodge, C., Felson, D., Gellar, K., Harvey, W. F., Hawker, G., Herzig, E., Kwoh, K., Nelson, A. E., Samuels, J., Scanzello, C., White, D., . . . Reston, J. (2020). 2019 American college of rheumatology/arthritis foundation guideline for the management of osteoarthritis of the hand, hip, and knee. *Arthritis & Rheumatology, 72*(2), 220–233. https:// doi.org/10.1002/art.41102

Mayo Clinic. (2020). *Stain intolerance clinic*. https://www.mayoclinic.org/departments-centers/ statin-intolerance-service/overview/ovc-20442137

Medscape. (n.d.a). *Acetaminophen*. https://reference.medscape.com/drugs/analgesics-other

Medscape. (n.d.b). *Antiplatelet agents*. https://reference.medscape.com/drugs/antiplatelet-agents-hematologic

Medscape. (n.d.c). *Cephalosporins.* https://reference.medscape.com/drugs/cephalosporins-other

Medscape. (n.d.d). *NSAIDs.* https://reference.medscape.com/drugs/nsaids

Medscape. (n.d.e). *Penicillins.* https://reference.medscape.com/drugs/penicillins-natural

Morris, M. (2020). *Medscape: Asthma medications.* Springer Publishing Company. https://emedicine.medscape.com/article/296301-medication\

NIH. (2020). *DailyMed: Spravato esketamine hydrochloride solution.* https://dailymed.nlm.nih.gov/dailymed/drugInfo.cfm?setid=d81a6a79-a74a-44b7-822c-0dfa3036eaed

Ouellette, D. (2020). *Pulmonary embolism medications: Direct thrombin inhibitors and factor Xa inhibitors.* https://emedicine.medscape.com/article/300901-medication#4

Owen, G. T., Bruel, B. M., Schade, C. M., Eckmann, M. S., Hustak, E. C., & Engle, M. P. (2018). Evidence-based pain medicine for primary care physicians. *Proceedings (Baylor University. Medical Center), 31*(1), 37–47. https://doi.org/10.1080/08998280.2017.1400290

Palaniyappan, L. (2009). Combining antidepressants: A review of evidence. *Advances in Psychiatric Treatment, 15*(2), 90–99. https://doi.org/10.1192/apt.bp.107.004820

Pisa, F. E., Reinold, J., Kollhorst, B., Haug, U., & Schink, T. (2020, June 22). Individual antidepressants and the risk of fractures in older adults: A new user active comparator study. *Clinical Epidemiology, 12*, 667–678. https://doi.org/10.2147/CLEP.S222888. PMID: 32606992; PMCID: PMC7319507.

Qaseem, A., McLean, R. M., O'Gurek, D., Batur, P., Lin, K., & Kansagara, D. L. (2020). Nonpharmacologic and pharmacologic management of acute pain from non-low back, musculoskeletal injuries in adults: A clinical guideline from the American college of physicians and American academy of family physicians. *Annals of Internal Medicine, 173*(9), 739–748.

Reddel, H. K., FitzGerald, J. M., Bateman, E. D., Bacharier, L. B., Becker, A., Brusselle, G., Cruz, A. A., Fleming, L., Inoue, H., Ko, F. W., Krishnan, J. A., Levy, M. L., Lin, J., Pedersen, S. E., Sheikh, A., Yorgancioglu, A., & Boulet, L. P. (2019). GINA 2019: A fundamental change in asthma management: Treatment of asthma with short-acting bronchodilators alone is no longer recommended for adults and adolescents. *European Respiratory Journal, 53*(6), 1901046. https://doi.org/10.1183/13993003.01046-2019

Remme, W. J., Torp-Pedersen, C., Cleland, J. G., Poole-Wilson, P. A., Metra, M., Komajda, M., Swedberg, K., Di Lenarda, A., Spark, P., Scherhag, A., Moullet, C., & Lukas, M. A. (2007). Carvedilol protects better against vascular events than metoprolol in heart failure: results from COMET. *Journal of the American College of Cardiology, 49*(9), 963–971. https://doi.org/10.1016/j.jacc.2006.10.059

Sandrock, C. (2019). *Medscape: Antiviral therapy.* https://emedicine.medscape.com/article/1966844-overview

Serban, M. C., Colantonio, L. D., Manthripragada, A. D., Monda, K. L., Bittner, V. A., Banach, M., Chen, L., Huang, L., Dent, R., Kent, S. T., Muntner, P., & Rosenson, R. S. (2017). Statin intolerance and risk of coronary heart events and all-cause mortality following myocardial infarction. *Journal of the American College of Cardiology, 69*(11), 1386–1395. https://doi.org/10.1016/j.jacc.2016.12.036

Shah, A., Hayes, C. J., & Martin, B. C. (2017). Characteristics of initial prescription episodes and likelihood of long-term opioid use—United States, 2006–2015. *MMWR. Morbidity and Mortality Weekly Report, 66*(10), 265–269. https://doi.org/10.15585/mmwr.mm6610a1

Singh, M. (2020). *Medscape: Chronic pain syndrome management.* https://emedicine.medscape.com/article/310834-medication#1 Springer Publishing Company.

Strawn, J. R., Mills, J. A., Cornwall, G. J., Mossman, S. A., Varney, S. T., Keeshin, B. R., & Croarkin, P. E. (2018). Buspirone in children and adolescents with anxiety: A review and Bayesian analysis of abandoned randomized controlled trials. *Journal of Child and Adolescent Psychopharmacology, 28*(1), 2–9. https://doi.org/10.1089/cap.2017.0060

Sweeney, M. E. (2019). *Medscape: Hypertriglyceridemia.* https://emedicine.medscape.com/article/126568-overview

Wedemeyer, R. S., & Blume, H. (2014). Pharmacokinetic drug interaction profiles of proton pump inhibitors: An update. *Drug Safety, 37*(4), 201–211. https://doi.org/10.1007/s40264-014-0144-0

Whelton, P. K., Carey, R. M., Aronow, W. S., Casey, D. E., Jr., Collins, K. J., Himmelfarb, D. C., DePalma, S. M., Gidding, S., Jamerson, K. A., Jones, D. W., MacLaughlin, E. J., Muntner, P., Ovbiagele, B., Smith, S. C., Jr., Spencer, C. C., Stafford, R. S., Taler, S. J., Thomas, R. J., Williams, K. A., Sr., . . . Williamson, J. D. (2018). 2017 ACC/AHA/AAPA/ABC/ACPM/AGS/APhA/ASH/ASPC/NMA/PCNA guideline for the prevention, detection, evaluation, and management of high blood pressure in adults: executive summary: A report of the American College of Cardiology/American Heart Association Task Force on clinical practice guidelines. *Journal of the American College of Cardiology, 71*(19), 2273–2275. https://doi.org/10.1161/HYP.0000000000000066

Yang, E. (2018). *Medscape: Lipid management guidelines.* https://emedicine.medscape.com/article/2500032-overview

Zafari, M. (2019). *Medscape: Myocardial infarction.* https://emedicine.medscape.com/article/155919-overview

3
NERVOUS SYSTEM

THE NEUROLOGICAL EXAM AND CRANIAL NERVE REVIEW

Overview

- The neurological examination begins with history taking to elicit subjective data. Observe the patient's behavior, speech, and paralanguage while conducting the interview.
- The physical examination consists of the following:
  - Mental status assessment
  - Cranial nerve examination
  - Motor examination
  - Muscle strength
  - Gait and coordination
  - Sensation
  - Reflexes
- Perform examination components and techniques relevant to the patient's reason for seeking care in the order that maximizes efficiency and patient comfort.

Mental Status Assessment

- Introduce yourself to the patient, explain the purpose of the examination, obtain permission, and conduct the interview. Assess the level of consciousness, wakefulness, thought processes, appearance, behavior, and speech.
  - Provide the name of three objects at the start of the exam.
  - Ask the patient to identify themselves, ask them to state their current location or place, and the time of day or date.
  - Ask the patient to recall the objects named at the start of the interview and record.
  - Ask the patient to identify an object and name other items in the group that they can think of in 1 min to evaluate their thought process further if indicated.
  - Consider evaluating the patient's ability to follow simple commands if comprehension is a concern.
- Note if the patient appears confused and use assessment tools such as the MMSE, SAGE, or Mini-Cog® screen during this part of the examination if confusion is present.
- Perform a depression screen routinely and an in-depth evaluation for depression if the patient has a positive screen or if the patient appears apathetic, sad, or withdrawn.

Cranial Nerve Examination

- Make observations and test the cranial nerves that arise from the forebrain (CN I and CN II) and brainstem (CN III–XII). See Table 3.1 for more information.

Table 3.1 Cranial Nerves I–XII

Nerve	Name	Technique
CN I	Olfactory	**Nares patency, odor identification** If the patient has an altered sense of smell, determine if the nares are patent and ask the patient to identify odors in each naris using scratch cards.
CN II	Optic (sensory)	**Pupillary light reflex, swinging light test, fundoscopy, visual fields by direct confrontation, and visual acuity** • Inspect pupils for equality in size, shape, and pupillary constriction in swinging light test. Determine if the response is consensual. • Track pupillary constriction and convergence bilaterally. Have the patient track a penlight from a distance to the tip of their nose. • Perform fundoscopy to assess for red reflex, optic disc color, margins, size, shape, and blood vessels. • Assess visual fields to assess peripheral vision. • Test visual acuity with Snellen chart.
CN III	Oculomotor (motor)	**Smooth pursuit, EOM, oculocephalic maneuver** • Examine palpebral fissure for symmetry and absence of ptosis. • Use H shape to examine smooth pursuit to evaluate EOMS. Note if nystagmus is present.
CN IV	Trochlear	
CN VI	Abducens	• Examine eyes for forward gaze when the head is turned from side to side, and the neck is flexed and hyperextended.
CN V	Trigeminal (sensory and motor)	*Sensory*: **Light touch and pinprick** • Perform the sensory exam using a cotton ball and pin to test the three branches of the nerve: ophthalmic, maxillary, and mandibular. *Motor*: **Mastication (masseter, temporalis, and pterygoid muscles)** • Examine the jaw for muscle atrophy and test the strength of chewing muscles. Palpate the angle of the jaw, ask the patient to clench their teeth, and observe muscle effort by touch. Instruct the patient to open their mouth against resistance. Determine if the jaw deviates when opening. *Sensory*: **Corneal reflex testing** • Observe for involuntary blink with a light touch to the cornea.
CN VII	Facial	**Motor testing** • Inspect the face for symmetry. Ask the patient to raise their eyebrows, smile, frown, and puff out their cheeks. *Sensory*: **Taste, lacrimation, and salivation, if indicated** • Test the sense of taste in the anterior two-third of the tongue using sweet, sour, and bitter solutions applied with a cotton swab.

Nerve	Name	Technique
CN VIII	Vestibulocholear	**Hearing** • Test hearing loss using the whisper or sound test in each ear. • *Weber test* (evaluates type of hearing loss): Place an active tuning fork on top of the head. The buzzing sensation should not lateralize to either side. • *Sensorineural loss*: Weber test lateralizes to *undamaged ear with loss*. (Remember, "It makes sense to go to the good ear.") • *Conduction loss*: Weber test lateralizes to *damaged ear with loss*. (Conduction is an opposite sensorineural loss.) • *Rinne test* (evaluates conduction; does not detect sensorineural loss): Activate the tuning fork and place the end on the mastoid process. Ask the patient to report when the buzzing stops. When it stops, hold the tuning fork over the ear and ask the patient to report when the sound stops. • *Sensorineural loss*: AC > BC **(normal)** • *Conduction loss*: BC > AC **Vestibular function** • Specialized testing to elicit nystagmus and vertigo
CN IX	Glossopharyngeal	**Soft palate and uvula symmetry without deviation** • Inspect for the symmetric elevation of palate and uvula with phonation without deviation. **Gag reflex in suspected brainstem pathology** • Touch the posterior oropharynx with a tongue blade. Observe for tongue elevation and constriction of oropharyngeal muscle if the gag reflex is present.
CN X	Vagus	**Phonation** • Assess articulation and strength of voice.
CN XI	Accessory	**Manual muscle test** • Test sternocleidomastoid and trapezius muscles for a range of motion and strength.
CN XII	Hypoglossal	**Tongue strength** • Assess tongue bulk and observe for the presence of fasciculations at rest. • Assess movements of the tongue; observe if tongue is midline or deviates to right or left.

Motor Examination

Muscle examination includes bulk, tone, strength, and pronator drift.
- Inspect for general and limb postures, muscle bulk, and involuntary movements such as tremor or fasciculation.
- Assess for pronator drift with arms extended and palms facing upward for 15 sec and eyes closed.
- Assess the tone of extremities, during passive ROM to identify catching (spasticity), resistance (rigidity), and weakness (flaccidity).

(continued)

Motor Examination (*continued*)

- Assess strength against resistance in all limbs and grade on a scale 0 to 5.
  - *Upper extremities*: Check resistance to shoulder abduction (deltoid; C5, C6), elbow flexion (biceps; C5, C6), elbow extension (triceps; C6, C7, C8), wrist extension (*wrist extensor muscles*: C6, C7, C8), finger abduction (C8, T1), thumb abduction (C8, T1).
  - *Lower extremities*:
    - Assess clonus in ankle using brisk dorsiflexion and observe for the presence of beats of clonus.
    - Check resistance to hip abduction, extension, flexion. Assess knee flexion, extension, and ankle dorsiflexion bilaterally.

Sensation Examination

Sensation examination evaluates sensation to light touch and pinprick, position sense, and vibration in all extremities.
- Assess light touch/pinprick.
  - Examine upper and lower extremities for sensation using a cotton ball and pin and compare bilaterally. Ask the patient to close their eyes to facilitate the exam. Start distally and move proximally, moving from areas of impairment to sites without impairment. Focus on nerve distribution associated with the patient's subjective report.
  - Perform testing for stereognosis, graphesthesia, two-point discrimination, extinction, and point location if a deviation from normal is found.
- Evaluate position sense.
  - Demonstrate MTP joint movement up and down. Ask the patient to close eyes and report a change in position, up or down, in response to your random repositioning of the joint. Start distally and move proximally and confirm if patient can identify direction of movement correctly.
- Evaluate vibration sense.
  - Activate the tuning fork and check if the patient can feel the vibration and feel when it stops. Proceed to evaluate vibration in each extremity on a distal bony prominence. Ask the patient to close their eyes and report when they sense vibration has stopped.

 ALERT

Abnormal motorsensory results require a referral to a neurologist.

Coordination and Gait

- *Coordination*: Assess the patient's ability to perform rapid alternating or point-to-point movements to evaluate cerebellar function.
  - Demonstrate a select rapid alternating movement and instruct the patient to perform the activity:
    - *Finger-to-finger test, finger-to-nose test, heel-to-shin test*: Observe for dysdiadochokinesis or dysmetria
- *Gait*: Assess the patient walking across the room normally and observe arm swing. Follow with instructions to walk heel-toe (tandem gait) and on heels alone.
- *Balance (Romberg) test*: Have the patient stand with heels together and eyes closed and assess for loss of balance. Conduct further inquiry and repeat the test if the patient loses their balance. If the patient maintains balance with eyes open, record a positive Romberg test.

Reflexes

Testing reflexes helps to distinguish between upper and lower motor neuron disease. LMN disease depresses reflexes while UMN disease increases reflexes. Test for clonus if hyper reflexes are noted. The intensity of reflexes can decrease with age. Compare all reflexes bilaterally. Record findings according to objective scale.

- *DTR*: Upper extremity reflexes
  - Biceps (C5, C6), triceps (C7), brachioradialis (C6)
- *DTR*: Lower extremity reflexes
  - Quadriceps (L4), Achilles/ankle jerk (S1), plantar (S1 and tibial nerve)
- Superficial reflexes
  - *Abdominal*: Light stroking of all four quadrants of the abdomen near the umbilicus cause muscle contraction; the absence of a response indicates spinal injury.
  - *Cremasteric*: Stroke the inner thigh below the inguinal crease in males. The ipsilateral testes will rise (L2).
- Pathological reflexes are a reversion to primitive reflexes due to loss of cortical inhibition.
  - *Rooting reflex*: Stroke lateral lip cause movement of mouth to stimulus.
  - *Grasping reflex*: Stroke the palm; the fingers attempt to flex and grasp.
  - *Plantar (Babinski)*: Stroke from the heel to the ball of the sole. Observe the great toe dorsiflex and the remaining toes fan.

Patient Population Considerations

Geriatric

- Obtain history of dizziness, impaired cognition, executive function, tremors, falls risk, anxiety, visual changes, recent losses, personal supports.
- Perform cognitive and depression screens.

Pediatric

- Obtain history of prenatal care, delivery, Apgar scores, congenital defects, presence of seizures, developmental milestones, contact sports participation, use of safety helmets and car seats, exposure to lead, learning difficulties, change in the home or family structure, and family history of neurologic disease.
- Perform an anxiety and depression screen.

ACUTE BACTERIAL MENINGITIS

Overview

- Acute bacterial meningitis is an infection of the leptomeninges of the brain and spinal cord. Inflammation of the subarachnoid space occurs as a result of hematogenous spread, invasive procedures, vaginal delivery, surgery, or direct extension along nerves or proximate structures.

CLINICAL PEARL

Reflex Scale

4+—very brisk, hyperactive
3+—brisker than average
2+—average, normal
1+—diminished, low normal
0—no response

POP QUIZ 3.1

A 69-year-old female with a history of hypothyroidism presents to the primary care provider and reports that she recently has had several episodes of jaw pain, described as burning in character, that last a few seconds to 30 min whenever she exercises. What is the most appropriate approach to the neurological component of the examination?

COMPLICATIONS

Acute: Sepsis, seizures, stroke, hypoventilation, brain herniation, DIC, SIADH, brain abscess

Chronic: Hydrocephalus, hearing loss, blindness, paresis/paralysis, cognitive dysfunction, learning issues

(continued)

Overview (*continued*)

- Inflammation from highly active leukocytes present in CSF cause increased ICP, seizure, neurological deficits, neuronal loss, coma, Waterhouse–Friderichsen syndrome, and death.

Etiology

- Exposure to an infected or colonized patient, vaginal delivery, or consumption of contaminated food
- Recent sinusitis, mastoiditis, otitis media, pneumonia, UTI
- Immunosuppression, chronic disease
- Head trauma, surgical/invasive procedure, contaminated ventriculoperitoneal shunt
- Extremes of age, congregate residential setting, occupation exposure, travel to an endemic region: Sub-Saharan Africa, and Mecca during Hajj and Umrah pilgrimages

 ALERT

Common Causative Bacteria

Young infants: Group B *Streptococcus, Escherichia coli, Listeria moncytogenes*

Older infants, children, and young adults: *Streptococcus pneumoniae* and *Neisseria meningitides*

Middle age and older adults: *Streptococcus pneumoniae*

Healthcare associated: *Staphylococcus aureus, Pseudomonas aeroginosa*

Signs and Symptoms

- Headache, fever, nuchal rigidity
- Petechial rash, nausea, or vomiting
- Change in mental status progressing to coma
- Kernig's or Brudzinski's signs may be present.
- *Infants*: Bulging fontanelles, high pitched cry, and hypotonia

Differential Diagnosis

- *NEURO*: Aseptic meningitis, brain abscess, brain tumor, brain cancer or metastasis, CNS vasculitis, ehrlichiosis, encephalitis, fungal disease, HIV, herpes virus, Lyme disease, West Nile virus, GBS, intracranial hemorrhage, mycobacterium tuberculosis, MS, neurosarcoidosis, neurosyphilis, stroke
- *Other*: APLA syndrome, SLE, DTs, overdose, medication-induced, poisoning

 CLINICAL PEARL

Primary Prevention
- MenB and MenACWY vaccines prevent *Neisseria meningitidis.*
- PPSV23 and PCV13 vaccines protect against *Streptococcus pneumoniae.*
- Hib vaccine protects against *Haemophilus influenzae* type B.

Diagnosis

Labs

- Blood cultures
- Urine or sputum c/s, if indicated
- CBC to evaluate for leukocytosis (may be normal); thrombocytopenia may be present with sepsis/DIC
- BMP, LFTs, PT/INR to assess electrolytes for SIADH; serum glucose to compare to CSF glucose, hepatorenal function, and coagulation

Additional Diagnostic Testing

- Head CT
- Lumbar puncture after head CT

Treatment and Management

Treatment Goals

- Prevent infection in high-risk groups, eradicate infection when present, deter transmission of disease, and prevent acute and chronic complications.

- Transfer patients with acute symptoms to the ED immediately for head CT, blood cultures, lumbar puncture, and treatment with dexamethasone, third-generation cephalosporins, and vancomycin.

Drug Treatment
- ABM is a reportable infection to the state DOH. Treat all close contacts and asymptomatic carriers with PEP:
  - MenACWY vaccine to ages >2 months, revaccinate in age >7 years if it is more than 5 years since their last dose. Revaccinate in age <7 years if it is more than 3 years since their previous dose.
  - MenB vaccines in persons aged ≥10 years who are at increased risk during meningococcal outbreaks.
  - Close contacts are prescribed chemoprophylaxis with ciprofloxacin when indicated.

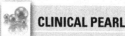

CLINICAL PEARL

MenACWY vaccine may be administered to high-risk contacts whose age is >56 years during outbreaks.

Interventions
- Complete report to the DOH, if necessary.
- Monitor results of microbiology. Beta-lactam and fluoroquinolone resistance has been observed.
- Observe close contacts for the emergence of resistant infection.
- Observe discharged patients for complications of neurological sequela.

Patient Education
- Discuss the risk of infection with resistant strains.
- Discuss ABM prophylaxis and follow-up.
- Review s/s of complications and adverse effects of medication to report.

Patient Population Considerations

Women (conception/pregnancy/lactation)
- Vaccinate close contacts of meningococcal infections in patients who are pregnant with MenACWY. MenB vaccination is generally deferred unless the risk of infection is present. Discuss risks and benefits using a shared decision-making model.

Geriatric
- Currently, the CDC does not recommend the use of MenACWY or MenB vaccination in the geriatric population to prevent meningitis caused by *Neisseria meningitidis*.

Pediatric
- Administer meningitis vaccines using the IM route. Do not combine MenACWY and MenB vaccines in a single syringe. Administer in vastus lateralis in children and infants. Select the deltoid site for older children.

Referring Patients
- Infectious disease consult
- Neurology consult

BELL'S PALSY

Overview
- Idiopathic facial paralysis is a peripheral nerve palsy affecting CN VII. This common disorder is acute in onset, self-limiting in course, with a risk of chronic sequela.

COMPLICATIONS

Acute: Corneal abrasion, posterior auricular pain

Chronic: Refractory facial paralysis, synkinesis, hemifacial spasm, crocodile tears syndrome

(continued)

Overview (*continued*)

- Neuritis secondary to inflammation of unknown etiology impedes motor function. Subsequent nerve entrapment leads to ischemia and nerve damage that may resolve over 3 to 6 months.

Etiology

- Unknown exact etiology
- *Infection*: HSV 1, herpes zoster infection, Lyme disease
- Positive family history and DM increase risk
- Pregnancy
- Autoimmunity, ischemia, and metabolic hypotheses

Signs and Symptoms

- Unilateral facial muscle weakness that progresses to facial paralysis over 48 hr
- Smooth forehead on affected side
- Dry eye on the affected side, decreased tearing, and inability to close the eyelid completely
- Mouth droop, drooling
- Earache and hypersensitivity to sound without evidence of effusion or otitis media
- Change in taste

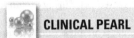

CLINICAL PEARL

House–Brackmann Grading of Faces
Grade I: Normal facial function
Grade II: Mild dysfunction
Grade III: Moderate dysfunction
Grade IV: Moderately severe dysfunction
Grade V: Severe dysfunction
Grade VI: Total paralysis

Differential Diagnosis

- *HEENT*: Scoustic neuroma, acute/chronic otitis media, herpes simplex, nasopharyngeal cancer, parotid tumor, Lyme disease, meningitis, Ramsey Hunt syndrome, Sjogren's syndrome
- *NEURO*: Cancer, CNS vasculitis, Guillain–Barré syndrome, immune-mediated polyneuropathy, intracranial hemorrhage, MS, stroke

Diagnosis

Labs
- No definitive diagnostic labs; exclude alternative causes of paralysis
- *Immune panel*: ESR, TSH, cANCA
- *Metabolic*: CBG, HbA1c, BMP, folate, vitamin B_{12}
- *Infectious*: CBC, tick-borne disease panel, HIV, HSV, RPR, VDRL

Additional Diagnostic Testing
- Head CT to rule out lesion, tumor, bleed
- MRI to evaluate immune-mediated inflammation
- EMG to evaluate prognosis
- Lumbar puncture is certain cases
- Lesion biopsy

Treatment and Management

Treatment Goals
- Protect eye from injury, promote comfort, reduce inflammation, and manage acute/chronic complications.
- Transfer patients with acute symptoms of unilateral facial paralysis with cerebrovascular disease risk factors to the ED for evaluation of stroke.

Drug Treatment

- Prescribe prednisone 1 mg/kg or 60 mg/d for 6 days, followed by a taper for 4 days. (Start within 72 hr of symptom onset.)
- Consider acyclovir 400 mg PO five times per day for 10 days for patients with HSV, 800 mg for patients with VZV.
- Offer artificial tears as needed.
- Consider acetaminophen 650 to 1,000 mg PO every 6 to 8 hr PRN for pain.
- Consider botulism toxin or muscle relaxants for overactive eye muscles.

Interventions

- Grade palsy using the House–Brackmann grading system.
- *Promote eye protection*: Forced blinking, patching for sleep, eyelid weights, and sunglasses outdoors
- Encourage facial muscle retraining exercises.
- Reevaluate the patient in 3 to 4 days and at 2 weeks to monitor progress.

Patient Education

- Explain that prednisone offers modest recovery of symptoms and that complete recovery may take 3 to 6 months.
- Discuss the small risk for recurrence.
- Review s/s of complications and adverse effects of medication to report.

Patient Population Considerations

Women (conception/pregnancy/lactation)

- There is an increased risk of Bell's palsy in pregnancy. Treat pregnant patients with prednisone in consultation with the obstetrician.

Geriatric

- Older patients are more likely than children to develop Bell's palsy.

Pediatric

- Bell's palsy is less common in children under age 15 years. Distinguish Bell's palsy from congenital facial paralysis, trauma, immune-mediated mass, or infection.

Referring Patients

- Neurology consult
- Ophthalmology

POP QUIZ 3.2

A 23-year-old female with no medical history presents to the primary care provider for evaluation of facial weakness. She reports that she had a recent tick bite and viral syndrome. What disorders should be included in the differential diagnosis?

DEMENTIA

Overview

- Dementia is a disorder of progressive decline in cognition, executive function, and social interaction leading to disuse syndrome. It is attributed to vascular disease, metabolic disease, neurodegenerative disorders, infection, drugs, and alcohol.
- Alzheimer's subtype has a genetic component that is believed to be caused by amyloid deposition and cerebral atrophy.

COMPLICATIONS

Acute: Acute complications of immobility, anxiety/depression

Chronic: Disuse syndrome

Etiology

- *Alzheimer's*: Age, APOE 4 genotype, brain injury, depression, diabetes, Down syndrome, family history, mid-life HTN, infection
- *Dementia*: Advancing age, alcoholism, atherosclerosis, CKD, depression, diabetes, drug abuse, hyperlipidemia, diseases (HIV, syphilis), neurodegenerative disorders, obesity, smoking

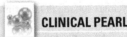 **CLINICAL PEARL**

The incidence of Alzheimer's is increased in patients who used NSAIDs earlier in life.

Signs and Symptoms

- Memory impairment
- Change in behavior, apathy, social withdrawal
- Inability to perform ADLs, manage finances, travel

Differential Diagnosis

- *CV*: Dehydration
- *ENDO*: Hypo/hyperthyroidism, ketoacidosis
- *GI*: Hepatotoxicity
- *GU*: Uremia
- *HEM*: Anemia, vitamin B_{12} deficiency, paraneoplastic syndrome infections, sepsis
- *NEURO*: Acute stroke, cerebral bleed, depression, neurodegenerative disease, normal pressure hydrocephalus, Creutzfeldt–Jakob disease, TBI
- *Other*: Medications, Wilson disease

 ALERT

Screening tools should be used early geriatric patients to detect mild neurocognitive disfunction.

- SAGE Test
- GPCOG
- Mini-Cog©
- Memory impairment screen
- Geriatric depression screen

Diagnosis

Labs

- No definitive diagnostic labs; exclude reversible causes of dementia
- *Netabolic*: HbA1c, BMP, folate, vitamin B_{12}, vitamin D
- *Infectious*: CBC; HIV; RPR; septic workup, if indicated
- *Other*: Toxicology screens, alcohol, genetic testing

Additional Diagnostic Testing

- Head CT to rule out lesion, tumor, bleed
- MRI to evaluate immune-mediated inflammation
- EEG
- PET scan
- Lumbar puncture to evaluate neurodegenerative disease and CJD

Treatment and Management

Treatment Goals

- Prevent progressive cognitive loss, reverse metabolic causes, protect the patient from harm, and minimize complications of disuse syndrome.

Drug Treatment

- Prescribe antidepressants according to depression screen results.
- *Prescribe centrally acting ChEI to improve cognition*: Donepezil, rivastigmine, or galantamine.

 ALERT

Many medications used to treat symptoms of neurocognitive disorders may increase the **risk for falls**. Compare the patient's medications against the Beer's list. Start low and titrate slowly to optimize effect while preventing harm. ChEIs may reduce risk of falls.

- Add NMDA antagonists to ChEI in more advanced disease.
- Treat symptoms of dementia with antiparkinsonian agents, beta blockers, anticonvulsants, and neuroleptics as indicated.

Interventions
- Integrate early detection methods in patients at risk for dementia and control risk factors through medication and recommendations for lifestyle changes (smoking cessation, the MIND diet, blood pressure control, and lipid management).
- Employ cognitive retraining and behavioral therapy early in the diagnosis.
- Prescribe occupational therapy, speech pathology, and physical therapy as necessary.

Patient Education
- Discuss strategies to promote autonomy end-of-life planning with patient and family.
- Review the safety plan and risk of falls.
- Review s/s of complications and adverse effects of medication to report.
- Encourage family members/caregivers to attend caregiver support programs.

Patient Population Considerations

Women (conception/pregnancy/lactation)
- Preeclampsia and maternal hypertension increase the risk of dementia in later life.

Geriatric
- The primary cause of death in patients with dementia is an illness or exacerbation of associated disorders, especially pneumonia. Ensure that the risk for aspiration is evaluated and immunizations are updated.

Pediatric
- Neuronal ceroid lipofuscinoses (Batten disease) are a group of inherited disorders that are associated with dementia in children that lead to shortened life expectancy.

Referring Patients
- Neurology consult

HEADACHE

Overview
- Pain in the head that can be primary or secondary to another disorder such as stroke, aneurysm, infection
- Primary headaches are tension (TTH), migraine, cluster, MOH, NDPH.

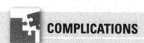

COMPLICATIONS

Acute: Pain, status migrainosis
Chronic: Migraine, stroke

Etiology
- Family history, inherited disorders (MELAS and CADASIL)
- *HEENT:* Obstructive sleep apnea
- *MSK:* Injury to the vertebral column, head
- *Environmental:* Alcohol, bright light (fluorescent), caffeine, cold stimulus, cough, exertion, fasting, food, herbs, hormonal changes, insufficient sleep, medications (NTG, vasodilators, OBC), sexual activity, smoking, stress

Signs and Symptoms

Table 3.2 outlines the symptoms of various headache types.

Differential Diagnosis

- *HEENT*: Sinusitis
- *NEURO*: Acute stroke, brain mass, cerebral aneurysm or bleed, encephalitis, internal carotid dissection, meningitis, temporal/giant cell arteritis, TMJ, TN, TBI
- *Other*: Carbon monoxide poisoning

Diagnosis

Labs
- No definitive diagnostic labs unless an infection is suspected.

Additional Diagnostic Testing
- CT or MRI with severe symptoms or focal neurological deficit
- Sleep study in the presence of daytime sleepiness

Treatment and Management

Treatment Goals
- Minimize recurrence, manage pain, and minimize the development of chronic complications.
- Refer any patient presenting with warning signs of a HA or manifesting a new focused neurological deficit to the ED.

Drug Treatment
- *Acute nonurgent pain management*: Ibuprofen 400 to 1,000 mg, acetaminophen 650 to 100 mg. May consider aspirin 650 mg.
- *Preventive medications, according to HA type*:
  - *TTH*: TCAs, botulism toxin
  - *Migraine*: ACEIs, angiotensin II receptor blockers, anticonvulsants, botulism toxin, calcium channel blockers, erenumab, fremanezumab-vfrm or galcanezumab-gnlm subcutaneous injection monthly (CGRP antagonist), propranolol, topiramate, TCAs (off label), triptans
  - *Cluster*: Anticonvulsants, calcium channel blockers (most effective), galcanezumab subcutaneous injection monthly (CGRP antagonist), mood stabilizers (lithium), oxygen therapy for 10 min (avoid TCAs or beta blocker in cluster HA)
  - *Complementary therapy*: CoQ10, feverfew, melatonin, omega-3, vitamin B2, and vitamin B6

Interventions
- Encourage patients to maintain a headache journal.
- Prescribe cognitive behavioral therapy, meditation, and physical therapy as indicated.
- Reevaluate the patient's response in 2 weeks.

ALERT

Headache Warning Signs
- Worst HA of life
- HA with pregnancy, systemic illness, signs of infection, cancer, immunocompromised state
- HA symptoms will not subside
- New onset HA after age 50 years
- HA with meningeal signs
- Change in the characteristics of HA
- HA after head injury
- Sudden HA with BEFAST signs
- Papilledema
- HA worsens with Valsalva or increased intraabdominal pressure, postural changes, or exertion

Refer patient with any of these signs to ED.

CLINICAL PEARL

New onset progressive headache in patients age >50 years should be evaluated for temporal arteritis. Examine for temporal artery swelling and pulselessness.

CLINICAL PEARL

Diagnostic Criteria for Migraine
- **Five or more HA lasting 4 to 72 hr (must be present) PLUS**

  Any two of:
  1. Unilateral location
  2. Throbbing/pulsating
  3. Worsened by movement
  4. Moderate to severe intensity

  Any one of:
  1. Nausea or vomiting
  2. Phonophobia or photophobia

Table 3.2 Headache Types and Descriptions

Types	Description
TTH	Episodic band-like head pain lasting 30 min to several days, radiating to the neck, bilateral presentation that is not aggravated by activity, **mild to moderate pain**
Migraine	Throbbing pain one side of the head lasting 4–72 hr after exposure to a trigger, associated with or without aura/prodrome, photophobia, and nausea; central or spotty scotoma, visual loss, homonymous hemianopsia or visual field defect, meningismus, hemiparesis, aphasia, confusion, paresthesia may be present, **moderate to severe pain**
Cluster	Episodic severe eye pain lasting 15–180 min, associated with possible eyelid droop and nasal congestion on the ipsilateral side, **severe pain**
MOH	Daily headache that varies in the timing of day and characteristic (symptoms are like TTH or migraine) cause of chronic migraine; uses medication ≥10–15 d/mo for >3 months

Patient Education

- Teach the patient to avoid triggers and encourage daily exercise (PT), CBT, and meditation.
- Review acute management using ergotamine and triptans and discuss criteria for urgent referral.
- Review s/s of complications and adverse effects of medication to report.

Patient Population Considerations

Women (conception/pregnancy/lactation)

- Preeclampsia and maternal hypertension increase the risk of dementia in later life. Avoid ergot derivatives and triptans in pregnant patients with migraine or cluster HA.

Geriatric

- Hypnic headaches are benign headaches that wake patients from their sleep and occur in the older adult population. Do not administer ergot derivative to older adults.

Pediatric

- Children ages 10 to 17 receiving TCAs and CBT were likely to have a 50% reduction in HA frequency.

Referring Patients

- Neurology consult

CLINICAL PEARL

Instructions for migraine medication:

Sumatriptan: Take at first sign of HA and repeat in 2 hr, if needed.

Ergotamine: Sublingual at first sign of HA and repeat twice as needed in 24 hr, not to exceed three doses in 24 hr.

Can cause serotonin syndrome when combined with antidepressants.

PARKINSON'S DISEASE

Overview

- PD is a chronic, progressive neurodegenerative disorder of dopamine deficiency and the presence of Lewy bodies.
- Dopaminergic neurons in the basal ganglia and substantia nigra responsible for processing movement signals start to degenerate, resulting in a dopamine deficiency. Nonmotor symptoms arise from alterations in acetylcholine and dopamine signaling throughout the brain.

COMPLICATIONS

Acute: Complications of immobility, aspiration pneumonia, UTI, wound infections, DVT/PE, anxiety/depression

Chronic: Disuse syndrome, chronic pain, psychosis

Etiology

- Exact etiology unknown
- Advancing age, family history, genetic predisposition, type A encephalitis
- Anticonvulsants, antidepressants, antipsychotics (phenothiazines), and prokinetics (metoclopramide)
- Atherosclerosis, diabetes, TBI, oxidative stress
- Manganese and carbon monoxide exposure

Signs and Symptoms

- Motor symptoms
  - Akinesia, bradykinesia, cogwheel rigidity, mask-like faces, resting tremor (pill-rolling), shuffling gait, postural instability
- Nonmotor symptoms
  - Anosmia, apathy, constipation, dementia, depression, dysphagia, erectile dysfunction, fatigue, hallucinations, hoarseness, hypersalivation, insomnia, orthostatic hypotension, stuttering speech, urinary incontinence

CLINICAL PEARL

Young Onset Parkinson's
Dystonia is a common initial symptom in patients age <40 years with PD.

Differential Diagnosis

- *ENDO*: Hypothyroidism
- *GI*: Hepatotoxicity
- *HEM*: Infections, sepsis
- *NEURO*: Acute stroke, Alzheimer disease, Lewy body dementia, cerebral bleed, chorea, depression, dystonia, essential tremor, Huntington disease, normal pressure hydrocephalus, vascular dementia
- *Other*: Alcoholism, Wilson disease in onset in patients aged <40 years; MPTP exposure, manganese exposure, medications

ALERT

Employ screening tools to identify mild neurocognitive disfunction and depression.
- SAGE Test
- GPCOG
- Mini-Cog©
- Memory impairment screen
- Geriatric depression screen

Diagnosis

Labs
- No definitive diagnostic labs; exclude reversible causes of dementia
- *Metabolic*: HbA1c, BMP, folate, vitamin B_{12}, vitamin D
- *Infectious*: CBC; HIV; RPR; VDRL; septic workup, if indicated
- *Other*: Toxicology screens, alcohol, genetic testing

Additional Diagnostic Testing
- Head CT to rule out lesion, tumor, bleed
- MRI to evaluate immune-mediated inflammation
- Speech pathology evaluation

Treatment and Management

Treatment Goals
- Prevent progressive cognitive loss, preserve mobility, protect the patient from harm, and minimize complications of disuse syndrome.

ALERT

Risk for falls is a major potential complications due to postural instability and impaired motor function.

Compare the patient's medications against the Beer's list. Start low and titrate slowly to optimize effect while preventing harm. ChEIs may reduce risk of falls.

Drug Treatment
- First-line therapy
  - Prescribe levodopa/carbidopa PO daily. Titrate to individual response or consider amantadine as monotherapy in patients <60 years.
  - Prescribe MAO BI (selegiline) in early disease as an adjunct to levodopa, which is neuroprotective.
- Second-line therapy
  - Prescribe dopamine agonists (ropinirole) as an adjunct to primary therapy.
  - Add COMT inhibitors (opicapone) to improve movement and reduce off episodes.
- Symptomatic therapy
  - Consider sildenafil citrate for erectile dysfunction.
  - Prescribe pimavanserin for hallucinations.
  - Anticholinergics (trihexyphenidyl) can be prescribed for resting tremor. Monitor for urinary retention.
  - *Prescribe centrally acting ChEI to improve cognition*: Donepezil, rivastigmine, or galantamine.
  - Add NMDA antagonists to ChEI in more advanced disease.

Interventions
- Monitor the patient's response to medication. Evaluate for periods of on/off syndrome when levodopa inadequately manages motor symptoms.
- Employ cognitive retraining and behavioral therapy early in the diagnosis.
- Prescribe occupational therapy, speech pathology, and physical therapy, as necessary.

Patient Education
- Discuss strategies to promote autonomy end-of-life planning with patient and family.
- Review the safety plan and risk of falls.
- Review s/s of complications and adverse effects of medication to report.
- Encourage family members to join a caregiver support program.

Patient Population Considerations

Women (conception/pregnancy/lactation)
- Provide preconception counseling to women of childbearing age with early-onset PD. Explain that there is a greater risk of disease progression with pregnancy.

Geriatric
- Drooling is a symptom of Parkinson's disease that can increase the risk of pneumonia. Discuss the use of medications and care needed to reduce aspiration of saliva.

Pediatric
- Parkinsonian symptoms in childhood are not PD, but Parkinsonian-like symptoms of neurologic or metabolic disease.

Referring Patients
- Neurology consult

STROKE AND TRANSIENT ISCHEMIC ATTACK

Overview
- TIA is a transient narrowing of cerebral circulation that produces stroke-like symptoms. TIA is the most significant predictor of a stroke.
- A stroke is a sudden cerebrovascular event of decreased circulation. It can be thrombotic, embolic, or hemorrhagic.

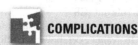

COMPLICATIONS

Acute: Cerebral edema, increased ICP, aspiration PNU, hypoxia, DVT/PE, paralysis, UTI, decubitus, malnutrition

Chronic: Chronic complications of immobility

(continued)

Overview (*continued*)

- Decreased blood circulation distal to the occlusion, embolus, or vascular disruption leads to cellular hypoxia and tissue death. In intracerebral hemorrhage, ischemia is aggravated by elevated ICP, increasing infarct size.

Etiology

- Thrombotic
  - Age, atherosclerosis, DM, ethnicity, family history, hyperlipidemia. HTN, migraine, obesity, sedentary lifestyle, smoking, stimulants, stress (TIA is a predictor for stroke)
- Embolic
  - Atrial fibrillation, AV septal defects, carotid artery stenosis, estrogen therapy, SERM medications, HF, hypercoagulability syndromes, preeclampsia, pregnancy, contraceptive use, rheumatic heart disease, tamoxifen, valve disease
- Hemorrhagic
  - Aneurysm, anticoagulation, arteriovenous malformation, cranial surgery, head trauma, recent stroke

 CLINICAL PEARL

Primary Prevention of Stroke
Risk reduction of modifiable risk factors of stroke and prothrombotic medications

Secondary Prevention of Stroke
Management of atherosclerosis, DM, hyperlipidemia:
- Antiplatelets
- Blood pressure control
- Cigarette smoking cessation
- Cholesterol management
- Carotid revascularization
- Diet
- Exercise

Signs and Symptoms

- Sudden change in a BEFAST assessment
- Altered mental state, cranial nerve deficit, decreased deep tendon reflexes, dizziness, headache, nausea or vomiting, paresthesia, seizure, urinary incontinence, visual loss
- Any new focal neurological deficit

Differential Diagnosis

- *CV*: Aortic dissection
- *ENDO*: DM emergency, hypothyroidism, thyrotoxicosis
- *NEURO*: Brain mass, CNS infection, GBS, intracranial hemorrhage, MS, stroke/TIA of alternative etiology
- *Other*: Intoxication, medication overdose

 ALERT

Acute Symptoms of stroke/TIA
Acute stroke/TIA symptoms require immediate evaluation with head CT in the ED. Thrombotic strokes may be offered alteplase if criteria are met within 4.5 hr.

Diagnosis

Labs
- BMP, CBG, CBC, LFTs, lipid panel, PTT, PT/INR
- Anticardiolipin antibody, protein S, protein C, antithrombin III test
- Toxicology screen

Additional Diagnostic Testing
- Head CT to rule out ICB
- 12-lead EKG to rule out atrial fibrillation
- MRI/MRA to evaluate cerebral circulation
- Carotid artery duplex scan
- TEE
- Lumbar puncture to rule out subarachnoid hemorrhage

Treatment and Management

Treatment Goals

- Restore cerebral perfusion, modify risk factors for stroke, and minimize complications.
- **Transfer patients with acute symptoms of stroke to ED.**

Drug Treatment

- Thromboembolic
  - Prescribe aspirin 75 to 100 mg daily and clopidogrel 75 mg PO daily to reduce thrombus formation.
  - Prescribe antihypertensives according to compelling conditions to maintain SBP between 130 and 149 mmHg. (*Note*: BP parameters may be lower in some instances.)
  - Initiate statins to lower LDL cholesterol.
  - Achieve glycemic control in DM using antidiabetic therapy to target random glucose between 140 and 180 mg/dL and HbA1c <7%.
  - Initiate antidysrhythmic therapy for atrial fibrillation.
- Hemorrhagic
  - Hold antiplatelets and anticoagulants but continue BP, cholesterol, and glucose management.
  - *Administer antidotes*: Vitamin K and FFP for warfarin, andexanet for rivaroxaban, and idarucizumab for apixaban
  - Prescribe anticonvulsant and titrate according to drug levels, if indicated.

Interventions

- *Monitor patient progress with rehabilitation*: PT, OT, speech pathology, smoking cessation, depression, and diet
- Periodically evaluate BP, lipid panel, HbA1c, CBC, PT/INR to titrate medication.
- Prescribe assistive devices as indicated to prevent injury.

Patient Education

- Discuss safety requirements for driving.
- Employ shared decision-making to define goals for medication therapy.
- Review s/s of complications and adverse effects of medication to report.

Patient Population Considerations

Women (conception/pregnancy/lactation)

- Provide preconception counseling to women with HTN about the increased risk for stroke.
- Older females have the highest risk of ischemic stroke.

Pediatric

- Infants and children are at risk for arterial ischemic, venous thrombotic, and hemorrhagic stroke. Atherosclerosis is not a factor in pediatric stroke.

Referring Patients

- Neurology consult
- Cardiology consult

 POP QUIZ 3.3

An 87-year-old female with a history of hypertension, peripheral arterial disease, and hyperlipidemia is taking amlodipine, clopidogrel, and simvastatin. She presents to the primary care clinic complaining of a sudden headache that has gotten progressively worse over 24 hr despite taking acetaminophen and ibuprofen. She denies recent falls, trauma, or history of headache in the past. Vital signs are BP 162/88, HR 122, RR 22, temp 100.2°F (37.9°C). Pertinent positive findings include left homonymous hemianopsia, slight facial droop, weakness LUE and LLE. DTR: 1+/4 LUE and LLE compared to 2+/4 RUE and RLE. Babinski absent. What is the most appropriate next step?

TEMPORAL ARTERITIS

Overview

- Temporal or GCA is a self-limiting inflammatory disorder of medium and large blood vessels of the head, neck, and arms, including the temporal artery.
- PMR is linked to GCA and may be manifestations of the same disease.
- In both disorders, macrophage and T cell activation triggers systemic inflammation. Inflammation in synovial tissue and bursae cause shoulder, neck, or hip pain associated with morning stiffness in PMR. Vessel injury and hyperplasia in temporal arteritis cause ischemia.

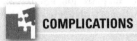 **COMPLICATIONS**

Acute: TIA/stroke, pain

Chronic: Relapse of GCA, aortic aneurysm

Etiology

- Unknown exact etiology
- Advancing age, autoimmunity, genetic predisposition, northern European ethnicity are risk factors.

 ALERT

Refer to ED if abrupt symptoms are present. GCA symptoms may mimic stroke symptoms and require immediate evaluation with a head CT in the ED.

Signs and Symptoms

- Abrupt or insidious blurred vision, cough, headache, tongue or jaw pain (claudication), scalp pain, fatigue, weight loss, fever
- Scalp tenderness, reduced or absent temporal artery pulse

Differential Diagnosis

- *HEENT*: Acute angle-closure glaucoma, herpes zoster, iritis, persistent idiopathic facial pain, retinal artery occlusion, TMJ, uveitis
- *NEURO*: TIA/stroke, migraine
- *Other*: RA, PMR, granulomatosis with polyangiitis

Diagnosis

Labs
- Elevated C-reactive protein and ESR >50 to 100 mm/hr.
- *CBC*: Normochromic normocytic anemia, mild thrombocytosis
- BMP, elevated LFTs

Additional Diagnostic Testing
- Head CT to rule out stroke
- Temporal artery biopsy
- Automated visual fields
- Doppler ultrasound of temporal artery

Treatment and Management

Treatment Goals
- Restore perfusion through immunosuppression and minimize complications.
- *Transfer patients with acute symptoms of stroke to ED.*

Drug Treatment
- Prescribe corticosteroids immediately. For patients with visual symptoms, do not delay for biopsy results to avoid irreversible damage.
- Prescribe aspirin 81 mg PO daily to prevent stroke.

Interventions
- Monitor for resolution of symptoms within 72 hr with an associated decline in inflammatory markers.
- Implement risk modification for stroke using ABCDE management.
- Schedule periodic reevaluation of ESR and for s/s of claudication.

Patient Education
- Explain to the patient that there is an increased risk of stroke with GCA.
- Teach the patient to monitor for s/s of relapse.
- Review s/s of complications and adverse effects of medication to report.

Patient Population Considerations

Women (conception/pregnancy/lactation)
- GCA presents in perimenopausal women.

Geriatric
- Caucasian women between 70 and 80 years are at the highest risk for GCA.

Pediatric
- Juvenile temporal arteritis is a rare disorder affecting only the temporal artery in children.

Referring Patients

- Neurology consult
- Ophthalmology consult

TRIGEMINAL NEURALGIA

Overview

- TN is a chronic neuropathic pain disorder of the CN V that is characterized by exacerbation and remission. There are two forms.
  - Type 1 is characterized by sudden, severe, spasmodic facial pain, lasting a few seconds to 2 min.
  - Type 2 manifests with less pain but is constant.
- One hypothesis is that compression of CN V causes demyelination, that when triggered, causes paroxysmal pain.

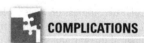

COMPLICATIONS

Acute: Social isolation, depression
Chronic: Excessive weight loss

Etiology

- Unknown exact etiology
- AV malformation, female gender, herpes zoster, HTN, Lyme disease, MS, sarcoidosis, stroke, and tumor compression are all risk factors

Signs and Symptoms

- Abrupt onset of unilateral burning pain along with the distribution of the trigeminal nerve initiated by light touch, chewing, brushing teeth, exposure to heat or cold, shaving, applying makeup, or washing face.

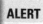

ALERT

Refer to ED if abrupt symptoms are present.
TN symptoms may mimic stroke symptoms and require immediate evaluation with head CT in the ED.

Differential Diagnosis

- *HEENT*: Cavernous sinus syndrome, hemifacial spasm
- *NEURO*: Migraine, cerebral aneurysm, cluster headaches, hydrocephalus, intracerebral hemorrhage, herpes zoster, postherpetic neuralgia

Diagnosis

Labs
- No labs are required to diagnose TN.

Additional Diagnostic Testing
- MRI

Treatment and Management

Treatment Goals
- Manage pain, prevent acute and chronic complications.
- *Transfer patients with acute symptoms of stroke to ED.*

Drug Treatment
- Prescribe carbamazepine or oxcarbazepine as first-line therapy. Consider baclofen, lamotrigine, or other anticonvulsants as second-line therapy.

Interventions
- Monitor the patient's pain response and for the development of depression and sleep disturbance.
- Collaborate with neurology on titration and maintenance of medication.
- Discuss alternative therapies to complement medication therapy.
- Refer patients with refractory pain to a surgeon for decompression.

Patient Education
- Discuss disease process and management.
- Review s/s of complications and adverse effects of medication to report.

Patient Population Considerations

Women (conception/pregnancy/lactation)
- Evaluate for MS when women of childbearing age present with symptoms of TN.

Geriatric
- Microvascular decompression is well tolerated in older patients who have an incomplete response to pharmacological therapy and should be considered in refractory pain.

Pediatric
- TN does not present in pediatric patients.

Referring Patients

- Neurology consult
- Neurosurgical consult

 POP QUIZ 3.4

A 70-year-old male presents to the primary care clinic accompanied by his spouse for evaluation of a recent change in behavior. He has a medical history of TBI from military service and epilepsy for which he takes gabapentin. In the general survey, the nurse practitioner notices that the patient appears apathetic and withdrawn, and a fine hand tremor is noted as he awaits examination. What diagnoses should the nurse practitioner suspect based on this information alone?

RESOURCES

Basit, S., Wohlfahrt, J., & Boyd, H. A. (2018). Preeclampsia and risk of dementia later in life: A nationwide cohort study. *BMJ, 363*, k4109. https://doi.org/10.1136/bmj.k4109.

Blanda, M. (2019). *Medscape: Cluster headache.* https://emedicine.medscape.com/article/1142459-overview#:~:text=Cluster%20headache%20%28CH%29%2C%20also%20known%20as%20histamine%20headache%2C,headaches%2C%20usually%20over%20a%20period%20of%20several%20weeks.

Cash, J. C., & Glass, C. A. (Eds.). (2019). *Adult-gerontology practice guidelines* (2nd ed.). Springer Publishing Company.

CDC. (2019). *Guidance for the evaluation and public health management of suspected outbreaks of meningococcal disease.* https://www.cdc.gov/meningococcal/downloads/meningococcal-outbreak-guidance.pdf

Chang, C. (2017). *Medscape: Neuronal ceroid lipofuscinoses.* https://emedicine.medscape.com/article/1178391-overview#a5

Chawla, J. (2020). *Medscape: Migraine headache.* https://emedicine.medscape.com/article/1142556-overview

Clinical Resource. (2019). *Potentially harmful drugs in the elderly: Beers list. Pharmacist's letter/prescriber's letter.* https://www.pharmacyquality.com/wp-content/uploads/2019/05/Beers-List-350301.pdf.

Codina Leik, M. T. (2018). *Family nurse practitioner certification: Intensive review* (3rd ed.). Spring Publishing Company.

de Assis Aquino Gondim, F. (2019). *Medscape: Meningococcal meningitis.* https://emedicine.medscape.com/article/1165557-overview.

Department of Veterans Affairs. (2020). *Headache algorithm.* https://www.healthquality.va.gov/guidelines/pain/headache/VADoDHeadacheCPGPocketCardFinal508v2.pdf

Ferriero, D. M., Fullerton, H. J., Bernard, T. J., Billinghurst, L., Daniels, S. R., DeBaun, M. R., & Smith, E. R. (2019). Management of stroke in neonates and children: A scientific statement from the American heart association/American stroke association. *Stroke, 50*(3), e51–e96. https://doi.org/10.1161/STR.0000000000000183

Hauser, R. (2020). *Medscape: Parkinson's disease.* https://emedicine.medscape.com/article/1831191-overview

Hoover, L. E. (2020). Migraines in children: Recommendations for acute and preventive treatment. *American Family Physician, 101*(9), 569–571.

Jarvis, C. (2019). *Physical examination and health assessment. E-Book.* Elsevier Health Sciences.

Lakhan, S. (2019). *Medscape: Alzheimer disease.* https://emedicine.medscape.com/article/1134817-overview#a1

Nandha, R., & Singh, H. (2012). Renin angiotensin system: A novel target for migraine prophylaxis. *Indian Journal of Pharmacology, 44*(2), 157–160. https://doi.org/10.4103/0253-7613.93840

National Institutes of Health. (2020). *GARD: Juvenile temporal arteritis.* https://rarediseases.info.nih.gov/diseases/3068/juvenile-temporal-arteritis

Saad, E. (2020). *Medscape: Polymyalgia rheumatica.* https://emedicine.medscape.com/article/330815-clinical

Sekula, R. F., Frederickson, A. M., Jannetta, P. J., Quigley, M. R., Aziz, K. M., & Arnone, G. D. (2011). Microvascular decompression for elderly patients with trigeminal neuralgia: A prospective study and systematic review with meta-analysis. *Journal of Neurosurgery, 114*(1), 172–179. https://doi.org/10.3171/2010.6.JNS10142

Seretharaman, M. (2020). *Medscape: Giant cell arteritis (temporal arteritis).* https://emedicine.medscape.com/article/332483-overview

Silver, B. (2019). *Medscape: Stroke prevention.* https://emedicine.medscape.com/article/323662-overview#showall

Singh, M. (2019). *Medscape: Trigeminal neuralgia.* https://emedicine.medscape.com/article/1145144-treatment#d19

Sorenson, M., Quinn, L., & Klein, D. (2019). *Pathophysiology: Concepts of human disease* (1st ed.). Pearson Education.

Taylor, D. (2019). *Medscape: Bell palsy.* https://emedicine.medscape.com/article/1146903-overview

EYES, EARS, NOSE, AND THROAT DISORDERS

BLEPHARITIS

Overview

- Blepharitis is a chronic inflammatory disease of the eyelid margin due to inflamed, blocked meibomian glands.
- Seborrhea sheds cells that block the glands, and bacteria colonize the lid margin causing recurrent inflammation.

COMPLICATIONS

Acute: Pain, chalazion, conjunctivitis, corneal injury

Chronic: Recurrent conjunctivitis, recurrent blepharitis, lid scar, trichiasis

Etiology

- Allergies, dry eyes, infection, mites
- Herpes, rosacea, seborrheic dermatitis

Signs and Symptoms

- A foreign body or gritty sensation with pain in both eyes (unilateral presentation should be monitored closely for neoplasm)
- Excessive tearing
- Conjunctival injection, corneal erosion
- Lid erythema, crusting, collarette (staph) or sleeving (mites), chalazion
- Blurred vision, photophobia
- Signs and symptoms of associated seborrhea or rosacea

Differential Diagnosis

- *HEENT:* Chalazion, conjunctivitis, dry eye disease, hordeolum, keratitis, ocular rosacea, skin cancer
- *INT:* Allergic or contact dermatitis
- *Other:* Sinusitis with periorbital involvement

Diagnosis

Labs
- *N/A:* Diagnosis based on clinical examination

Additional Diagnostic Testing
- Visual acuity exam to rule out visual changes
- Slit-lamp examination
- Microscopic examination of the lash base to identify mites

Treatment and Management

Treatment Goals
- Manage pain, eradicate the infection, promote lid hygiene, and prevent complications.

Drug Treatment
- Prescribe topical erythromycin or bacitracin ointment at bedtime to reduce bacterial colonization and infection.
- Consider oral doxycycline in patients with comorbid rosacea or acne vulgaris.
- Encourage artificial tears as needed for dry eyes.

Interventions
- Prescribe warm soaks and lid massage to the eye for comfort as needed.
- Evaluate the patient's response to therapy and reevaluate in 2 to 6 weeks.
- Manage comorbid allergies, seborrhea dermatitis, and rosacea.

Patient Education
- Discuss lid hygiene to prevent a recurrence.
- Review s/s of complications and adverse effects of medication to report.

 CLINICAL PEARL

Lid Hygiene
- Wash with warm water and mild soap after a warm soak.
- Apply a mixture of water and baby shampoo to a cotton-tipped applicator and gently scrub along the lid margin to remove softened crusts, sleeves, and collarettes.

Patient Population Considerations

Women (conception/pregnancy/lactation)
- Hormone changes in pregnancy aggravate acne and rosacea, which can trigger blepharitis. Encourage lid hygiene to prevent the onset of disease.

Geriatric
- Demodex infestations increases with age, dry skin, skin pH of 5.6 to 7, and elevated skin temperature. Investigate mites as a cause of recurrent blepharitis in older adults.

Pediatric
- The management of blepharitis in infants and children mirror that of an adult.

Referring Patients

- Ophthalmology consult
- Dermatology consult

CHALAZION AND HORDOLEUM

Overview

- A *chalazion* is a chronic sterile granulatomous inflammatory nodule of the eyelid. Blocked meibomian glands release lipid-rich meibum into the tarsal plate and surrounding lid tissue, causing a painless or painful lump.
- A *hordeolum* or *stye* is an acute localized infection of the eyelid at the follicle and glands of Zeis (external) or meibomian gland (internal) and may be associated with blepharitis.

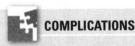 **COMPLICATIONS**

Hordeolum: Pain, cellulitis, recurrent hordeolum

Chalazion: Corneal injury, recurrent chalazion

Etiology

- Chalazion
  - Meibomian gland dysfunction (thick secretions)
  - Blepharitis, rosacea, seborrheic dermatitis
- Hordeolum
  - *Staphylococcus aureus*

Signs and Symptoms

- Chalazion
  - Diffuse erythema and edema that becomes localized to the eyelid as a nodule
  - Tearing, foreign body sensation
  - May or may not be painful
  - Lasting 2 to 8 weeks
- Hordeolum
  - Painful erythema and swelling at the lid margin
  - Associated with tearing, photophobia, and foreign body sensation

Differential Diagnosis

- *HEENT*: Blepharitis, conjunctivitis, keratitis, orbital cellulitis, ptosis
- *INT*: Allergic or contact dermatitis, skin cancer

Diagnosis

Labs
- Diagnosis based on clinical examination

Additional Diagnostic Testing
- Visual acuity exam to rule out visual changes
- Slit-lamp examination to rule out corneal injury

Treatment and Management

Treatment Goals
- Manage pain, treat contributing factors, and prevent complications.
- Hordeola may resolve spontaneously or evolve into chalazia.

ALERT

Refer large chalazion that does not improve to ophthalmology for fine needle aspiration and incision and curettage.

Drug Treatment (Chalazion)
- Refer to ophthalmology for corticosteroid, as indicated.
- Refer to ophthalmology for lesions requiring drainage and systemic antibiotics.
- Prescribe oral cephalexin, erythromycin, or augmentin if periorbital cellulitis is present.

Interventions
- Prescribe warm soaks, lid massage, and lid hygiene to the eye for comfort 2 to 4 times daily.
- Evaluate the patient's response to therapy, reevaluate in 1 week, then every 2 weeks.
- Manage comorbid allergies, seborrhea dermatitis, and rosacea.

Patient Education
- Discuss lid hygiene to prevent a recurrence.
- Review s/s of complications to report.

Patient Population Considerations

Women (conception/pregnancy/lactation)
- As in blepharitis, hormone changes in pregnancy that aggravate acne and rosacea can trigger chalazion and hordeolum. Encourage lid hygiene to prevent the onset of disease.

Geriatric
- Refer older patients with lid lesions that do not improve to dermatology for evaluation of skin cancer.

Pediatric
- Frequent eye infections in children should alert the provider to check for diabetes and immunocompromised states.

Referring Patients
- Ophthalmology consult
- Dermatology consult

CONJUNCTIVITIS

Overview
- Conjunctivitis is a common eye disease that is characterized by inflammation of the conjunctiva by cellular infiltration and exudate.

Etiology
- Close contact with an infected person, sexual activity
- Allergens or mechanical or chemical injury
- *Viral*: Adenovirus with recent URI, ECHO viruses, herpes simplex in newborns of infected mothers, herpes zoster
- *Bacterial*: *Staphylococcus aureus*, *Streptococcus pneumoniae*, *Neisseria gonorrhoeae*, *Chlamydia trachomatis*
- Fungal, parasitic, toxic, chemical, and allergic agents
- Newborn of mother with STI

Signs and Symptoms
- Unilateral progressing to bilateral erythema and injection
- Associated with eye discharge, and tearing
- Vesicular skin eruption in chickenpox, herpes simplex, and zoster
- Bilateral presentation in infection and allergy

Differential Diagnosis
- *HEENT*: Acute angle-closure glaucoma, blepharitis, corneal injury, scleritis, uveitis, subconjunctival hemorrhage, iritis
- *Other*: Kawasaki disease

Diagnosis

Labs
- Diagnosed by clinical examination

COMPLICATIONS

Acute: Severe eye infection, neonatal conjunctivitis due to maternal transmission

Chronic: Recurrent conjunctivitis; blindness in untreated neonatal infection

CLINICAL PEARL

Localized itchiness or pain in the distribution of the bridge of nose, eye, and forehead of the first division of trigeminal nerve with abrupt termination at the midline is the prodrome of herpes zoster opthalmicus.

Additional Diagnostic Testing

- Fluorescein stain with a yellow filter and slit-lamp examination to evaluate for conjunctive damage
- Eye gram stain and culture in corneal ulceration or orbital cellulitis

Treatment and Management

Treatment Goals

- Eradicate infection and prevent infection transmission and recurrence.

Drug Treatment

- Treat conjunctivitis according to suspected cause.
  - *Bacterial*: Prescribe topical quinolones, macrolides, gentamycin, or sulfacetamide.
  - *Allergic*: Prescribe topical antihistamines or ketorolac in allergic.

 ALERT

Newborn presentation in ambulatory care with gonococcal conjunctivitis requires admission to hospital.

Interventions

- Monitor for reinfection and cross contamination.
- Follow up in 2 to 3 days to evaluate response. Failure to recognize herpes simplex keratitis and other causes can lead to ocular injury.

Patient Education

- Teach the patient proper eye hygiene, risks of sharing a pillow, and to avoid swimming pools and touching eyes.
- Counsel the patient to use eyeglasses instead of contact lenses and discard all makeup worn at the time of the infection.

Patient Population Considerations

Women (conception/pregnancy/lactation)

- Conduct screening for gonorrhea, chlamydia, and genital herpes during pregnancy. Genital herpes in pregnancy is a consideration for cesarean delivery when there are active lesions or risk for viral shedding.

Geriatric

- Offer shingles vaccine to immunocompetent patients age 50 and older who are varicella positive. Encourage patients, especially those patients who are anticipating immunosuppression or have recovered from an immunosuppressing illness, to get the live vaccine.

Pediatric

- Erythromycin ointment is applied to newborns' eyes according to state regulation. It prevents conjunctivitis from maternal transmission of STIs.

Referring Patients

- Ophthalmology consult

GLAUCOMA

Overview

- Glaucoma is a chronic eye disorder characterized by increased IOP from increased aqueous humor in the anterior chamber that damages the optic nerve.
- It leads to decreased peripheral vision, followed by decreased central vision, and is the second leading cause of blindness.

COMPLICATIONS

Acute: Impaired vision, acute angle-closure glaucoma

Chronic: Blindness, risk for injury

(continued)

Overview (*continued*)

- Types of glaucoma
  - *Open-angle glaucoma:* Insidious onset where drainage through the trabecular meshwork is decreased over time (most common)
  - *Closed-angle glaucoma:* Abrupt disruption of drainage that causes acute symptoms
  - *Normal-tension glaucoma:* Occurs in the presence of physiologic cupping of the optic nerve, with normal IOP
  - *Unilateral glaucoma:* Can occur with trauma and chronic conditions

Etiology

- Increasing age; genetics; and African American, Middle Eastern, Hispanic, or Asian descent
- *Diseases:* Vasculitis, MS, SLE, infection, ischemia, Behçet's disease, DM, HTN, giant cell arteritis
- *Acute angle-closure:* Prone surgical positioning, sympathomimetics, anticholinergic, SSRI, anticonvulsant, sulfonamides, cocaine, botulism toxin, rapid correction of hyperglycemia
- *Unilateral:* Head trauma, thyroid disease, vasculitis, malignancy, surgery, benign tumor

Signs and Symptoms

- All types of glaucoma
  - Cupping of the optic nerve on fundoscopic exam
  - Decreased vision with peripheral field testing
- *Open-angle:* Asymptomatic in early disease, decreased vision, peripheral vision over time
- *Closed-angle:* Acute pain, photophobia, blurred vision, farsightedness (hyperopia), irregular pupil shape, mid-dilated nonreactive pupil
- *Normal tension:* Cupping of the optic nerve with normal IOP

 ALERT

Acute angle-closure glaucoma, red eye with ciliary flush, hard globe, "silent blinders," and dilated pupil with no pupillary response with IOP >50, is a medical emergency. It requires same-day referral for intervention to prevent blindness.

Differential Diagnosis

- *HEENT:* Other glaucoma disorders, glaucoma suspect, hyphema, ocular ischemic syndrome, acute angle-closure glaucoma, acute orbital compartment syndrome, corneal laceration, orbital infection, UV keratitis, uveitis, vitreous hemorrhage
- *NEURO:* Carotid-cavernous fistula, neurosyphilis
- *Other:* Autoimmune disorders

Diagnosis

Labs
- ESR, serology for syphilis

Additional Diagnostic Testing
- Tonometry >20
- Dilated pupil examination
- Slit-lamp exam in acute angle-closure reveals corneal edema and cloudiness
- Visual field testing
- Fundus photography

Treatment and Management

Treatment Goals
- Maintain IOP <20, promote safety, and prevent progressive vision loss.

Drug Treatment

- *Refer to ophthalmology for elevated IOP and concomitant optic nerve damage, progressive cupping, or IOP >28 to 30 mmHg.*
- Open-angle
  - Prescribe beta blockers or carbonic anhydrase inhibitors to decrease the production of aqueous humor.
  - Prescribe prostaglandin analogs increase the outflow of aqueous humor.
  - Prescribe alpha agonists to decrease production and increase outflow.

Interventions

- Refer patients at increased risk for glaucoma to ophthalmology for a dilated pupil exam and tonometry.
- Monitor the patient's visual acuity, adherence to medications, and results of tonometry testing.
- Control risk factors for retinopathy caused by DM or HTN that can contribute to impaired vision.
- Review home safety and prevention of injury due to impaired vision.

Patient Education

- Instruct the patient in the correct use of eye drops to avoid systemic absorption.
- Discuss safety concerns and assistance needs with impaired vision and strategies to manage.
- Instruct the patient to seek consultation with acute eye pain, photophobia, and blurred vision.

Patient Population Considerations

Women (conception/pregnancy/lactation)

- Diagnosis of glaucoma occurs at earlier ages due to improved diagnostics. Most anti-glaucoma medications are category C. Preconception planning is essential to avoid fetal harm. Brimonidine, a category B, is the safest medication for the first trimester.

Geriatric

- The incidence of glaucoma increases after age 60 years and annually with each successive year. Screen for glaucoma every 1 to 2 years in this population.

Pediatric

- Congenital, infantile, and juvenile open-angle glaucoma constitutes primary childhood glaucoma. Cloudy cornea and buphthalmos are the most common presenting signs.

Referring Patients

- Ophthalmology consult
- OT consult for low vision aids
- Social services consult in advanced disease to obtain assistance for transportation and ADLs

---

HERPES KERATITIS

Overview

- Herpes keratitis is an acute latent or reactivated acute infection caused by HSV I (orofacial and ocular) and HSV II (sexual and perinatal).
- It affects eyelids, conjunctiva, and cornea, and can cause blindness if untreated.
- The virus migrates to the trigeminal ganglion and becomes latent following initial infection. On reactivation, the virus travels to the cornea, damaging the epithelial cells, causing opacities.
- The opacities coalesce into ulcers in a linear branching pattern.

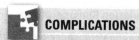

COMPLICATIONS

Acute: Severe eye infection, fatal encephalitis in newborn from HSV keratitis

Chronic: Recurrent keratitis, blindness with recurring infections

Etiology

- HSV 1 and 2 infection
- Maternal infection at the time of vaginal birth
- *Reactivation occurs with*:
  - Psychological or physical stress, sun exposure, medication
  - Use of latanoprost, an intravitreal triamcinolone injection, ophthalmic steroids

Signs and Symptoms

- Mild to moderate pain, photophobia, blurred vision
- Foreign body sensation, lacrimation, erythema
- Ciliary congestion
- Branching ulcer with staining

Differential Diagnosis

- *HEENT*: Acanthamoeba keratitis, conjunctivitis, contact lens complications, drug-induced keratitis, healing corneal injury, neurotrophic keratitis, recurrent corneal erosion, staphylococcus ulcer
- *INT*: Impetigo

Diagnosis

Labs
- Diagnosed by clinical examination
- Fluorescein staining reveals ulcers with linear branching pattern with clubbing or geographical ulcer

Additional Diagnostic Testing
- PCR testing for herpes simplex
- Viral culture

Treatment and Management

Treatment Goals
- Minimize scarring and damage and prevent recurrence and blindness.

Drug Treatment
- Prescribe ganciclovir ophthalmic gel 0.15% 5 times daily and/or oral acyclovir 400 mg BID for 10 days.

Interventions
- Refer to ophthalmology for debridement, if indicated.
- Follow up in 2 to 3 days to evaluate response to avoid ocular injury.

Patient Education
- Teach the patient to wash hands carefully during herpes breakouts and avoid touching eyes.
- Explain to the patient that this virus has no cure, and they can consider prophylactic antiviral therapy to reduce the frequency of recurrence.

Patient Population Considerations

Women (conception/pregnancy/lactation)
- Screen for the presence of herpes simplex in pregnant women.

Geriatric
- The shingles vaccine offers no protection to herpes simplex keratitis. The virus is more likely to reactivate in patients with more complex medical conditions, surgical interventions, and immunosuppressive therapy or disease.

Pediatric

- Transmission during vaginal delivery or eye contact with contaminated hands can transmit infection. Ensure infected caregivers use precautions.

Referring Patients

- Ophthalmology consult

UVEITIS

Overview

- Inflammation of the uveal tract; the iris, ciliary body, and choroid
- Anterior uveitis accounts for 60% to 90% of cases
- Parasympathetic tone constricts pupil and rounds pupil to increase acuity. Inflammation interferes with the parasympathetic tone, causing the pupil to become nonreactive, dilated, and develop synechia.

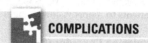

COMPLICATIONS

Acute: Pain, glaucoma, blindness

Chronic: Recurrent uveitis, cataracts

Etiology

- Exact etiology unknown
- *Autoimmune:* Ankylosing spondylitis, collagen vascular disease, inflammatory bowel disease, MS, psoriatic arthritis, Reiter's syndrome, sarcoidosis
- *Infections:* HSV, Lyme disease, syphilis, TB, VZV
- Trauma

Signs and Symptoms

- Dull aching eye pain, photophobia, decreased visual acuity
- Nonreactive, irregular pupil shape, and dilated in size with synechia

Differential Diagnosis

- *HEENT:* Acute angle glaucoma, central retinal artery occlusion, conjunctivitis, endophthalmitis, retinal detachment

Diagnosis

Labs

- VDRL
- IGRA to identify TB infection
- Lyme disease (intermediate uveitis)

Additional Diagnostic Testing

- Chest x-ray to reveal if sarcoidosis is present
- Slit-lamp examination
- Dilated fundoscopic exam

Treatment and Management

Treatment Goals

- Promote comfort, reduce inflammation, minimize transformation to cataracts, prevent blindness

Drug Treatment
- Treat infection if present.
- Collaborate with an ophthalmologist regarding the prescription of corticosteroids to reduce inflammation.

Interventions
- Refer the patient to an ophthalmologist to manage the event.
- Monitor response to therapy in 2 weeks.
- Monitor for s/s of inflammatory bowel disease flare that can occur with uveitis.

Patient Education
- Explain to the patient that uveitis may recur.
- Advise patients to report vision changes immediately.

Patient Population Considerations

Women (conception/pregnancy/lactation)
- Uveitis does not recur as frequently during pregnancy if it is autoimmune in origin.

Geriatric
- The shingles vaccine offers no protection to herpes simplex keratitis. The virus is more likely to reactivate in patients with more complex medical conditions, surgical interventions, and immunosuppressive therapy or disease.

Pediatric
- Pediatric patients with autoimmune mediations arthropathies and bowel disease may develop anterior uveitis. Early identification helps to reduce the lifelong burden of visual disturbance.

Referring Patients

- Ophthalmology consult

ALERT

Refer patients with uveitis to ophthalmology immediately due to risk of cataracts and blindness.

POP QUIZ 4.1

A mother and 1-week-old newborn present to the urgent care clinic for evaluation of the newborn's copious eye secretions starting 2 days ago. The mother states that the infant was delivered at home without complications. She expresses concern because she had pink eye the week before delivery and is worried that her home was not clean enough. On examination, bilateral lid edema with copious mucopurulent discharge and crusting at the lid margins is noted. What is the priority action?

EARS

ACUTE OTITIS MEDIA

Overview

- OM is the inflammation of the middle ear.
- It is more common in children, where the eustachian tube is smaller, more lateral, and flexible.
- SOM occurs when the tympanic membrane ruptures, which can lead to chronic OM and OME.
- Infections spread by direct extension into adjacent structures and through the bloodstream.

COMPLICATIONS

Acute: Persisting otitis media (>2 weeks), mastoiditis, intracranial abscess, seizures, increased ICP due to hydrocephalus, meningitis/sepsis, facial nerve palsy, conduction hearing loss, labyrinthitis, sigmoid sinus thrombosis

Chronic: Chronic otitis media, sensorineural hearing loss, and otitis media with effusion

Etiology

- *Viral*: Adenovirus with recent URI, herpes simplex in newborns of infected mothers
- *Bacterial*: *Haemophilus influenza, Moraxella catarrhalis, Staphylococcus aureus, Streptococcus pneumoniae*

- Exposure to tobacco
- Increased incidence in Down syndrome

Signs and Symptoms

- Anorexia, fever, hearing loss, irritability, otalgia, otorrhea
- Signs or symptoms of direct extension or bacteremia are an urgent concern

 ALERT

Newborn presentation with high fever requires admission to the hospital for a full septic workup.

Differential Diagnosis

- *HEENT*: Acute sinusitis, allergic rhinitis, hearing impairment, mastoiditis, nasal polyps, OE, OM with effusion, parainfluenza, pharyngitis, RSV
- *Other*: Bacteremia

Diagnosis

Labs
- Diagnosed by visual inspection and history taking.

Additional Diagnostic Testing
- Head CT for refractory OM and meningeal irritation
- MRI
- Lumbar puncture with suspected meningitis following imaging

Treatment and Management

Treatment Goals
- Eradicate infection, identify/prevent complications, and manage symptoms.

Drug Treatment
- Prescribe high-dose amoxicillin 80 to 90 mg/kg/d × 3 days. Otherwise, prescribe amoxicillin/clavulanic acid and evaluate response in 3 days.
- If no improvement with amoxicillin or amoxicillin/clavulanic acid, prescribe cefuroxime 30 mg/kg/d, or ceftriaxone IM.
- In patients with non–type 1 PCN sensitivity, consider cefuroxime, cefpodoxime, ceftriaxone.
- Prescribe antihistamine, decongestant, mucolytic to improve symptoms.
- Prescribe acetaminophen or NSAIDs for pain and fever.
- Prescribe intranasal steroids for middle ear effusion.

Interventions
- Follow up in 2 weeks to evaluate the response and revise therapy.
- Provide prompt referral to otolaryngology for surgical intervention in patients with Down syndrome, cleft palate, and refractory infection.

Patient Education
- Instruct caregivers and patients to avoid exposure to tobacco. Encourage breastfeeding beyond 3 months, discourage pacifier use to reduce the incidence. Explain that daycare increases risk of infection.
- Remind the patient and family to complete the entire antibiotic prescription.
- Teach s/s of complications and adverse medication effects to report.

Patient Population Considerations

Women (conception/pregnancy/lactation)
- Maternal use of antibiotics increases the risk for OM in children, especially late in term.

Geriatric

- OM in older adults are uncommon. Recurrent ear infections should be evaluated for risk of or experiencing nasopharyngeal cancer, especially in the presence of hearing loss, nasal stuffiness, and facial nerve palsy.

Pediatric

- Use shared decision-making with parents of children with OM who are >24 months in age and do not have a fever ≥102.2°F (39°C), moderate to severe otalgia, otalgia >48 hr, or otorrhea. In this subset, consider observation and delayed antibiotic prescription to reduce overall antibiotic use.

Referring Patients

- ENT consult

HEARING LOSS

Overview

- Hearing impairment is a sensory disorder described as complete or partial due to interference with air conduction of sound waves to the inner ear, nerve transmission from the inner ear to the brain, or processing of auditory information in the brain. It may affect one or both ears and can be temporary or permanent. Also, hearing loss can be insidious or sudden. Any sudden hearing loss requires immediate evaluation.
- Hearing loss is labeled conductive, sensorineural, central, or mixed.

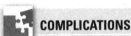

COMPLICATIONS

Permanent hearing loss, impaired verbal communication, social isolation

Etiology

- Genetics, congenital infections (CMV, herpes, rubella, syphilis, toxoplasmosis, varicella), fetal exposure to teratogens, prematurity at birth, low birth weight and low Apgar score, hyperbilirubinemia
- Headphone use
- Conductive
  - Cerumen impaction, cholesteatoma, chronic OME, foreign body OE, otosclerosis, trauma, tumor, tympanic scarring, or perforation
- Sensorineural
  - Anterior cerebral artery occlusion, acoustic neuroma, aging (presbycusis), atherosclerosis, chemical ototoxicants (solvents, asphyxiants, nitriles, metals, and compounds), cochlear otosclerosis, CV VIII damage, ototoxic medications, frequent infections, Meniere's disease, meningitis, mumps, noise-induced damage (sound >85–90 dB), tumor
- Central
  - Arising from CNS disorder
- Mixed
  - Combination of conductive and sensorineural losses

ALERT

Ototoxic Medications

Aminoglycoside antibiotics, aspirin, chemotherapy agents containing platinum, loop diuretics, NSAIDs, quinine, SSRIs, TCAs

Use the lowest possible dose for the shortest period and monitor drug levels if indicated.

Signs and Symptoms

- Report of difficulty hearing in noisy areas, occupational exposure to loud noise, brief exposure to deafening noise, tinnitus, dizziness, recent URI

ALERT

Universal Neonatal Screening

All newborns should be screened for hearing loss no later than age 1 month.

- *Ear exam*: Abnormality to the external ear canal, presence of a foreign body, impacted cerumen, otorrhea, perforated TM, bulging TM, tympanosclerosis
- Inability to hear soft sound on physical exam
- Positive Weber or Rinne tests

Differential Diagnosis

- *HEENT*: Acoustic neuroma, cerumen impaction, cholesteatoma, congenital hearing loss, ear infections, Meniere's disease, ototoxicity, presbycusis, traumatic hearing loss
- *NEURO*: Stroke

Diagnosis

Labs
- Genetic markers, serum drug levels, toxicology screen as indicated
- ESR, RH factor, and immune panel with bilateral loss

Additional Diagnostic Testing
- CT, MRI, MRA
- Audiometry
- Brainstem auditory evoked response testing

> **CLINICAL PEARL**
>
> **Interpreting Tuning Fork Tests in Unilateral Hearing Loss**
> - Sensorineural loss
>   - *Weber*: Lateralizes to good ear
>   - *Rinne*: AC > BC
> - Conductive loss
>   - *Weber*: Lateralized to bad ear
>   - *Rinne*: BC ≥ AC

Treatment and Management

Treatment Goals
- Treat reversible factors, provide hearing aids, promote safety, and prevent progressive vision loss.

Drug Treatment
- Treat primary condition as indicated.

Interventions
- Remove cerumen and simple foreign bodies.
- Perform screenings as appropriate and refer to audiologist for additional diagnostics.
- Promote lifestyle modifications to preserve hearing.

Patient Education
- Instruct the patient in the primary prevention of hearing loss.
- Discuss safety concerns and assistance needs with impaired hearing and strategies to manage.
- Teach strategies to avoid additional harm to remaining hearing.

Patient Population Considerations

Women (conception/pregnancy/lactation)
- Provide preconception counseling to women of childbearing age regarding factors that increase the risk of hearing loss in fetuses during pregnancy. Ensure immunizations are up to date to minimize congenital infections. Discuss limiting exposure to environmental toxins that may be harmful to the fetus.

Geriatric
- Screen geriatric patients for hearing loss as they advance in age.

Pediatric
- Monitor the social and linguistic development of children who are deaf.

Referring Patients

- Audiology consult
- ENT consult
- Otolaryngology consult

OTITIS EXTERNA

Overview

- OE, or swimmer's ear, is inflammation of the external auditory canal that can be found in patients throughout the life span.
- Chronic OE lasts >6 weeks.
- Eczematous OE may be seen in patients with atopic dermatitis or autoimmune SLE
- Necrotizing OE extends into neighboring structures and bones in patients who are immunosuppressed.
- Otomycosis is a fungal infection of the external ear.
- Osteomyelitis can occur with extension of inflammation to the bone.

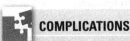

COMPLICATIONS

Acute: Necrotizing OE, meningitis/sepsis, osteomyelitis, conductive hearing loss, facial nerve palsy, cellulitis, and lymphadenopathy

Chronic: Chronic OE

Etiology

- Eczema, seborrhea, neurodermatitis, contact dermatitis from devices, purulent OM, reaction to topical medication, immunocompromised, DM
- Use of earplugs or devices, recent swimming, cleaning
- Consider *Pseudomonas* in immunocompromised patients

Signs and Symptoms

- Pruritus and pain, especially with mobility of tragus or pinna (deep severe pain suggests necrotizing OE)
- Erythema, edema, discharge, and extending cellulitis and lymphadenopathy
- Tinnitus and hearing loss
- History of exposure to water or recent trauma to the ear, like forceful cleaning

ALERT

Signs or symptoms of direct extension or higher level of pain than expected based on the clinical exam are an urgent concern.

Differential Diagnosis

- *HEENT*: Cerumen impaction, ear canal trauma, foreign body, malignant OE in DM, myringitis, OM, preauricular cyst, Ramsay Hunt syndrome (geniculate ganglia herpes), wisdom tooth eruption
- *NEURO*: Cranial nerve palsy

Diagnosis

Labs
- Diagnosed by clinical examination
- Gram stain and culture drainage
- Capillary BG to evaluate for hyperglycemia

Additional Diagnostic Testing
- Head CT to rule out extension of infection to adjacent bone
- Bone scan in refractory OE or severe pain
- MRI to rule out extension of infection to adjacent soft tissue

Treatment and Management

Treatment Goals
- Remove debris/foreign body to eradicate the infection, identify/prevent complications, and manage symptoms.

ALERT

Newborn presentation with high fever requires admission to hospital.

Patients with comorbidities and immunosuppression with severe pain should be referred to the ED for further evaluation and for IV antibiotics.

Drug Treatment

- Topical antibiotics with intact TM
  - Prescribe topical antibiotics or antifungal depending on presentation with or without corticosteroids after removal of debris.
  - Avoid aminoglycosides due to their ototoxicity adverse effect. Consider ciprofloxacin 0.3% with dexamethasone 0.1% otic solution.
  - Treat fungal infection with clotrimazole 1%.
  - Insert ear wick to facilitate antibiotic administration in severe edema.
- Oral antibiotics with perforated TM, fever, cellulitis, and comorbidity
  - Prescribe ciprofloxacin as an oral agent.
  - Consider acetaminophen or NSAIDs for pain and fever.

Interventions

- Follow up in 2 to 3 days to evaluate the response and revise therapy if needed.
- Provide prompt referral to otolaryngology for surgical intervention with persisting or worsening symptoms or fever.

Patient Education

- Instruct the caregiver and patient to keep the ear canal dry for 1 to 2 weeks. Use earplug to prevent water penetration.
- Remind the patient and family to complete the entire antibiotic prescription.
- Teach s/s of complications and adverse medication effects to report.

Patient Population Considerations

Women (conception/pregnancy/lactation)

- Avoid swimming in water with a high bacterial count, especially after storms, to avoid infections.

Geriatric

- Clean and dry hearing aids before and after use to minimize infection.

Pediatric

- OE is frequently a sign of foreign objects in the ear in young children. Caution caregivers and parents to remove items from a child's reach that could fit into the nose or ear.

Referring Patients

- Otolaryngology consult with hearing loss or worsening symptoms
- Speech therapy with hearing loss

 POP QUIZ 4.2

A 35-year-old male highway crewman reports for an annual work physical. He states he noticed that he has needed to turn the television volume up louder over the past few months. On examination the external ears are symmetric, no lesions, drainage or tenderness, cerumen, or foreign bodies. His TMs are intact and pearly gray and are not bulging. He is unable to detect soft sounds in his right ear. *Weber test:* Lateralized to left ear. *Rinne:* AC > BC bilaterally. What is the most likely diagnosis and appropriate next step?

NOSE

ACUTE BACTERIAL RHINOSINUSITIS

Overview

- Acute bacterial rhinosinusitis is an infection of the nasal mucosa and sinuses frequently following a recent URI. Ostial obstruction and inflammation impede sinus drainage which results in bacterial growth. It can be acute or subacute.
- Infection extension to orbit and intracranial structure require immediate referral.

 COMPLICATIONS

Acute: Preseptal cellulitis, intracranial abscess, increased ICP, cavernous sinus thrombosis, meningitis
Chronic: Chronic rhinosinusitis

Etiology

- *Disease risk*: Allergic rhinitis, autoimmune disorders, cystic fibrosis, COPD, DM, hypothyroidism, medication-induced rhinitis, pregnancy, URI, vascular headache
- *Structural risk*: Adenoid enlargement, chronic tonsillitis, deviated septum, foreign body, masses, nasal obstruction, trauma
- *Environmental*: Airplane travel, diving, swimming, tobacco, pollution

 CLINICAL PEARL

Streptococcus pneumoniae and *Haemophilus influenza* represent 50% of acute cases.

Moraxella catarrhalis, Streptococcus pyogenes, Staphylococcus aureus, gram-negative bacilli, and anaerobes are responsible for the remainder.

Signs and Symptoms

- Facial pain, pressure, tenderness above/below eyes, obstruction to nares, purulent discharge, and loss of sense of smell

Differential Diagnosis

- *HEENT*: Allergic rhinitis, cancer, chronic sinusitis, cystic fibrosis, dental abscess, drug-induced rhinitis, facial pain syndromes, foreign body hypertrophic turbinates, immotile cilia syndrome, granulomas, nasal obstruction due to polyps or deviation, viral rhinitis
- *NEURO*: Cluster headache, migraine, vasculitis

 ALERT

AMS, high fever, exophthalmos, orbital migraine, extraocular movement deficit, decreased visual acuity, loss of vision, and meningeal signs should be referred to ED.

Diagnosis

Labs
- Diagnosed by clinical examination.

Additional Diagnostic Testing
- CT of sinuses if alternative diagnosis likely
- Lumbar puncture for patients with meningeal signs

Treatment and Management

Treatment Goals
- Remove debris/foreign body, eradicate the infection, identify/prevent complications, and manage symptoms.

Drug Treatment
- Prescribe amoxicillin with or without clavulanate for 10 days.
- Prescribe doxycycline or fluoroquinolone if allergic to PCN.
- Prescribe acetaminophen or NSAIDs for pain and fever.
- Consider topical oxymetazoline for 3 days if no contraindication.
- Consider topical steroids daily or topical ipratropium bromide 0.06% to decrease rhinorrhea.
- Prescribe guaifenesin to thin secretions and nonsedating antihistamine to reduce secretions.

CLINICAL PEARL

Diagnostic criteria for children and adolescents

Persisting symptoms without improvement >10 days (consider an addition 3 days of observation)

OR

Worsening symptoms with fever daytime cough or nasal discharge after improvement from an URI

OR

Severe symptoms including temp ≥102.2°F (39°C), purulent discharge for 3 consecutive days

Interventions
- Clear debris and promote vasoconstriction with nasal saline irrigation or spray installation daily.
- Follow up in 2 to 3 days to evaluate the response and revise therapy if needed.
- Provide prompt referral to otolaryngology for surgical intervention with persisting or worsening symptoms or fever.

Patient Education

- Provide instructions for smoking cessation, hydration, warm compresses, and humidification.
- Remind the patient and family to complete the entire antibiotic prescription.
- Teach s/s of complications and adverse medication effects to report.

Patient Population Considerations

Women (conception/pregnancy/lactation)

- Prescribe amoxicillin/clavulanic acid during pregnancy.

Geriatric

- Evaluate persistent sinusitis risk of head and neck cancer, especially in those patients who smoke and drink alcohol. Monitor for sinusitis in patients with current or prior nasoentereic feeding tubes.

Pediatric

- Evaluate children who present with frequent URI and sinusitis for obstructive pathologies and chronic disease risk.

Referring Patients

- Otolaryngology consult

ALLERGIC RHINITIS

Overview

- Allergic rhinitis is an IgE-mediated type I hypersensitivity reaction to allergens.
- Allergens can be inhaled, ingested, injected, or by direct contact.
- Grass, mold, tree, and weed allergens, along with infection commonly trigger allergic rhinitis. Allergic rhinitis can be triggered by animal dander, cockroaches, dust mites, latex, medications, perfumes, pollution, rodents, strong odors, tobacco.
- The patient may have a concomitant risk for anaphylaxis and allergy to NSAIDs, aspirin, ACEIs, ARBs, or oral contraceptives.

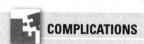

COMPLICATIONS

Acute: Obstructive sleep apnea
Chronic: Possible ADHD

Etiology

- Family or personal history of an allergic reaction to seasonal or perennial irritants
- Exposure to irritant
- *Disease risk*: Asthma, eczema

Signs and Symptoms

- *Acute*: Nasal congestion, rhinorrhea, postnasal drip, anosmia, watery eyes, red eyes, itchy throat headache, fatigue, drowsiness.
- *Chronic*: Allergic shiners, nasal crease, boggy, pale, blue-gray mucosa, allergic salute, Dennie–Morgan lines (prominent creases below the inferior eyelid), tonsillar hypertrophy, high, arched palate

Differential Diagnosis

- *HEENT*: CSF leak, hormonal rhinitis in pregnancy, medication-induced rhinitis, nonallergic rhinitis eosinophilic syndrome, granulomatous rhinitis, OM, sinusitis, structural defect
- *ENDO*: Hypothyroidism
- *Other*: Sarcoidosis

Diagnosis

Labs
- Allergy skin testing
  - RAST testing if skin testing is unavailable
- CBC elevated eosinophils
- IgE elevated
- Nasal smear

Additional Diagnostic Testing
If complications are suspected:
- Rhinoscopy
- Sleep study

Treatment and Management

Treatment Goals
- Treat acute allergy, implement environmental control measures and allergen avoidance, and manage symptoms/prevent reactions with immunotherapy.

Drug Treatment
- *First-line therapy*: Intranasal steroids daily with nonsedating long-acting oral antihistamine daily
- *Second-line therapy*: Intranasal antihistamine sprays, intranasal cromolyn, intranasal anticholinergic sprays
- *Third-line therapy*: Consider montelukast (*Note*: Black box warning for suicidality)
- Additional therapies
  - Pseudoephedrine 30 mg PRN for acute symptom management if no hypertension or cardiac comorbidity present
  - Short course of oral corticosteroids for severe acute symptoms if intranasal steroids are insufficient
  - Sublingual or subcutaneous immunotherapy in consultation with an allergist if the patient fails to respond to medications

Interventions
- *Environmental control*: Remove exposure to allergens, such as carpeting, pets, insect/rodent extermination, mold. Reduce exposure to respiratory irritants and decrease exposure to strong smells, detergents, and cleaners.
- Stop smoking and eliminate exposure to secondhand smoke. Wash bedding weekly in sanitize cycle to reduce allergens.
- Cover mattresses and pillows with allergen protectors. Use HEPA air filtration at home and HEPA filter mask when allergens are not avoidable.
- Encourage saline lavage to nares daily to remove irritants.
- Reevaluate at periodic intervals to determine response to therapy and adjust as needed.

Patient Education
- Review environmental control strategies.
- Discuss daily therapy to prevent acute events.
- Explain the management of acute events.
- Teach patients about medication adverse effects and symptoms to report.

Patient Population Considerations

Women (conception/pregnancy/lactation)
- Hormonal influences of pregnancy increase nasal congestion and can increase the risk of allergic rhinitis and subsequent acute sinusitis.

Geriatric

- Persistent allergic rhinitis refractory to therapy should be referred to otolaryngology for rhinoscopy and evaluated for risk of head and neck cancer, especially in patients who smoke and drink alcohol.

Pediatric

- Children with allergic rhinitis are at increased risk for OM, eustachian tube dysfunction, and acute and chronic sinusitis.

Referring Patients

- Allergist/immunologist consult
- Otolaryngology consult

EPISTAXIS

Overview

- Epistaxis is anterior or posterior bleeding from the nose. Most nosebleeds are benign, while others are a sign of an alteration in hemostasis and require additional evaluation.
- Anterior bleeds arise from the Kiesselbach's plexus.
- Posterior bleeds are more common in older adults and arise from the internal maxillary artery.

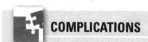

COMPLICATIONS

Acute: Bleeding, airway obstruction
Chronic: Anemia

Etiology

- Trauma, picking, dry air and irritants, topical medication, foreign body (e.g., batteries), poisonings, forceful blowing, surgery, polyp, or cancer
- Anal fissures, coagulopathies, chronic alcoholism, cirrhosis, colon polyps, GERD, hemorrhoids, inflammatory bowel disease, pancreatitis, platelet sequestration in splenomegaly, PUD, or thrombocytopenia due to cancer, radiation, or chemotherapy
- *Medications*: Aspirin, anticoagulants, antiplatelets, antithrombins, COX-2 inhibitors, NSAIDs
- *Nutraceuticals*: Anise, chamomile, clover, fish oil, ginger, garlic, ginkgo biloba, turmeric, vitamins C and E

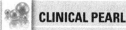

CLINICAL PEARL

Massive epistaxis can be confused with hemoptysis and hematemesis. Careful history taking and examination can help isolate the cause.

Signs and Symptoms

- *Anterior bleed:* Large amount of bleeding from the nose; elevated BP may aggravate bleeding
- *Posterior bleed:* Large amount of bleeding drains to the posterior oropharynx, increasing the risk for aspiration; may be confused with upper GI bleed

Differential Diagnosis

- *GI:* Esophageal varices, hepatic failure, leukemia, thrombocytopenia, upper GI bleeding
- *HEENT:* Foreign body, neoplasm, rhinitis, tumor
- *HEM:* DIC, Inherited bleeding diathesis
- *Other:* Accidental poisoning/toxicity, medication-induced coagulopathy

Diagnosis

Labs
- CBC to evaluate baseline Hgb, HcT, and platelet. Hgb <8 mg/dL and platelets <100,000 require additional inquiry; baseline reading reflects a Hgb level from 4 hr before the blood draw
- PT/INR: >1.5 or PTT >40 sec without warfarin or heparin, requires further inquiry for coagulation defect

ALERT

Labs do not need to be performed unless HPI indicates that an underlying problem is at root cause, recurrent bleeding is reported, or the patient is potentially unstable.

Additional Diagnostic Testing
If complications are suspected:
- DIC panel
- BMP, LFTs
- Blood type and screen
- Head CT of a foreign body is suspected

Treatment and Management

Treatment Goals
- Treat acute bleeding, protect the airway, and prevent rebleeding.

Drug Treatment
- Prescribe topical phenylephrine for vasoconstriction as needed.
- Prescribe topical lidocaine 4% for cautery or nasal packing.
- Prescribe reversal agents for anticoagulation, antithrombin agents if hemodynamically unstable.
- Prescribe antibiotics as prophylaxis if cautery or nasal packing is used.

Procedures
- *Manual hemostasis*
  - Sit upright with head elevated with neck neutral, patient leaning slightly forward to protect the airway.
  - Perform hemostasis with direct pressure to nasal septum and nostril pinched closed 5 to 10 min.

ALERT

Apply PPE with face shield, mask, impermeable gown, gloves, and shoe covers. Have suction available.

- *Chemical hemostasis*
  - If manual hemostasis is ineffective and the patient is not in a hypertensive emergency, prescribe topical phenylephrine to promote vasoconstriction.
  - Prescribe cool mist face tent to provide humidification and promote vasoconstriction.
- *Cauterization or nasal packing*
  - Perform silver nitrate cauterization or nasal packing with adequate topical lidocaine.

Interventions
- Monitor airway, vital signs, and CBC and bleeding times if indicated.
- Monitor for rebleeding after hemostasis.
- Discharge on antibiotics with otolaryngology referral.

Patient Education
- Instruct the patient to avoid physical activity that could disrupt hemostasis for 7 to 10 days.
- Review OTC medications and nutraceuticals that increase the risk of bleeding.
- Teach s/s of complications and adverse medication effects to report.

Patient Population Considerations

Women (conception/pregnancy/lactation)
- Increased abdominal pressure in pregnancy can increase the risk of epistaxis. It has also been associated with increased risk for postpartum hemorrhage.

Geriatric
- Persistent epistaxis in geriatric patients should be referred to otolaryngology and evaluated for neoplasm, especially in those patients who smoke and drink alcohol. Comorbid conditions requiring anticoagulation and antiplatelet therapy may require temporary interruption.

Pediatric
- Otolaryngologist should evaluate frequent nosebleeds in children.

Referring Patients

- Otolaryngology consult
- Hematology consult

POP QUIZ 4.3

A 45-year-old female presents to the urgent care center with epistaxis. The patient reports that she woke up in the night with blood on her pillow and oozing which resolved after 5 min of pressure. It restarted this morning, 2 hr ago, and continues to ooze despite interventions. She reports a history of perennial allergic rhinitis managed with fluticasone intranasal spray and ibuprofen daily for sinus headache. She denies headache, nausea, or vomiting or bleeding disorders. She drinks two to three alcoholic beverages per day and denies tobacco use. Relevant exam findings: BP 168/94, HR 101, RR 20, Temp: 98.7°F (37°C). Sinuses dull to percussion. Nasal speculum exam reveals anterior septal bleeding from septal erosion. No mass, polyp, or foreign body noted. Homeostasis is achieved in office. What factors contributed to the bleeding, and what are the next steps post homeostasis?

THROAT

INFECTIOUS MONONUCLEOSIS

Overview

- Infectious mononucleosis is a self-limiting viral syndrome transmitted through contact with the saliva and body secretions of an infected person.
- EBV virus infects B cells in the oropharyngeal epithelium causing exudative pharyngitis. It circulates systemically to the liver, spleen, and lymph nodes, causing lymphadenopathy and hepatosplenomegaly.
- Acute syndrome persists for 3 to 4 weeks. Fatigue lasts for several months.

Etiology

- Contact with an infected person
- Increased incidence in ages 15 to 25

Signs and Symptoms

- Flu-like syndrome 3 to 5 days with fever and fatigue
- *HEENT*: Cervical lymphadenopathy, edema, erythema, palatal petechiae, tonsillar enlargement, tonsillar exudates
- *GI*: Abdominal tenderness, nausea, hepatomegaly, splenomegaly
- *INT*: Jaundice, maculopapular rash

COMPLICATIONS

Acute: Airway obstruction secondary to compression from edema, splenic rupture, hepatic failure, myocarditis, pancytopenia, meningitis, infection transmission

Chronic: Risk for splenic injury, fatigue, multiple sclerosis

Differential Diagnosis

- *CV*: Bacterial endocarditis
- *HEENT*: Peritonsillar abscess, retropharyngeal abscess, streptococcal pharyngitis,
- *HEM*: Acute leukemia, coagulopathy, lymphoma
- *NEURO*: Bacterial meningitis
- *Other*:
  - *Infectious*: Acute HIV infection, acute cytomegalovirus, viral hepatitis, malaria, rubella, toxoplasmosis
  - *Immune*: SLE flare

Diagnosis

Labs
- Positive mononuclear spot test
- *CBC with differential*: Slight elevation in WBC with lymphocytes >50%, atypical >10%
- Elevated BMP, LFTs, and bilirubin
- If atypical lymphocytes <10%, order a rapid HIV test
- If EBV IgM negative, order CMV IgM
- If CMV IgM negative, evaluate for hepatitis, toxoplasmosis, herpesvirus

Additional Diagnostic Testing
- Lateral neck film to evaluate obstructive symptoms
- Head CT with CNS involvement
- Lumbar puncture with CNS involvement

Treatment and Management

Treatment Goals
- Prevent organ failure, provide supportive care, treat symptoms, and prevent infection transmission.

> **ALERT**
>
> Obstructive symptoms, meningeal irritation, and chest pain should be referred to ED immediately.

Drug Treatment
- Prescribe acetaminophen or NSAIDs for pain and fever. (Use lowest possible effective dose.)
- Provide corticosteroids for airway obstruction, autoimmune hemolytic anemia, severe thrombocytopenia, and myocarditis.

Interventions
- Monitor temperature, vital signs, and signs of dehydration.
- Encourage fluids, ice chips, and humidification to improve pharyngeal edema.
- Manage fever and pain by alternating acetaminophen and NSAIDs.
- Monitor for complications of myocarditis, encephalitis, GBS, pancytopenia.
- Implement bleeding, infection, and infection transmission precautions.
- Prevent splenic rupture through activity restriction.

Patient Education
- Instruct the patient to avoid sharing utensils or food until the fever has resolved.
- Take acetaminophen and NSAIDs as prescribed and monitor for adverse effects.
- Avoid heavy lifting and contact sports until cleared to return to activity.
- Teach signs and symptoms of complications to report.
- Call 911 if you note difficulty breathing, chest discomfort, abdominal pain or swelling, confusion, or seizure activity.

Patient Population Considerations

Women (conception/pregnancy/lactation)
- Pregnant women are at risk for EBV reactivation and infectious mononucleosis during pregnancy. Treatment is supportive care. Careful attention to protect the patient from hepatotoxicity and organ involvement is critical in reducing the risk of miscarriage.

Geriatric
- Infectious mononucleosis is not prevalent in geriatric patients.

Pediatric
- Monospot test may be inconclusive in young children, and EBV antibodies will need to evaluate.

Referring Patients
- Infectious disease consult

STREPTOCOCCAL PHAYRINGITIS

Overview
- Bacterial pharyngitis causes oropharyngeal edema, erythema, tonsillar exudate, cervical lymphadenopathy, and fever. Enzymes produced by Group A streptococcal bacteria release toxins while anti-M antibodies may cross-react with cardiac tissue, causing myocarditis.
- Contact with the saliva from an infected person or GABHS carrier transmits the infection.
- GABHS is classified as nonsuppurative or supportive.

> **COMPLICATIONS**
>
> *Acute*: Peritonsillar or retropharyngeal abscess, cervical lymphadenitis, sinusitis, mastoiditis, OM, pneumonia, rheumatic fever (endocarditis, septic arthritis, meningitis) sepsis, scarlet fever, post-streptococcal glomerulonephritis, PANDAs
>
> *Chronic*: Rheumatic heart disease, (mitral stenosis, AF, HF), HTN, CKD

Etiology
- Contact with oral or respiratory secretions of an infected person
- Family history of rheumatic heart disease, nasal colonization
- Crowded living conditions, poor sanitation, immunocompromised state
- Age (peak prevalence age 5–15 years)

> **CLINICAL PEARL**
>
> *Streptococcus pyogenes* is responsible for strep infection, transmissible by respiratory droplets or contact.

Signs and Symptoms
- *General*: Absent cough, fever >100.9°F (38.3°C)
- *HEENT*: Cervical lymphadenopathy, edema, erythema, palatal petechiae, tonsillar enlargement, tonsillar exudates
- *GI*: Abdominal pain, nausea, vomiting
- *INT*: Maculopapular rash
- *Centor score 4.25% (high risk of streptococcal pharyngitis)*

Differential Diagnosis
- *CV*: Acute rheumatic heart disease
- *ENDO*: Thyroiditis
- *HEENT*: Candida pharyngitis, croup, epiglottis, gonococcal pharyngitis, hand-foot-and-mouth disease, diphtheria, postnasal drip, SLE flare, postnasal drip, retropharyngeal or peritonsillar abscess, sinusitis, stomatitis
- *NEURO*: Lemierre syndrome
- *Other*:
  - *Infectious*: Acute HIV infection, acute cytomegalovirus, viral hepatitis, malaria, rubella, toxoplasmosis, coxsackie virus, herpes simplex, HIV infection, mononucleosis
  - *Immune*: Behcet's syndrome, Kawasaki syndrome, SLE flare

Diagnosis

Labs
- GABHG rapid antigen test
- Throat c/s
- Monospot
- Gonococcal culture according to history

Additional Diagnostic Testing
- Plain lateral neck x-ray to rule out an abscess

Treatment and Management

Treatment Goals
- Eradicate infection, prevent acute/chronic complications, provide supportive care, prevent infection transmission.

Drug Treatment
- Penicillin V potassium 250 mg tab every 8 to 12 hr; (pediatric) every 6 hr (adult) × 10 days, *OR*
- Amoxicillin 50 mg/kg (max 1,000 mg) tab daily × 10 days, *OR*
- Azithromycin 12 mg/kg × 1 day then 6 mg/kg tab (PCN allergy) × 4 days, *OR*
- Cephalexin (PCN nonimmediate hypersensitivity) 25 to 50 mg/kg every 1 to 2 hr. (pediatric) 500 mg tab every 12 hr (adult) × 10 days
- Routine testing or treatment of asymptomatic household contacts not required
- Acetaminophen or ibuprofen for fever or pain PRN

 ALERT

Small children who refuse to drink with signs of dehydration may require hospitalization for IV hydration.

Procedures
Prompt referral to otolaryngology for:
- Needle aspiration and drainage of peritonsillar abscess
- Tonsillectomy
- Surgical drainage of retropharyngeal abscess

Interventions
- Assess temperature, vital signs, and signs of dehydration.
- Encourage fluids, ice chips, and humidification to improve pharyngeal edema. In obstructive symptoms, observe in a clinical setting or refer to ED. Prescribe cool mist.
- Manage fever and pain with alternating acetaminophen and NSAIDs monitoring for adverse events of hepatotoxicity and bleeding.
- Monitor for complications of myocarditis, encephalitis, GBS, pancytopenia.
- Implement bleeding precautions, infection protection, infection transmission precautions, and energy management strategies.
- Prevent splenic rupture through activity restriction.

Patient Education
- Instruct the patient to avoid contact with others for 24 hr after antibiotics are initiated.
- Explain that symptoms that do not improve within 48 hr should return for reevaluation.
- Call 911 for difficulty breathing, chest discomfort, abdominal pain or swelling, confusion, or seizure activity.
- Take acetaminophen and NSAIDs as prescribed and monitor for adverse effects.
- Teach signs and symptoms of complications to report.

Patient Population Considerations

Women (conception/pregnancy/lactation)
- Antibiotics for streptococcal pharyngitis are safe for use in pregnancy.

Geriatric
- Advanced age increases the likelihood of severe, invasive GABHS with multi-organ system involvement, and death.

Pediatric
- Pharyngitis is the leading cause of office visits in ambulatory care. If untreated, GABHS can cause scarlet fever in children 5 to 15 years. A rash is the most common sign.

Referring Patients

- Otolaryngology consult

POP QUIZ 4.4

A 55-year-old female presents to the primary care office complaining of flu-like symptoms, activity intolerance, rash, and shortness of breath. The patient reports that she was treated for a sore throat in an urgent care clinic 2 weeks earlier and started on amoxicillin/clavulanic acid. After taking the antibiotic for 23 days, she noticed a rash getting progressively worse and stopped taking the medication. Following discontinuation, she developed fatigue, activity intolerance, and malaise that has gotten progressively worse. What is the priority intervention?

RESOURCES

American College of Obstetricians and Gynecologists. (2019). *Committee on obstetric practice: Prevention of group b streptococcal early-onset disease in newborns.* https://www.acog.org/clinical/clinical-guidance/committee-opinion/articles/2020/02/prevention-of-group-b-streptococcal-early-onset-disease-in-newborns

Altman, A. (2020). *Medscape: Acute otitis externa.* https://emedicine.medscape.com/article/994550-overview#:~:text=Practice%20Essentials.%20Otitis%20externa%20%28OE%29%20is%20an%20inflammation,all%20age%20groups.%20%20%5B4%5D%20See%20the%20image%20below

American Cancer Society. (n.d.). *Signs and symptoms of nasopharyngeal cancer.* https://www.cancer.org/cancer/nasopharyngeal-cancer/detection-diagnosis-staging/signs-and-symptoms.html

Badawi, A. H., Al-Muhaylib, A. A., Al Owaifeer, A. M., Al-Essa, R. S., & Al-Shahwan, S. A. (2019). Primary congenital glaucoma: An updated review. *Saudi Journal of Ophthalmology: Official Journal of the Saudi Ophthalmological Society, 33*(4), 382–388. https://doi.org/10.1016/j.sjopt.2019.10.002

Bessette, M. (2019). *Medscape: Hordeolum and stye in emergency medicine treatment & management.* https://emedicine.medscape.com/article/798940-treatment#d9

Biggerstaff, K. (2020). *Medscape: Primary open angle glaucoma.* https://emedicine.medscape.com/article/1206147-overview

Brooks, I. (2018). *Medscape: Acute sinusitis.* https://emedicine.medscape.com/article/232670-overview

Cash, J. C., & Glass, C. A. (Eds.). (2019). *Adult-gerontology practice guidelines* (2nd ed.). Springer Publishing Company.

Centers for Disease Control and Prevention. (2017). *Antibiotic prescribing and use in doctor's offices: Pediatric treatment recommendations.* https://www.cdc.gov/antibiotic-use/community/for-hcp/outpatient-hcp/pediatric-treatment-rec.html

Centor, R. M., Witherspoon, J. M., Dalton, H. P., Brody, C. E., & Link, K. (1981). The diagnosis of strep throat in adults in the emergency room. *Medical Decision Making, 1*(3), 239–246. https://doi.org/10.1177/0272989X8100100304

Codina Leik, M. T. (2018). *Family nurse practitioner certification: Intensive review* (3rd ed.). Springer Publishing Company.

Deschenes, J. (2019). *Medscape: Chalazion.* https://emedicine.medscape.com/article/1212709-overview

Ehrenhaus, M. (2018). *Medscape: Hordeolum.* https://emedicine.medscape.com/article/1213080-overview#a4

Freedman, J. (2018). *Medscape: Acute angle closure glaucoma in emergency medicine.* https://emedicine.medscape.com/article/798811-overview

Hoge, C. W., Schwartz, B., Talkington, D. F., Breiman, R. F., MacNeill, E. M., & Englender, S. J. (1993). The changing epidemiology of invasive group a streptococcal infections and the emergence of streptococcal toxic shock-like syndrome. A retrospective population-based study. *JAMA, 269*(3), 384–389. https://doi.org/10.1001/jama.1993.03500030082037

Intermountain Healthcare. (2019). *Diagnosis and management of pediatric acute otitis media, 2019 update.* https:// intermountainhealthcare.org/ckr-ext/Dcmnt?ncid=522927223#:~:text=Antibiotics%20are%20commonly%20 overprescribed%20for%20acute%20otitis%20media.&text=The%20following%20is%20a%20list,diagnosis%20 and%20treatment%20of%20AOM.&text=Only%20diagnose%20AOM%20if%20exam.criteria%20(see%20 page%202).&text=antibiotic%20resistance%20in%20pathogens%20that%20commonly%20cause%20it

Lowery, S. (2019). *Medscape: Adult blepharitis.* https://emedicine.medscape.com/article/1211763-overview

McKinney, K. (2020). Is it COVID-19 or allergies? *American Academy of Ophthalmology.* https://www.aao.org/ eye-health/tips-prevention/coronavirus-versus-allergies-pink-eye

Muchachuta, M. (2019). *Medscape: Iritis and uveitis.* https://emedicine.medscape.com/article/798323-overview

Nguyen, Q. (2020). *Medscape: Epistaxis.* https://emedicine.medscape.com/article/863220-overview

Occupational Safety and Health Administration. (2018). *Preventing hearing loss caused by chemical (ototoxicity) and noise exposure.* https://www.cdc.gov/niosh/docs/2018-124/pdfs/2018-124.pdf?id=10.26616/NIOSHPUB2018124

O'Dell, L. (2020). Cast a wide net for demodex to serve patients, practice. *Primary Care Optometry News.* https:// www.healio.com/news/optometry/20200819/cast-a-wide-net-for-demodex-to-serve-patients-practice

Omori, M. (2019). *Medscape: Infectious mononucleosis in emergency medicine.* https://emedicine.medscape.com/ article/784513-overview

Patel, S. (2020). *Bimatoprost implant a promising weapon in fight against glaucoma–Medscape.* https://www. medscape.com/viewarticle/932890

Pedersen, T. M., Stokholm, J., Thorsen, J., Mora-Jensen, A. R. C., & Bisgaard, H. (2017). Antibiotics in pregnancy increase children's risk of otitis media and ventilation tubes. *The Journal of Pediatrics, 183*, 153–158. https://doi. org/10.1016/j.jpeds.2016.12.046

Randel, A. (2013). IDSA updates guideline for managing group a streptococcal pharyngitis. *American Family Physician, 88*(5), 338–340.

Scott, I. (2020). *Medscape: Unilateral glaucoma.* https://emedicine.medscape.com/article/1207362-overview

Sethi, H. S., Naik, M., & Gupta, V. S. (2016). Management of glaucoma in pregnancy: Risks or choices, a dilemma? *International Journal of Ophthalmology, 9*(11), 1684–1690. https://doi.org/10.18240/ijo.2016.11.24

Sheikh, J. (2018). *Medscape: Allergic rhinitis.* https://emedicine.medscape.com/article/134825-overview#:~:text= Rhinitis%2C%20which%20occurs%20most%20commonly%20as%20allergic%20rhinitis%2C,anaphylaxis%29 %2C%20morbidity%20from%20the%20condition%20can%20be%20

Shulman, S. T., Bisno, A. L., Clegg, H. W., Gerber, M. A., Kaplan, E. L., Lee, G., Martin, J. M., & Van Beneden, C. (2014). Correction to infectious diseases society of clinical practice guideline for the diagnosis and management of group a streptococcal pharyngitis: 2012 update by the Infectious Diseases Society of America. *Clinical Infectious Diseases, 58*(10), 1496. https://doi.org/10.1093/cid/cis847. https://academic.oup.com/cid/ article/58/10/1496/287267

Silverman, M. (2018). *Medscape: Acute conjunctivitis.* https://emedicine.medscape.com/article/797874-overview#a1

Simon, H. (2019). *Medscape: Pediatric pharyngitis.* https://emedicine.medscape.com/article/967384-overview

Sorenson, M., Quinn, L., & Klein, D. (2019). *Pathophysiology: Concepts of human disease* (1st ed.). Pearson Education.

Wang, L. (2019). *Medscape: Herpes simplex keratitis.* https://emedicine.medscape.com/article/1194268-overview

Waseem, M. (2020). *Medscape: Acute otitis media.* https://emedicine.medscape.com/article/994656-overview

Yu Chan, J. Y., Choy, B. N. K., Ng, A. L. K., & Shum, J. W. H. (2015). Review on the management of primary congenital glaucoma. *Journal of Current Glaucoma Practice, 9*(3), 92–99. https://doi.org/10.5005/jp-journals-10008-1192

CARDIOVASCULAR SYSTEM

ABDOMINAL AORTIC ANEURYSM

Overview

- An aortic aneurysm is a form of PAD characterized by weakening and dilation of the aorta wall, making it vulnerable to tearing or dissection that results in life-threatening hemorrhage.
- There are two types of aortic aneurysms: thoracic and abdominal. This chapter will cover AAAs, which are more common.

Etiology

- Family history of AAA
- Marfan or Ehlers–Danlos Syndrome vascular type
- Men >65 years who have ever smoked
- Patients with COPD, previous aneurysm repair, or peripheral aneurysm
- HTN, hyperlipidemia
- Fluoroquinolone use in an at-risk patient

Signs and Symptoms

- Asymptomatic unless undergoing expansion
- Abdominal, back, or groin pain, pulsating mass
- Apprehension, AMS, nausea/vomiting
- Diaphoresis, pallor, blue toe syndrome
- Hemodynamic instability
- Abdominal distention, bruit, Grey Turner's sign

Differential Diagnosis

- *CV*: MI
- *GI*: Acute abdomen, gallbladder disease, diverticulitis, bowel obstruction, gastritis, pancreatitis, incarcerated hernia
- *GU*: Ascending UTI, renal colic
- *MSK*: Lumbar spine disease

Diagnosis

Labs

- BMP, LFTs, Ca, Mg, to evaluate electrolyte and hepatorenal function
- CBC to evaluate for baseline Hgb, HcT, and platelets
- Lipid profile, HbA1c
- Obtain PTT, PT/INR D-dimer

COMPLICATIONS

Acute: Hemorrhage, MI, bowel ischemia and obstruction, blue toe syndrome, AKI, spinal cord ischemia, arteriovenous fistula, HF

Chronic: Lower extremity amputation

CLINICAL PEARL

The USPSTF recommends a one-time screening for AAA with ultrasonography in men aged 65–75 years who have ever smoked.

ALERT

Do not touch pulsating masses in abdomen with acute abdominal or back pain. Keep NPO, hold all anticoagulants and antiplatelets, and send to ED.

Additional Diagnostic Testing
- 12-lead EKG
- Chest x-ray, which may suggest enlarged thoracic aorta in TAA
- CT to evaluate aneurysm size; annual increase in aneurysmal expansion >1 cm or absolute size >5.5 cm require surgical referral

Treatment and Management

Treatment Goals
- No chest pain, no evidence of bleeding, no increase in aneurysm size or risk factors for aortic dissection with HR <60, SBP 90 to 120 mmHg, ensure no changes in urinary pattern
- Equal and present peripheral pulses

Drug Treatment
- Asymptomatic AAA <5 cm: Prescribe beta blocker or ACEI to control stress on aneurysm wall, antilipemic therapy, and antiplatelet with comorbid ASCVD to reduce risk factors for aneurysm and its expansion.

Interventions
- Assess abdominal girth, vital signs, ankle-brachial index, and annual evaluation of aneurysm ≥3 cm by CT versus ultrasound or with symptoms.
- Initiate ASCVD risk factor modification and manage HR and BP.
- Evaluate for the presence of adverse medication effects.

Patient Education
- Counsel patient on alcohol and tobacco cessation, lipid management, and BP monitoring.
- Instruct the patient to avoid OTC NSAIDs and nutraceuticals.
- Review strategies to manage modifiable risk factors, heart rate, and blood pressure control for AAA.
- Review s/s of complications and adverse effects of medication to report.

Patient Population Considerations

Women (conception/pregnancy/lactation)
- Do not screen women who have never smoked and have no family history of AAA.

Geriatric
- Older men who have never smoked do not need to participate in screening.

Pediatric
- Pediatric patients with Marfan or Ehlers–Danlos syndrome vascular type require close monitoring and risk factor modification.

Referring Patients
- Vascular surgery consult

ARRHYTHMIAS

Overview
- Arrhythmias are transient or persisting irregularities in HR, rhythm, or conduction. Arrhythmias result from a conduction tract anomaly, ectopic foci, structural change to the heart, or a symptom of a noncardiac condition.

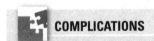

COMPLICATIONS

Acute: ACS, HF, stroke, PE
Chronic: Recurrent arrhythmia, refractory HF, CVHD, recurrent PE

- Patients with no acute symptoms of ischemia and HF, electrolyte imbalances, or thromboembolism who are under a cardiologist's care can be managed in the outpatient setting. All patients with new-onset arrhythmias and acute symptoms require immediate referral.

Types of Arrhythmias

- *Atrial fibrillation:* Most common arrhythmia that has an atrial rate >400 and ventricular response that varies: slow (<60), moderate (60–100), or rapid (>100). Key features include a ventricular response (QRS) that is irregular in rhythm and a fibrillatory line replacing the p wave (Figure 5.1).
- *Paroxysmal supraventricular tachycardia:* Narrow QRS tachycardia of sudden onset that is regular in rhythm with rate >100 (Figure 5.2).

(continued)

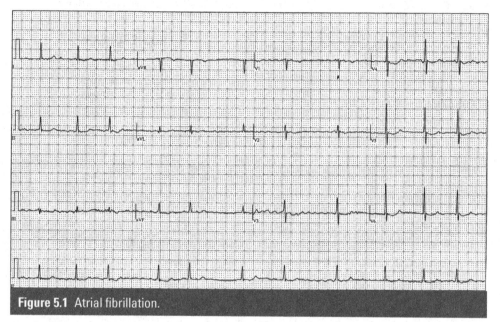

Figure 5.1 Atrial fibrillation.

aVF, augmented voltage foot; aVL, augmented voltage left-arm; aVR, augmented voltage right-arm.
Source: From Knechtel, M. A. (2021). *EKGs for the nurse practitioner and physician assistant* (3rd ed.). Springer Publishing Company.

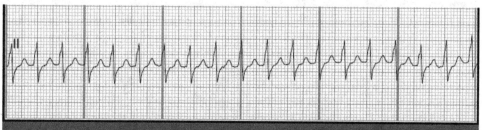

Figure 5.2 Paroxysmal supraventricular tachycardia.

Source: From Roberts, D. (2020). *Mastering the 12-lead EKG* (2nd ed.). Springer Publishing Company.

Types of Arrhythmias (continued)

- *Ventricular tachycardia:* Wide QRS tachycardia that is regular in rhythm with rate >100 (Figure 5.3).
- *Premature atrial contractions:* Ectopic atrial beat that presents early before the next sinus complex (Figure 5.4).
- *Sinus bradycardia:* Sinus rhythm that has a heart rate of less than 60. It may be a normal variant or symptomatic. The rhythm may present with or without a low-grade heart block (Figure 5.5).

Etiology

- Family history of sudden premature death, personal history of prolonged QT syndrome, WPW syndrome, congenital heart disease, HF, CVHD, ASCVD, stroke, hyperlipidemia, pericarditis, valvular disease
- Sepsis, COVID-19, thyrotoxicosis, sleep apnea, COPD, DM, CKD, anemia, proarrhythmic medication
- Obesity, sedentary lifestyle, increasing age, female gender, organophosphate poisoning, displaced implanted device or catheter, substance abuse, alcohol, tobacco, stimulants, herbal supplements, vasovagal, anxiety, panic disorder, electrolyte imbalance (hypokalemia, hyperkalemia, hypocalcemia, hypomagnesemia)

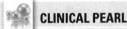 **CLINICAL PEARL**

- Perform medication reconciliation to identify proarrhythmic agents.
- Perform rhythm strip analysis and 12-lead EKG.

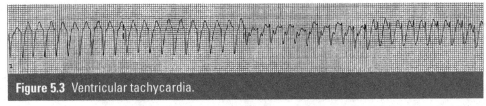

Figure 5.3 Ventricular tachycardia.

Source: From Knechtel, M. A. (2021). *EKGs for the Nurse Practitioner and Physician Assistant* (3rd ed.). Springer Publishing.

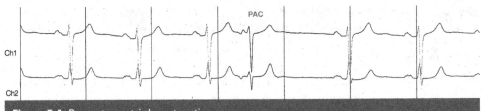

Figure 5.4 Premature atrial contractions.

Source: From Green, J. M., & Chiaramida, A. J. (2015). *12-lead EKG confidence.* Springer Publishing Company.

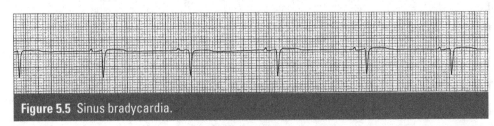

Figure 5.5 Sinus bradycardia.

Source: From Knechtel, M. A. (2021). *EKGs for the nurse practitioner and physician assistant* (3rd ed.). Springer Publishing Company.

Signs and Symptoms

- May be asymptomatic
- Palpitations, apprehension, dizziness
- S/s of HF, ACS, PE, or stroke
- Tachy-bradycardia, hypotension, tachypnea
- Displaced PMI, thrill, heave, murmur, S3, S4, decreased intensity of peripheral pulses
- Sudden death

Differential Diagnosis

- *CV*: ACS, CVHD, HF, cardiac structure anomalies, cardiac conduction disorders, cardiac device malposition/malfunction
- *ENDO*: DM, metabolic conditions
- *GU*: AKI, CKD
- *HEM*: Bleeding, anemia, coagulopathy, infections
- *PULM*: Hypoxia, COPD, pulmonary embolism
- *Other*: Poisoning, stimulants, proarrhythmic medications, alcohol, or substance abuse

Diagnosis

Labs
- Stat CBG if patient has diabetes
- BMP, Mg, Ca, LFTs to evaluate electrolyte imbalance and hepatic and renal function
- CBC to evaluate for anemia and infection
- TSH to evaluate for hyperthyroidism
- BNP level to evaluate for HF
- *Drug levels*: Digoxin, amiodarone, lithium, quinidine, procainamide, theophylline, anticonvulsant, if indicated

Additional Diagnostic Testing
- Chest x-ray to evaluate heart size and for pulmonary congestion
- 12-lead EKG to evaluate for atrial fibrillation, ischemia, conduction anomaly, LBBB, LVH
- Echocardiogram to evaluate systolic, diastolic function, thrombus formation, valve function, and EF
- Holter monitoring
- Toxicology screen for abuse/poisoning, if indicated

Treatment and Management

- Hemodynamically unstable patients or patients with ischemia require ACLS. Refer to ED immediately.

Treatment Goals
- Correction of underlying cause when possible, control of arrhythmias, and reduction of recurrence to preserve cardiac output, prevention/management of complications (thromboembolism, ischemia, and HF)

Drug Treatment
- *Atrial fibrillation*
  - *Rate control with HF*: Prescribe digoxin or cardioselective beta blocker (may convert rhythm to NSR).
  - *Rate control without HF*: Prescribe nondihydropyridine calcium channel blockers (diltiazem or verapamil) or beta blocker.
  - *Anticoagulation*: Prescribe DOAC or warfarin based on CHA_2DS_2-VAS.

(continued)

Drug Treatment (continued)

- *Paroxysmal supraventricular tachycardia*
  - Encourage vagal maneuvers and prescribe beta blockers or calcium channel blockers (diltiazem or verapamil) to prevent recurrent PSVT and refer to cardiology for EPS study.
- *Ventricular tachycardia*
  - Hold all medications that prolong the QT interval. Correct potassium, magnesium, and calcium levels.
  - Prescribe beta blockers to prevent recurrent runs of VT and refer to cardiology for AICD.
  - Prescribe amiodarone, the drug of choice for acute VT refractory to cardioversion.
- *Premature ventricular contractions*
  - Review diuretics, sympathomimetics, beta agonists, and methylxanthines for proarrhythmic effect.
  - Prescribe potassium replacement in the presence of hypokalemia or add ACEI, ARB, or aldosterone antagonist in HTN management to avoid depletion.
- *Premature atrial contractions*
  - Review sympathomimetics, beta agonists, and methylxanthines, and explore prescribing alternative agents for improved tolerance.
- *Sinus bradycardia*
  - Withhold all medications that in symptomatic bradycardia and/or cause hyperkalemia.
  - Prescribed sodium zirconium cyclosilicate 10 g 3 times per day × 48 hr if hyperkalemia is present.

Interventions

- Assess the progression of ACS, HF, and for the presence of refractory arrhythmias.
- Monitor hepatic function and estimate eGFR for medication dosing.
- *Monitor electrolytes*: Mg, K, Ca, and keep at the high side of the normal range. Review medication changes that can alter electrolytes, especially insulin.
- Monitor for bleeding, thromboembolism, and reevaluate the need for anticoagulation in AF annually.

Patient Education

- Counsel patients on alcohol and tobacco cessation and weight loss in overweight or obese patients.
- Teach patient to avoid agents, factors, and activities that can trigger arrhythmia.
- Review s/s of complications and adverse effects of medication to report.

Patient Population Considerations

Women (conception/pregnancy/lactation)

- Preconception planning is essential in patients with underlying congenital heart disease, HTN, and valve disorders, as these changes could exacerbate symptoms of arrhythmias.

Geriatric

- Polypharmacology and dehydration secondary to decreased thirst reflex can exacerbate AKI and increase the risk for medication-induced arrhythmia.

Pediatric

- Calculate QT intervals with pediatric patients to identify prolonged QT syndrome. Do not rely on computer interpretations of QT interval duration, as they may be for a normal adult range.

Referring Patients

- Cardiology consult

BACTERIAL ENDOCARDITIS

Overview

- BE is an infection of the endothelium. Damage from turbulent blood flow, bacteria from invasive procedures, or immune-mediated inflammation cause endothelial injury.
- Thrombi and vegetation build at the site impeding cardiac output. It can be acute (BE) or subacute (SBE).

Etiology

- *Streptococci*, *staphylococcus*, or *enterococci* (most cases)
- Immunosuppression, hypercoagulability
- Congenital or degenerative heart disease, rheumatic heart disease, valve disorder, prosthetic valve replacement
- IV drug abuse, CVC, shunts, invasive procedures, hemodialysis, recent hospitalization, dental work

Signs and Symptoms

- *SBE*: Nonspecific indolent fever × 2 weeks splenomegaly
- *BE*: Acute onset of fever, chills myalgia, fatigue, weight loss, anorexia, joint pain, cough, petechiae, increased pulse pressure
- *Both SBE and BE*:
  - Osler's nodes, splinter hemorrhages, Janeway lesions, Roth spots
  - New murmur of valvular regurgitation, pericardial or pleural friction rub
  - S/s of HF
- *S/s of septic embolism*: Aching bone pain, meningeal signs, pleuritic chest pain

Differential Diagnosis

- Antiphospholipid syndrome, SLE myocarditis, polymyalgia rheumatica, RA flare, Lyme disease, HIV

Diagnosis

Labs
- *Blood cultures*: Continuous sets over time to document bacteremia
  - SBE: Draw three to five sets of blood cultures over 24 hr
  - BE: Draw three sets over 30 min
- CBC to evaluate for anemia and leukocytosis
- Elevated ESR; positive Rh factor
- BMP, LFTs, PT/INR to assess electrolytes, hepatorenal function, and coagulation
- UA for protein and hematuria

Additional Diagnostic Testing
- TEE for all cases to detect the presence of an abscess, mass on valves, or dehiscence to prosthetic valves
- 12-lead EKG and chest x-ray
- CT head with meningeal signs
- Bone scan with signs of osteomyelitis

COMPLICATIONS

Acute: Sepsis, HF, AKI, septic embolism (osteomyelitis, pneumonia, meningitis), ACS

Chronic: CVHD, HF, valvular disease

CLINICAL PEARL

- **HACEK** occur in neonates and immunoincompetent children. Fungal disease is found in patients with IV drug abuse and those in the ICU.

ALERT

Acute symptoms should be referred to ED immediately.

Treatment and Management

Treatment Goals

- Eradication of infection, restoration of cardiac output to maintain tissue perfusion and supplement gas exchange, and prevention of acute and chronic complications

Drug Treatment

- Use empiric antibiotics according to clinical situation for 2 to 6 weeks (PCN, aminoglycoside, MSSA PCN, third-generation cephalosporin, vancomycin), adjusted according to microbiology report.
- Evaluate the effectiveness of HF therapy.
- Adjust antidiabetic therapy to maintain HbA1c <7%, if indicated.
- Update vaccinations to prevent respiratory infections.

Interventions

- Assess hydration status, weight changes, DVT score, and evaluate eGFR for s/s of HF.
- Order periodic bloodwork to evaluate hepatic function, CBC, and electrolytes for antibiotic therapy.
- Prescribe BE prophylaxis.

> 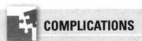 **CLINICAL PEARL**
>
> Use a validated DVT prediction tool to calculate risk for DVT and determine the need for IPC and chemical prophylaxis with UFH or LMWH.
>
> Use a validated PE scoring tool to determine risk. Do initial testing with CT angiography.

Patient Education

- Instruct in the importance of dental hygiene and avoidance of body piercing or tattooing.
- Discuss BE prophylaxis.
- Review s/s of complications and adverse effects of medication to report.

Patient Population Considerations

Women (conception/pregnancy/lactation)

- Provide BE prophylaxis for vaginal delivery in women with congenital heart disease, prosthetic valves, prior infective endocarditis, cardiac transplant.

Geriatric

- Provide BE prophylaxis to high-risk older patients with cardiac disease before all invasive dental procedures, invasive respiratory tract procedures, and skin or musculoskeletal procedures.

Pediatric

- The incidence of BE has increased due to a larger number of invasive procedures in infancy and childhood. Septic embolism is more frequently seen in neonates.

Referring Patients

- Cardiothoracic surgery consult
- Infectious disease consult
- Home care evaluation for IV antibiotics

DEEP VEIN THROMBOSIS AND PULMONARY EMBOLISM

Overview

- DVT is characterized by thrombus formation caused by Virchow's triad: venous stasis, vessel injury, and hypercoagulability.
- PE is a pulmonary vascular occlusion from embolized thrombi.

> **COMPLICATIONS**
>
> *Acute*: PE/cardiogenic shock, pulmonary infarct, superior vena cava syndrome
>
> *Chronic*: recurrent DVT/PE, postthrombotic syndrome

Etiology

- *Major*: Orthopedic trauma or surgery stroke, major surgery or trauma, SCI
- *Intermediate*: Prior DVT/PE, malignancy, chemotherapy, CVC, HF, MI, stroke, pregnancy, prothrombotic medications, prothrombotic disorders, dehydration
- *Low*: Advanced age, obesity, bed rest >3 days; car or air travel >8 hr, chronic venous insufficiency

Signs and Symptoms

- *DVT*: Calf swelling >3 cm compared to other leg, edema along the length of the leg, leg pain, or tenderness
- *PE*: Sudden onset anxiety, chest pain, dyspnea, hemoptysis, rales, pleural rub, S3, S4, cough, fever, hemodynamic instability, oxygen desaturation

 CLINICAL PEARL

Silent PE in DVT occurs in >8% of AF patients. Patients with high CHA_2DS_2-VASc score that are not anticoagulated are at greatest risk.

Differential Diagnosis

DVT

- *GI*: Hepatic disease
- *INT*: Soft tissue injury, hematoma
- *MSK*: Compartment syndrome
- *NEURO*: CRPS with edema
- *PV*: Dependent edema, acute peripheral arterial occlusion, postphlebitic syndrome, lymphedema, chronic venous insufficiency

PE

- *CV*: ACS, CHF, pericarditis, aortic dissection
- *GI*: GERD
- *PULM*: Pneumonia
- *Other*: Panic disorder; other embolism

Diagnosis

Labs

- Calculate DVT/PE probability score.
- Obtain D-dimer (remains elevated for 7 days), PT/INR, PTT, CBC, BMP to evaluate platelets and calculate eGFR.

ALERT

Acute signs and symptoms of PE require immediate referral to ED.

Additional Diagnostic Testing

- DVT
  - D-dimer test and venous ultrasonography
- PE
  - D-dimer test for patients with low or intermediate risk
  - CT peripheral angiography in high-probability patients; may consider VQ scan if not available
  - *Hypercoagulability panel if indicated*: Anticardiolipin antibody, antithrombin III prothrombin, factor V gene mutation homocysteine level, lupus anticoagulant

Treatment and Management

Treatment Goals

- Pain management and prevention of PE and postthrombotic syndrome in a patient with DVT
- No s/s of PE, no tachycardia, tachypnea, SBP >100 mmHg, UO >0.5 mL/kg/hr.

Drug Treatment
- DVT/PE treatment
  - Prescribe weight-adjusted LMWH with warfarin or direct oral anticoagulants.
  - *Do not use direct oral anticoagulants in patients requiring medications that are P-gp inhibitors or CVP 450 inducers. No pediatric dosing is available.*
- Pain and comfort
  - Prescribe acetaminophen 325 mg one to two tablets PO q6h PRN for mild pain (1–3/scale 1–10).

Interventions
- Consider a falls-risk screening, bleeding precautions, and dietary teaching if patient is starting warfarin.
- Monitor CBC PT/INR periodically.
- If DVT is present, remove compression device or stocking from affected extremity and elevate leg for edema until anticoagulated.
- When ambulatory, prescribe elastic wraps when standing to reduce the postthrombotic syndrome.
- Evaluate for the presence of adverse medication effects, use of OTC medications, and nutraceuticals.

Patient Education
- Counsel patient on alcohol and tobacco cessation and weight and diet management.
- Instruct the patient to avoid NSAIDs, herbal supplements, and nutraceuticals while on anticoagulants.
- Inform the patient that DVT/PE can recur and review strategies to manage modifiable risk factors.
- Review s/s of complications and adverse effects of medication to report.

Patient Population Considerations

Women (conception/pregnancy/lactation)
- Pregnant women diagnosed with DVT require admission to a hospital. Warfarin is contraindicated in pregnancy.

Geriatric
- Careful evaluation of falls risk is needed to ensure safety while anticoagulated.

Pediatric
- The safety and efficacy of direct oral anticoagulants have not been established in children.

Referring Patients

- Vascular surgery
- Hematology consult

POP QUIZ 5.1

An 82-year-old male with history of rheumatoid arthritis, HTN, and type 1 DM presents to the HCP following left total knee replacement for medication renewal. Edema is noted on the right lower extremity. What is the nurse practitioner's assessment priority?

HEART FAILURE

Overview

- HF is a chronic progressive disorder characterized by decreased cardiac output that reduces tissue perfusion to target organs and decreases activity tolerance.
- It is classified as systolic or diastolic. Stressors trigger SNS and RAAS stimulation, which decreases cardiac output, increases venous congestion, and thrombus formation.

COMPLICATIONS

Acute: Pulmonary edema, cardiogenic shock, MI, arrhythmia, VTE, PE, stroke, AKI, hepatic failure

Chronic: Advanced stage HF, ESRD, cirrhosis

Etiology

- Advanced age
- Congenital heart disease, HTN, MI, valvular disease, pericarditis, cardiomyopathy
- COPD, pulmonary fibrosis
- Hyperthyroidism, DM
- Alcohol, chemotherapy, and medications

Signs and Symptoms

- PND or activity intolerance with dyspnea on exertion progressing to dyspnea at rest over several days associated with weight gain
- *Left-sided*: AMS, PND, orthopnea, dyspnea, rales, S3
- *Right-sided*: JVD, hepatomegaly, ascites, peripheral edema

Differential Diagnosis

- *CV*: Lymphatic obstruction, CVI
- *GI*: Hepatomegaly
- *GU*: CKD
- *PULM*: ARDS, pneumonia, respiratory failure, COPD exacerbation, pulmonary embolism, obesity, hypoventilation syndrome

ALERT

NYHA Classification of HF
- *Class I*: No limitation of physical activity
- *Class II*: Slight limitation of physical activity
- *Class III*: Marked limitation of physical activity
- *Class IV*: Symptoms occur even at rest; discomfort with any physical activity

Stages of HF
- *Stage A*: High risk; no structural disease; no symptoms
- *Stage B*: Structural disease without symptoms
- *Stage C*: Structural disease with symptoms
- *Stage D*: Refractory disease requiring specialized intervention

Diagnosis

Labs
- BMP, Ca, Mg, to evaluate electrolyte and renal function
- LFT to evaluate liver function
- CBC to evaluate for anemia and infection
- TSH to evaluate for hyperthyroidism
- BNP level elevates in HF
- Lipid profile, HbA1c
- PT/INR for baseline

Additional Diagnostic Testing
- 12-lead EKG to evaluate for atrial fibrillation, MI, LBBB, LVH
- Pulse oximetry to assess oxygenation
- Chest x-ray to assess heart size and for pulmonary congestion
- Echocardiogram to evaluate systolic, diastolic function, thrombus formation, valves function, and EF
- Cardiac MRI and nuclear imaging (consider)
- Cardiac catheterization with angiography to evaluate perfusion

Treatment and Management

Treatment Goals
- Absence of HF symptoms, no progression of systolic or diastolic function, no acute hospital readmissions, mitigation of arrhythmias, VTE prophylaxis, prevention of acute and chronic complications increase in EF >50%

Drug Treatment

Refer patients with acute HF to the ED.

- *Stage A*: Prescribe ACEI or ARB to inhibit RAAS stimulation and statins to reduce atherosclerotic risk.
- *Stage B*: Prescribe beta blockers or alpha beta blockers to reduce heart rate, cardiac workload, and promote peripheral vasodilation.
- *Stage C*: Prescribe loop diuretics to reduce preload in symptom management.
  - Consider digitalis to improve cardiac output in atrial fibrillation.
  - Consider hydralazine and/or nitrates to promote vasodilation, as indicated in the patient situation.
  - Consider aliskiren with EF <35% to reduce mortality.
- *Stage D*: Refer to cardiology for chronic inotrope therapy.
  - Prescribe aspirin or anticoagulant based on risk for VTE.
  - *Order immunization updates*: Influenza, pneumonia

Interventions

- Assess hydration status, monitor daily weights, and evaluate eGFR for fluid management.
- Review the patient's dietary intake, sodium intake, activity tolerance, and ADLs.
- Monitor BMP, CBC, LFTs, Ca, Mg, digoxin levels to evaluate for rising azotemia, hepatic dysfunction, and electrolyte balance.
- Review 12-lead EKG to assess for the presence of changes.
- Evaluate for the presence of adverse medication effects, use of OTC medications, and nutraceuticals.

Patient Education

- Counsel patient on alcohol and tobacco cessation.
- Review HF action plan to avoid readmission.
- Instruct the patient to avoid OTC NSAIDs and nutraceuticals.
- Answer questions regarding bleeding precautions, falls prevention, and infection protection.
- Review s/s of complications and adverse effects of medication to report.

Patient Population Considerations

Women (conception/pregnancy/lactation)

- Inform patients with a history of cardiomyopathy, HTN, advancing age with an EF <30% to seek consultation regarding pregnancy due to an increased risk of poor outcome.

Geriatric

- The frequency of HF with preserved systolic function has increased in the older population.

Pediatric

- Diaphoresis, grunting, and difficulty feeding are signs of HF in infants. In older children, HF can be mistaken for asthma.

Referring Patients

- Cardiology consult
- Cardiac rehabilitation referral

HEART MURMURS

Overview

- A murmur indicates turbulent blood flow at the auscultatory site that is congenital or acquired. Sites are aortic, pulmonic, tricuspid, and mitral valves, and Erb's point. Document the location, timing, radiation, configuration, grade, pitch, quality, and *correlate to the patient's clinical condition.*

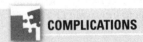

COMPLICATIONS

Acute: ACS, stroke, PE, HF, BE
Chronic: BE prophylaxis

- Diastolic murmurs are always pathologic.
- Murmurs can be categorized as:
  - Narrowing or constricting blood flow (Table 5.1)
  - Abnormal blood flow or regurgitation between chambers (Table 5.2)

Etiology

- Congenital defects, valve abnormalities, papillary muscle rupture, HF, cardiomyopathy, infection, rheumatic fever, infective endocarditis, injury, inflammation
- Increased blood flow (systolic murmur of anemia, thyrotoxicosis, and sepsis), increased resistance to blood flow (stenosis, coarctation), or abnormal blood flow between chambers (regurgitation, PDA, ASD, VSD)

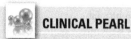

CLINICAL PEARL

- Innocent murmurs tend to disappear with standing, sitting, or on inspiration.
- Murmurs can be seen in pregnancy and childhood.

Table 5.1 Murmurs With Increased Resistance

Condition	Location	Timing/Description
Aortic stenosis	Aortic region, upright	**Systolic,** following ejection click, crescendo–decrescendo
Coarctation of the aorta	Back, between scapula	**Systolic,** harsh, or continuous, machine-like
Mitral stenosis	Apex, left side	**Diastolic,** following opening snap, rumbling
Pulmonic stenosis	Pulmonic region	**Systolic,** following ejection click, crescendo–decrescendo

Table 5.2 Murmurs Caused by Abnormal Flow Between Chambers

Condition	Location	Timing/Description
Aortic regurgitation	Left 2nd–4th intercostal space leaning forward	**Diastolic (early),** decrescendo, blowing in quality
Atrial septal defect	Pulmonic region	**Wide split S2** with systolic ejection murmur, diastolic murmur at lower left sternal border
Hypertrophic cardiomyopathy	Apex and axilla on left side	**Mitral valve regurgitation, aortic regurgitation** displaced PMI laterally
Mitral valve regurgitation	Apex, on left side, squatting	**Holosystolic,** blowing or shushing in quality
Mitral valve prolapse	Apex	**Late systolic,** following midsystolic click, plateau
Patent ductus arteriosus	Pulmonic region	**Continuous**
Transposition of the great vessels	All sites	**No S1,** with or without systolic ejection murmur
Tricuspid regurgitation	Tricuspid region	**Holosystolic,** blowing in quality
Ventricular septal defect	Left sternal border edge	Pansystolic murmur with thrill

Signs and Symptoms

- Auscultatory sites
  - *Aortic*: Right sternal border, 2nd intercostal space
  - *Pulmonic*: Left sternal border, 2nd intercostal space
  - *Tricuspid*: Left sternal border, 4th to 5th intercostal space mitral: left MCL 5th intercostal space
- May be asymptomatic
- S/s of HF or ischemia
- Cyanosis, palpitations, clubbing

Differential Diagnosis

- *Other*: Transmitted sound from abdomen or carotid artery, normal finding

Diagnosis

Labs
- CBC to evaluate for anemia and infection
- TSH to evaluate for hyperthyroidism
- BNP level to evaluate HF

Additional Diagnostic Testing
- Echocardiogram to evaluate systolic, diastolic function, thrombus formation, valve function, and EF
- 12-lead EKG to evaluate for atrial fibrillation, MI, LBBB, LVH
- Chest x-ray to evaluate heart size and for pulmonary congestion
- 24-hr Holter monitoring

Treatment and Management

Treatment Goals
- Mitigation of arrhythmia, prevention of progression to HF, BE prophylaxis, if indicated, infection protection; initiate primary prevention of acquired cardiac disease

Drug Treatment
- Prescribe metoprolol 25 mg PO for palpitations to provide symptomatic relief, if necessary.
- Prescribe IE prophylaxis: Amoxicillin 2 g PO 30 to 60 min before procedure or clindamycin 600 mg PO if allergic to penicillin.

Interventions
- Assess cardiovascular risk factors at diagnosis and evaluate for progression of abnormal blood flow every 3 to 5 years and more frequently as indicated.

Patient Education
- Counsel patient on alcohol and tobacco cessation.
- Discuss lifestyle recommendations for primary prevention of cardiac disease.

ALERT

Grading Intensity
- *Grade I*: Heard by expert
- *Grade II*: Heard with careful attention
- *Grade III*: Heard without difficulty
- *Grade IV*: Loud sound with a thrill
- *Grade V*: Thrill with a very loud murmur audible with stethoscope placed lightly or with one side of the diaphragm lifted
- *Grade VI*: Thrill with a very loud murmur audible even with the stethoscope away from the chest

Acute symptoms of hypoxia, HF, or ACS should be evaluated in the ED.

CLINICAL PEARL

Conditions/Procedures Indicated for Endocarditis Prophylaxis

Conditions
- Prosthetic cardiac valve
- Cardiac transplant with valvular disease or regurgitation
- Cyanotic congenital heart disease
- Prosthetic repair, implanted device, or shunt in congenital heart disease

Procedures
- Manipulation of gingival tissue or periapical tooth, or oral mucosa perforation in dental procedures
- Invasive respiratory tract procedures
- Surgery involving infected skin, skin structure, or musculoskeletal tissue

Prophylaxis is no longer indicated for mitral valve prolapse.

- Teach patients to avoid caffeine, OTC stimulants, and nutraceuticals to minimize events of palpitations in presence of mitral valve prolapse.
- Review s/s of complications and adverse effects of medication to report.

Patient Population Considerations

Women (conception/pregnancy/lactation)
- Evaluate CBC and ferritin, especially in women who experience hyperemesis that could contribute to high output murmurs.

Geriatric
- New-onset murmurs in older patients with comorbidities require careful clinical correlation.

Pediatric
- Venous hums are functional murmurs in children, heard continuously when the child is sitting. They should disappear when supine with light pressure to the jugular vein and do not require a cardiology referral.

Referring Patients

- Cardiology consult

HYPERLIPIDEMIA

Overview

- Hyperlipidemia is a disorder characterized by elevated cholesterol, TGs, LDL, and/or low circulating HDL.
- It can be primary or secondary to medications or disease.

Etiology

- Family history of premature CVHD, familial hypertriglyceridemia, familial combined hyperlipidemia, South Asian ancestry
- Tobacco use, alcohol use, marijuana use, obesity, sedentary lifestyle, pregnancy, and diets high in saturated fat, trans fat, and simple carbohydrates
- Pituitary, adrenal, thyroid, and pancreatic disorders, hyperuricemia, PCOS, SLE, RA, hemolytic uremic syndrome
- Medication-induced

Signs and Symptoms

- Asymptomatic
- Upper abdominal pain if pancreatitis is present
- Xanthomas, xanthelasma, corneal arcus in severe long-standing disease
- Presence of risk factors

Differential Diagnosis

- *ENDO*: Hypothyroidism, DM
- *GI*: Pancreatitis

 COMPLICATIONS

Acute: Atherosclerosis, pancreatitis

Chronic: Metabolic syndrome, fatty liver disease, HTN, type 2 diabetes

 CLINICAL PEARL

Lipid Screening
- Recommendation is a screening lipid profile for all adults age 20 years or older.
- AAP recommends screening school-age children and in late adolescence.
- Fasting or nonfasting on 2 separate days confirm positive results.

 ALERT

Metabolic Syndrome
1. Patients with **TG >150 mg/dL** and **HDL <40 to 50 mg/dL based on gender** should be evaluated for metabolic syndrome.
2. **African American women** and **Mexican Americans** are especially at risk.
3. Waist circumferences should be <40 inches in males, <35 inches in females.
4. FBG ≥100 mg/dL or on antidiabetic therapy.
5. BP ≥130/85 mmHg or on antihypertensive therapy.

Diagnosis when 3/5 criteria are present.

(continued)

Differential Diagnosis (*continued*)

- *GU*: Renal failure
- *Other*: Alcohol abuse, hormone replacement therapy

Diagnosis

Labs
- Lipid profile
- BMP, LFTs, Ca, Phos, LFTs, serum uric acid, C-reactive protein
- TSH, amylase, lipase, HbA1c

Additional Diagnostic Testing
- Coronary artery calcium test in a patient with no risk factors
- Genetic testing of LDLR, APOB, PCSK9 with risk for familial hypercholesterolemia
- *Additional standard testing based on associated disorders*: ASCVD, PAD, HTN, HF, stroke
- Calculate risk for ASCVD event

Treatment and Management

Treatment Goals
- Compliance with lifestyle modifications, diet, and medication to modify lipids
- Target lab results
  - Total cholesterol <200 mg/dL
  - *Patients with no risk factors*: TG <150 mg/dL or LDL <100 mg/dL
  - Patients with CVHD, DM, PAD, HF, *stroke*: LDL <70 mg/dL
  - Target HDL males >40 mg/dL, women >50 mg/dL

Drug Treatment
- Prescribe statins, ezetimibe, ACL inhibitors (targeted therapy for genetic disorders), bile acid sequestrants, niacin to *lower LDL*.
- Prescribe fibrates, statins, omega three fatty acids, ezetimibe, niacin to *lower triglycerides*.
- Prescribe niacin (will increase BG), statins, fibrates, bile acid sequestrants, ezetimibe to *raise HDL*.
- Prescribe evolocumab SC to patients to lower LDL in genetic hyperlipidemia.
- Consider low-dose aspirin in a patient with intermediate risk for a cardiac event.
- *To avoid rhabdomyolysis, do not combine fibrates and statins.*

Interventions
- Reassess effect and tolerance of medications at 12 weeks and periodic intervals after that.
- Monitor for risk of cardiovascular events and perform relevant diagnostic testing.
- Control BG and blood pressure and evaluate the need to add or discontinue aspirin at each visit.
- Evaluate for the presence of adverse medication effects, use of OTC medications, and nutraceuticals.

Patient Education
- Counsel patient on alcohol and tobacco cessation, exercise, and diet management.
- Instruct the patient to avoid herbal supplements and nutraceuticals.
- Review strategies to manage modifiable risk factors.
- Review s/s of complications and adverse effects of medication to report.

Patient Population Considerations

Women (conception/pregnancy/lactation)
- Dyslipidemia is associated with adverse outcomes for the mother and fetus during pregnancy. However, antilipemic therapy prescribed may be teratogenic. Provide preconception counseling for women at risk.

Geriatric

- Statins are prescribed for geriatric patients up to age 75 for primary prevention. Statins can be used at a lower intensity in patients aged >75 years. Patient should be monitored carefully for adverse effects.

Pediatric

- Perform routine lipid screening between ages 9 to 11 and 17 to 21 years. Consider earlier screening in patients with a family or personal history of risk factors.

Referring Patients

- Cardiology consult

HYPERTENSION

Overview

- HTN in a cardiovascular condition of sustained elevated BP obtained on separate visits and averaged (*adult*: two visits; *children*: three visits). It can be primary or secondary to another cause.

COMPLICATIONS

Acute: MI, stroke, AKI, aortic dissection, hypertensive urgency, hypertensive emergency

Chronic: Retinopathy, nephropathy, PAD

Etiology

Primary HTN

- Family history, African American ethnicity, age
- Tobacco use, excessive sodium intake, alcohol intake, sedentary lifestyle, obesity, stress
- Hyperlipidemia, DM, metabolic syndrome

CLINICAL PEARL

Staging of Hypertension

Prehypertension: *SBP*: 120–139 mmHg
DBP: 80–89 mmHg

Stage 1: *SBP*: 140–159 mmHg
DBP: 90–99 mmHg

Stage 2: *SBP*: > 160 mmHg
DBP: > 100 mmHg

Secondary HTN

- *CV*: Coarctation of the aorta, vasculitis
- *GU*: CKD, PKD, renal artery sclerosis
- *ENDO*: Primary aldosteronism, hyperthyroidism, hypercalcemia, hyperparathyroidism, pheochromocytoma, Cushing's syndrome, pituitary disorder
- *REPRO*: Pregnancy, eclampsia
- *Other*: Medications, nutraceuticals, stimulant use and abuse, sleep apnea, SLE, RA

Signs and Symptoms

- Asymptomatic with elevated blood pressure taken in both arms
- Evidence of target organ damage
  - *CNS*: TIA/stroke, encephalopathy, dementia
  - *Eyes*: Retinopathy (AV nicking, hemorrhages), papilledema
  - *CV*: ASCVD, CVHD, LVH, HF
  - *Abdomen*: Aortic aneurysm
  - *GU*: Nocturia, nephropathy
  - *Extremities*: PAD, decreased pulses, rubor, ischemic ulcers; bilateral edema in HF, unilateral edema in DVT/CVI

Differential Diagnosis

- *CV*: Coarctation of the aorta
- *GU*: CKD, PKD, renal artery sclerosis
- *ENDO*: Primary aldosteronism, hyperthyroidism, hypercalcemia, hyperparathyroidism, pheochromocytoma, Cushing's syndrome, pituitary disorder
- *REPRO*: Pregnancy, eclampsia
- *Other*: SLE, vasculitis, RA medications, nutraceuticals, stimulant use and abuse, sleep apnea

Diagnosis

Labs

- BMP, Ca, Phos, uric acid, CBC, LFT, HbA1c, lipid profile, BNP level, TSH
- U/A for microscopic albumin

Additional Diagnostic Testing

- Additional workup for secondary HTN based on history
  - 12-lead EKG
  - Ten-year risk calculation for a coronary event
  - Ambulatory BP monitoring and home BP monitoring (consider)
  - *CNS*: CT head, MRI, MRA brain, carotid Doppler
  - *Eyes*: Ophthalmic exam
- *CV*: Chest x-ray, echocardiogram, CT angiography
- *Abdomen*: Abdominal ultrasound, abdominal CT
- *GU*: UA for microscopic albumin, stage CKD with estimated GFR
- *Extremities*: Ankle-brachial index, angiography

Treatment and Management

Treatment Goals

- Target SBP <130 to 140 and DBP <90 in most adults especially with CVHD, HF, CKD <80 years.
- Mitigate/minimize the risk of complications of target organ damage, engage patient compliance in risk factor modification and lipid management.

Drug Treatment

- One or two antihypertensives in combination according to compelling indications to reduce complications and reevaluate in 8 to 12 weeks
- Statin therapy for LDL ≥70 mg/dL with 10-year risk ≥10%
- Low-dose aspirin 81 PO daily based on CVHD, thrombotic stroke, and PAD risk factors, and for patients who are high risk for preeclampsia at 12 to 28 weeks' gestation

Interventions

- Evaluate for target organ damage every 3 to 6 months in low-risk patients and refer for an annual ophthalmology exam.
- In a patient whose 10-year risk ≥10%, reevaluate in a month.
- Initiate counseling for alcohol use and tobacco cessation, DASH diet, exercise recommendations, glycemic control, nephroprotection, and stimulant avoidance.

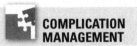

COMPLICATION MANAGEMENT

Recommended Medication to Minimize Complications

Pregnancy: Labetalol and nifedipine
Avoid ACEIs, ARBs, and renin inhibitors.

Black: Thiazide diuretics, CCBs, or combination

Older women: Thiazide or loop diuretics, ACEIs, CCBs
Avoid alpha-1 blockers and central acting agents.

HF: ACEIs, ARBs, beta blockers, diuretics, spironolactone (note risk for hyperkalemia with ACEIs or ARBs)
Avoid CCB.

TIA/Stroke: Thiazide diuretics, ACEIs or ARBs, or combination; target SBP <140

DM: ACEIs, ARBs, CCBs, diuretics
Note diuretics and CCBs raise BG.

CKD: ACEIs, ARBs

CVHD: ACEIs, ARBs, beta blockers
Avoid potassium depleting diuretics in patients with arrythmia. Avoid CCBs in patients with MI.

ALERT

Hypertensive urgency: BP >180/120 with elevated blood pressure with no signs of target organ damage

Malignant hypertension: BP >180/120 with papilledema and retinal hemorrhages

Hypertensive emergency: BP >180/120 with symptoms of target organ damage, dyspnea, chest pain, blurred vision, pulsating abdomen, acute limb ischemia, or focal CNS deficit

Patient Education
- Explain the importance of alcohol and tobacco cessation and diet management.
- Review the impact of lifestyle modifications on BP control.
- Inform patients of the risk associated with stimulant use, especially caffeine.
- Explain s/s of complications and adverse effects of medications to report.

Patient Population Considerations

Women (conception/pregnancy/lactation)
- Perform yearly assessment of BP, lipids, BG, BMI in patients with a history of preeclampsia with preterm delivery or recurrent preeclampsia.

Geriatric
- Consider target lower BP target <130/80 with high-risk comorbidities and risk for coronary events in patients age 65 or older.
- Weigh the risk of orthostatic hypotension, adverse effects, and falls against polypharmacology.

Pediatric
- Begin BP screening at 3 years of age.

Referring Patients

- Cardiology consult
- Ophthalmology consult

POP QUIZ 5.2

A 78-year-old female with a history of HTN and type 2 DM presents to the primary care provider for routine evaluation of hypertension. The patient has been prescribed metformin, HCTZ, and diltiazem. BP averages 108/64 mmHg. Heart rate is 82. The patient denies any syncope but reports increased urination and incontinence. Which lab/diagnostics should the nurse practitioner prioritize and why?

MYOCARDIAL INFARCTION

Overview

- Ischemia occurs when an unstable plaque in coronary arteries is injured and ruptures. Thrombus formation is triggered, which occludes the vessel. MI is necrosis to myocardial tissue distal to the occlusion in the presence of persisting ischemia.

Etiology

- Tobacco use, obesity, substance abuse, psychological stress, sedentary lifestyle
- Male gender, advancing age, family history of premature CVHD
- *Ethnicity*: African American, Mexican American, Pacific Islander, Asian American, Native American
- Personal history of DM, CKD, HTN, hyperlipidemia, angina, previous MI, valve disease, HF, cardiomyopathy, obesity, PAD, stroke, vasospasm, immune-mediated vasculitis, hyperthyroidism, infections

Signs and Symptoms

- Substernal or epigastric chest discomfort that may radiate to the jaw and arm described as constant and persists for 30 to 60 min
- Associated with dyspnea, anxiety, syncope, nausea, indigestion, diaphoresis, and activity intolerance

COMPLICATIONS

Acute: Acute pain, arrythmia, HF/shock, DVT/PE, pericarditis, infarct extension, activity intolerance, premature death

Chronic: Ventricular remodeling/refractory HF, recurrent MI, recurrent arrhythmia, depression, disability, stroke, DVT/PE

CLINICAL PEARL

African American patients have a higher mortality rate than White patients. Females, older adults, and patients with DM and HF may have more atypical presentation: nausea, shortness of breath, vague chest discomfort, and indigestion during coronary events.

A high index of suspicion must be maintained with these symptoms in the presence of risk factors.

Differential Diagnosis

- *CV*: Aortic dissection, pericarditis, HF/cardiogenic shock
- *GI*: Abdominal compartment syndrome, GERD, esophagitis, PUD, biliary disease, cholelithiasis, pancreatitis
- *NEURO*: Herpes zoster, anxiety disorders
- *PULM*: Asthma, COPD, pneumothorax, pulmonary embolism, pneumonia

Diagnosis

Labs
- Elevation in serial troponin enzymes, CKMB, myoglobin
  - First set of enzymes collected that are negative do not exclude infarction
- BNP level indicates comorbid CHF
- CBC to evaluate for contributing factors
- CMP with LFTs to evaluate hepatorenal function and possible organ ischemia
- CBG elevated in DM
- PT/PTT/INR and fibrinogen for baseline
- Lipid profile, HbA1c should be collected

Additional Diagnostic Testing
- 12-lead EKG with chest pain (Figure 5.6)
  - ST elevation in two contiguous leads indicates an acute injury.
  - ST depression indicates ischemia.
  - Q waves indicate infarction, age undetermined.
  - A normal EKG does not exclude MI.
- Chest x-ray to evaluate for pulmonary edema
- Echocardiogram in the presence of heart murmur or friction rub and if pulmonary edema is present on x-ray
- Percutaneous coronary angiography in acute MI that meets EKG criteria
- Exercise stress testing as a follow-up in low-risk patients with no EKG changes and negative cardiac enzymes
- Myocardial perfusion imaging, pharmacological stress testing, and stress echocardiography ordered in the absence of acute MI
  - The purpose of testing is to evaluate for the presence of ischemia in response to stress in a controlled environment. *The presence of chest discomfort at rest precludes the need for stress testing.*

Treatment and Management

- Patients with symptoms of MI require immediate referral to the ED.

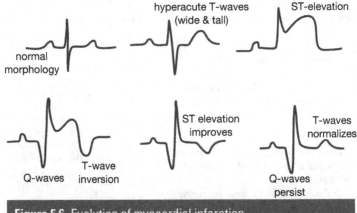

Figure 5.6 Evolution of myocardial infarction.

Source: Courtesy of Oldblueday.

Treatment Goals

- Absence of chest discomfort, restoration of tissue perfusion through revascularization, mitigation of arrhythmias, and medications to reduce myocardial oxygen demand and improve years and quality of life
- Prevention of acute and chronic complications
  - Target LDL <70 to 100; SBP >90 to 100 mmHg; HR 50 to 75; no arrhythmias; no weight gain, peripheral edema, or nocturia; no activity intolerance; HbA1c <7% if patient has diabetes

Drug Treatment

- Outpatient
  - Evaluate the effectiveness of aspirin, antiplatelet, ACEIs or ARBs, beta blockers, statins.
  - Adjust antidiabetic therapy to maintain HbA1c <7%.
  - Update vaccinations to prevent respiratory infections.

Interventions

- Assess for the presence of ischemic complications and HF.
- Evaluate understanding of cardiac diet, lipid management, and activity.
- Order periodic bloodwork to evaluate hepatic function, CBC, and electrolytes.

Patient Education

- Review strategies to manage modifiable risk factors for stroke and PAD.
- Discuss concerns about sexual function and activity post-MI.
- Explain bleeding precautions, fall prevention, infection protection, and sublingual nitroglycerin use.
- Review s/s of complications and adverse effects of medication to report.

Patient Population Considerations

Women (conception/pregnancy/lactation)

- CVHD is the third-leading cause of death in women. Discuss risk factors, primary and secondary prevention in female patients to prevent disease.

Geriatric

- Review safety and fall risk with patients on aspirin, antiplatelets, beta blockers, ACEIs, or ARBs.

Pediatric

- Marfan syndrome, Kawasaki disease, and Takayasu arteritis are seen in pediatric coronary artery disease.

Referring Patients

- Cardiology consult
- Cardiac rehabilitation referral

PERIPHERAL ARTERIAL DISEASE

Overview

- PAD is a chronic vascular disorder of progressive atherosclerosis that narrows the lumen of peripheral arteries over time, causing ischemia. Plaque rupture can cause acute symptoms that can result in the need for amputation.
- Without intervention, critical limb ischemia can occur over time due to chronic injury to peripheral arteries. The disease causes chronically decreased perfusion, resulting in ischemic ulcers and limb amputation.

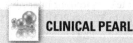

CLINICAL PEARL

PAD Stages
- *Stage I*: No limitation of physical activity
- *Stage IIa*: Mild claudication
- *Stage IIb*: Moderate to severe claudication
- *Stage III*: Symptoms occur even at rest
- *Stage IV*: Ulceration or gangrene

Etiology

- Tobacco use, obesity, stimulants, substance abuse, psychological stress, sedentary lifestyle
- Male gender, advancing age, family history of premature CVHD, stroke, ethnicity
- Personal history of DM, CKD, HTN, hyperlipidemia, CVHD, obesity, stroke, immune-mediated vasculitis, APLA syndrome
- Musculoskeletal or vascular trauma

Signs and Symptoms

- Asymptomatic, developing ischemic pain, and paresthesia
- Muscle atrophy, thickened nails, loss of hair, paresthesia, cooler temperature, dependent rubor, delayed capillary refill, dry, nonhealing ulceration
- Presence of new-onset six P signs is a medical emergency.

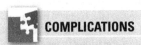

COMPLICATIONS

Acute: Acute arterial thrombosis, aortic aneurysm

Chronic: Advanced stage HF, ESRD, cirrhosis

Differential Diagnosis

- *MSK*: Osteoarthritis, chronic compartment syndrome, lumbar radiculopathy
- *NEURO*: Neuropathy
- *CV*: Venous disease, popliteal entrapment syndrome, DVT, chronic venous insufficiency, thromboangiitis obliterans

Diagnosis

Labs

- BMP, LFTs, Ca, Mg, to evaluate electrolyte and hepatorenal function
- CBC
- lipid profile, HbA1c
- PTT, PT/INR for baseline

Additional Diagnostic Testing

- 12-lead EKG
- Peripheral transluminal angiography, CT angiography, MRA, and duplex ultrasonography for PAD
- Ankle-brachial index <0.9 indicates PAD

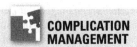

COMPLICATION MANAGEMENT

Acute Arterial Occlusion

In the presence of abrupt onset of new six P assessment; pain, pallor, pulselessness, poikilothermia, paresthesia, and paralysis:

- Keep leg neutral.
- Protect from injury.
- Obtain surgical consult to get emergency intervention within 6 hr.

Treatment and Management

Treatment Goals

- No report of six P's, no extremity injury, skin intact, increasing tolerance of physical activity

Drug Treatment

- *PAD*: No acute symptoms or intermittent claudication
  - Aspirin 81 to 325 mg PO daily
  - Clopidogrel 75 mg PO daily
  - Statins and antihypertensive therapy
- Intermittent claudication
  - Add pentoxifylline 400 mg PO every 8 hr
  - Consider cilostazol in place of clopidogrel
- *Order immunization updates*: Influenza, pneumonia for all stages

Interventions

- Assess BP and heart rate, ankle-brachial index, stage PAD, and evaluate eGFR.
- Assess the patient's dietary fat intake, sodium intake, tobacco use.
- Order BMP, CBC, LFTs to evaluate for rising azotemia, hepatic dysfunction, and electrolyte balance.
- Evaluate for the presence of adverse medication effects and use of OTC medications and nutraceuticals.

Patient Education

- Counsel patient on alcohol and tobacco cessation, proper diet and BP.
- Review BG if diabetes is present.
- Review strategies to manage modifiable risk factors for PAD.
- Explain foot care to prevent injuries, nail care, and the importance of an annual exam by podiatry.
- Answer questions regarding bleeding precautions, falls prevention, and infection protection.
- Review s/s of complications and adverse effects of medication to report.

Patient Population Considerations

Women (conception/pregnancy/lactation)

- APLA syndrome is a frequent cause of fetal loss. It manifests with nontraumatic thrombosis or thromboembolism (venous or arterial) in women of childbearing age. Provide preconception counseling to avoid adverse maternal and fetal outcomes.

Geriatric

- Exercise programs, cilostazol, and statins improve exercise time in patients with intermittent claudication and should be employed in the older adult population to enhance the quality of life.

Pediatric

- PAD is not commonly reported in pediatric patients. APLA syndrome manifests more frequently as DVT.

Referring Patients

- Cardiology consult
- Vascular surgery consult

? POP QUIZ 5.3

A 55-year-old female presents to the ambulatory care complaining of upper back pain, nausea associated with dizziness, and malaise that started suddenly this morning. She has a history of HTN, chronic lower back pain, and familial hyperlipidemia. She reports tobacco use one pack per day for 30 years, drinks one alcoholic beverage daily, and denies illicit drug use. Father died of MI at age 74. Medications at home are olmesartan 20 mg daily, NSAID for back pain PRN, and simvastatin 40 mg PO daily. BP 110/70, HR 59, RR, 22, T 97.1°F (36.2°C), HT 5'6", WT 170 lb. Which lab or diagnostic test should the nurse practitioner prioritize?

RESOURCES

Agency for Healthcare Research and Quality. (n.d.). *Preventing hospital-associated venous thromboembolism.* https://www.ahrq.gov/patient-safety/resources/vtguide/guide4.html

Alexander, M. (2020). *Hypertension.* https://emedicine.medscape.com/article/241381-overview

American College of Cardiology. (2019). *AHA/ACC/HRS focused update of the 2014 guideline for management of patients with atrial fibrillation.* https://wwwaccorg/~/media/Non-Clinical-Files-PDFs-Excel-MS-Word-etc/Guidelines/2019/2019-Afib-Guidelines-Made-Simple-Toolpdf

American Heart Association. (2020). *ACLS cardiac arrest algorithm for suspected or confirmed covid-19 patients.* https://cprheartorg/-/media/cpr-files/resources/covid-19-resources-for-cpr-training/english/algorithmacls_cacovid_200406pdf?la=en&hash=C8D69AA2B4226798CA5D293CC5A36A5D57697D1C

Berg, T. (2020). *Medscape: Abdominal aortic aneurysm.* https://emedicine.medscape.com/article/261691-overview

Beyerbach, D. (2019). *Medscape: Pacemakers and implantable cardioverter-defibrillators.* https://emedicinemedscape com/article/162245-overview#a6

Cash, J. C., & Glass, C. A. (Eds.). (2019). *Adult-gerontology practice guidelines* (2nd ed.). Springer Publishing Company.

Codina Leik, M. T. (2018). *Family nurse practitioner certification intensive review: Fast facts and practice questions* (3rd ed.). Springer Publishing Company.

Compton, S. J. (2017). *Ventricular tachycardia.* https://emedicine.medscape.com/article/159075-overview

Dominguez, J. A. (2019). *Peripheral arterial occlusive disease.* https://emedicine.medscape.com/article/460178-overview.

Gewtiz, M. (2016). *Medscape: Pediatric bacterial endocarditis.* https://emedicinemedscapecom/article/896540-overview#a2

Green, J. M., & Chiaramida, A. J. (2015). *12-lead EKG confidence.* Springer Publishing Company.

Gugneja, M. (2017). *Medscape: Paroxysmal supraventricular tachycardia.* https://emedicinemedscapecom/article/156670-treatment#showall

Guler, G. B., Can, M. M., Guler E., Akinci, T., Sogukpinar, O., Hatipoglu, S., Killicaslan, F., & Serebruarny, V. L. (2016). Asymptomatic pulmonary embolism after ablation. *Cardiology, 134*(4), 426–432. https://doi.org/10.1159/000444440

Henneman, A., Guirguis, E., Grace, Y., Patel, D., & Shah, B. (2016). Emerging therapies for the management of chronic hyperkalemia in the ambulatory care setting. *American Journal of Health-System Pharmacy, 73*(2), 33–44. https://doi.org/10.2146/ajhp150457

Hopkins, C. (2018). *Medscape: Hypertensive emergencies.* https://emedicinemedscapecom/article/1952052-overview

Hughes, M. J., Stein, P. D., & Matta, F. (2014). Silent pulmonary embolism in patients with distal deep venous thrombosis: Systematic review. *Thrombosis Research, 134*(6), 1182–1185. https://doi.org/10.1016/j.thromres.2014.09.036

Knechtel, M. A. (2021). *EKGs for the nurse practitioner and physician assistant* (3rd ed.). Springer Publishing Company.

Krausei R. (2019). *Medscape: Cardiac tests.* https://emedicinemedscapecom/article/811577-overview#a1

Lauer, B. R., Nelson, R. A., Adamski, J. H., Janko, M. R., Ravi, G., & Barcelona, R. A. (2019). Protamine sulfate for the reversal of enoxaparin associated hemorrhage beyond 12 h. *The American Journal of Emergency Medicine, 37*(1), e174–e175. https://doi.org/10.1016/j.ajem.2018.09.043

Mangla, A. (2014). *Medscape: Heart sounds.* https://emedicinemedscapecom/article/1894036-overview

McConnell, M. E., & Adkins, S. B. (1999). Heart murmurs in pediatric patients: When do you refer? *American Family Physician, 60*(2), 558–564.

Nguyen, V. (2020). *Medscape: Endocarditis prophylaxis.* https://emedicinemedscapecom/article/2172262-overview

National Institutes of Health. (2020). *DailyMed: Sodium zirconium cyclosilicate powder.* https://dailymednlmnihgov/dailymed/drugInfocfm?setid=90bf8e28-748d-4e4b-a19f-9cf483370eff

Patel, K. (2019). *Medscape: Deep vein thrombosis.* https://emedicinemedscapecom/article/1911303-overview

Quellette, D. (2019). *Medscape: Pulmonary embolism.* https://emedicinemedscapecom/article/300901-overview

Rahimi, S. (2019). *Medscape: Abdominal aortic aneurysm.* https://emedicine.medscape.com/article/1979501-overview.

Roberts, D. (2020). *Mastering the 12-Lead EKG* (2nd ed.). Springer Publishing Company.

Satou, G. (2019). *Medscape: Pediatric heart failure.* https://emedicinemedscapecom/article/2069746-overview

Schünemann, H., Cushman, M., Burnett, A., Kahn, S., Beyer-Westendorf, J., Spencer, F. Rezende, S. M., Zakai, N. A., Bauer, K. A., Dentali, F., Lansing, J., Balduzzi, S., Darzi, A., Morgano, G. P., Neumann, I., Nieuwlaat, R., Yepes-Nuñez, J. J., Zhang, Y., & Wiercioch, W. (2018). American Society of Hematology 2018 guidelines for management of venous thromboembolism: Prophylaxis for hospitalized and nonhospitalized medical patients. *Blood Advances, 2*, 3198–3225. https://doi.org/10.1182/bloodadvances.2018022954

Sorenson, M., Quinn, L., & Klein, D. (2019). *Pathophysiology: Concepts of human disease* (1st ed.). Pearson Education.

Sweeney, M. E. (2019). *Medscape: Hypertriglyceridemia.* https://emedicinemedscapecom/article/126568-overview

USPFTF. (2019). *Final recommendation statement: Abdominal aortic aneurysm: Screening.* https://www.uspreventiveservicestaskforce.org/uspstf/recommendation/abdominal-aortic-aneurysm-screening.

Wang, S. (2020). *Medscape: Metabolic syndrome.* https://emedicinemedscapecom/article/165124-overview

Yang, E. (2018). *Medscape: Lipid management guidelines.* https://emedicinemedscapecom/article/2500032-overview

Zafari, M. (2019). *Medscape: Myocardial infarction.* https://emedicinemedscapecom/article/155919-overview

RESPIRATORY SYSTEM

ACUTE BRONCHITIS

Overview

- Acute bronchitis is a lower respiratory disorder characterized by inflammation and excess mucous production of the tracheobronchial tree. The inflammation inhibits ciliary action, causing stasis of secretions, which impedes air conduction.
- Bronchial irritation can trigger bronchospasm. Repeated exposure to irritants, such as tobacco, can lead to chronic bronchitis.

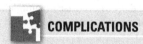

COMPLICATIONS

Acute: Bronchitis, bronchopneumonia, status asthmaticus

Chronic: COPD

Etiology

- Allergens, irritants, aspiration
- Dysphagia, GERD
- *Viral infection*: Adenovirus, influenza, parainfluenza, RSV
- *Bacterial infections*: Bordetella pertussis, Corynebacterium diphtheriae, Mycobacterium tuberculosis, Mycoplasma pneumoniae

Signs and Symptoms

- Anorexia, fever, malaise, nasal congestion, nausea, pleuritic chest discomfort, productive cough, sore throat, tachypnea
- Adenopathy, conjunctivitis, rhinorrhea
- Use of accessory muscles and tachypnea with activity
- Rhonchi and wheezing on auscultation

Differential Diagnosis

- *GI*: GERD, hiatal hernia
- *HEENT*: Acute sinusitis, pharyngitis, upper respiratory infection
- *PULM*: Alpha1-antitrypsin deficiency, asthma, bronchiectasis, bronchiolitis, COPD, cystic fibrosis, pneumonia
- *Other*: Group A streptococcal infection, influenza

Diagnosis

ALERT

AMS, cyanosis, peak flow <50%, pulse oximetry <90% or 88% in patients with COPD requires immediate referral to the ED.

Labs

- Diagnosis made by physical examination
- Sputum c/s in persistent cough

Additional Diagnostic Testing

- Pulse oximetry to identify hypoxia
- Peak flow to identify airflow limitation

(continued)

Additional Diagnostic Testing (continued)
- Chest x-ray to rule out pneumonia
- PFTs with asthma/COPD

Treatment and Management

Treatment Goals
- Manage pain and cough, promote ventilation and gas exchange, treat infection, if indicated, and prevent complications.

Drug Treatment
- Prescribe inhaled SABA bronchodilator one to two puffs every 4 hr PRN for wheezing.
- Consider inhaled corticosteroids or oral prednisone 6 to 20 mg daily to decrease inflammation.
- Offer guaifenesin to manage cough and thin secretions.
- Prescribe acetaminophen or NSAIDs for the pain to promote adherence to pulmonary hygiene.
- Update vaccinations to prevent respiratory infections.

CLINICAL PEARL

Antibiotic Recommendations

Consider antibiotics for patients >65 years with multiple chronic conditions (COPD, DM, HF):

Amoxicillin with clavulanic acid, doxycycline, levofloxacin, or trimethoprim/sulfamethoxazole

Interventions
- Evaluate hydration and encourage thin liquids.
- Monitor response to therapy and reevaluate in 3 to 5 days.
- Encourage cough and deep breathing and energy conservation strategies.

Patient Education
- Promote tobacco and alcohol cessation and review GERD instruction if indicated.
- Discuss pulmonary hygiene to promote recovery.
- Review s/s of complications and adverse medication effects to report.

Patient Population Considerations

Women (conception/pregnancy/lactation)
- Update vaccinations for diphtheria, pertussis, and influenza in women of childbearing age to reduce the incidence of respiratory infection during pregnancy.

Geriatric
- Provide vaccinations for all respiratory infections and encourage handwashing, avoiding crowds, and distancing from people who are ill.

Pediatric
- Children with pediatric bronchitis can return to school if they are afebrile, and signs of infection have decreased. A cough may persist for 10 days to 3 weeks.

Referring Patients

- Pulmonology consult
- Gastroenterology consult
- Infectious disease consult

POP QUIZ 6.1

A 79-year-old male with a history of DM type 2 and atrial fibrillation presents to the primary care providers office with complaints of a cough and low-grade fever. As the nurse practitioner applies the pulse oximeter, she notices the nail bed of the digit is spongy with a loss of nail curvature. What is the significance of this finding and what diagnoses should be considered?

ASTHMA AND CHRONIC OBSTRUCTIVE PULMONARY DISEASE

Overview

- Asthma, emphysema, and chronic bronchitis are respiratory disorders of airflow limitation.
- Asthma manifests in childhood in response to allergens or irritants that trigger a cascade of acute and chronic inflammation. Acute inflammation, combined with reversible bronchoconstriction, reduce airflow. Chronic airway remodeling results from continued exposure to irritants and poor management. Evidence-based treatment halts progression.
- COPD is a chronic progressive respiratory disorder. Emphysema and chronic bronchitis are two subtypes of COPD that can present alone or are mixed.
  - Emphysema occurs when there are permanent distention and damage to alveoli from chronic exposure to irritants or insufficient alpha1-antitrypsin activity.
  - Chronic bronchitis occurs when bronchiole thickening and mucous gland hypertrophy narrows the airway.
  - In each instance, chronic complications occur when risk factors that can worsen gas exchange and airflow persist. In some cases, advanced COPD can lead to chronic hypercapnia, resulting in fully compensated respiratory acidosis with hypoxemia and secondary polycythemia.
- Tobacco cessation is the first step in each of these disorders to control progression and severity.
- Asthma-COPD overlap syndrome can occur in patients with asthma who smoke tobacco and is diagnosed when features of all disorders are present.

Etiology

- Asthma
  - Family history, immune excess, allergies, obesity
  - Exposure to allergens, animal dander, exercise, infections, irritants, medications (aspirin, ACEIs, beta blockers, and NSAIDs), mold, occupational irritants, pests, pollen, stomach aspirate in GERD, strong odors, temperature change, tobacco use
- COPD
  - Increasing age, recurrent respiratory infections beginning in childhood, or poorly controlled asthma
  - Alpha-1-antitrypsin deficiency
  - Tobacco smoking or exposure to second-hand smoke
  - Occupation exposure to dust, chemicals, pollution

Signs and Symptoms

- Asthma
  - Episodic shortness of breath, cough, chest tightness, and wheeze due to tracheobronchial constriction and worsening inflammation in response to a trigger (see etiology)
  - Increased use of accessory muscles

 COMPLICATIONS

Acute: Exacerbation of asthma/COPD, arrhythmia, respiratory failure

Chronic: ACOS, advanced COPD, atrial fibrillation, right-sided HF, respiratory infections, protein calorie malnutrition

 ALERT

Work-related asthma is highest in ages 45 to 64 years and account for 15.7% of asthma cases.

CLINICAL PEARL

Classification Criteria for Asthma

Age: ≥12 years

- **Step 1: Mild**—PEFR >80% predicted with SABA use ≤2/week, nighttime symptoms ≤2/month; 20% variability day to day
- **Step 2: Mild persistent**—PEFR >80% predicted with SABA use >2 days/week but not daily, nighttime symptoms 3 to 4 per month; 20% to 30% variability day to day
- **Step 3: Moderate**—PEFR = 60% to 80% predicted; SABA use daily, nighttime symptoms >1 time per week but not daily; 30% variability day to day
- **Step 4: Severe**—<60% predicted; SABA use throughout the day <2/week, nighttime symptoms often daily; 30% variability day to day

(continued)

Signs and Symptoms (*continued*)

- Wheeze on auscultation
- A silent chest does not exclude asthma; all that wheezes is not asthma
- COPD
  - Reports chronic productive cough, wheezing, dyspnea on exertion progressing to dyspnea at rest, activity intolerance, hypoxemia
  - Headache from hypercapnia, sleep disturbance, and protein-calorie malnutrition with advanced disease
  - AP diameter increased, hyperresonance to percussion, decreased chest excursion
  - Distant breath sounds with rhonchi and wheezing present; increased use of accessory muscle
  - S1, S2 distant, irregular rhythm, increased JVD, central cyanosis
  - Ascites may be present
  - Extremity edema and clubbing

 CLINICAL PEARL

Staging Criteria for COPD
- *Stage 1*: Mild FEV$_1$ >80% of predicted value
- *Stage 2*: Moderate FEV$_1$ = 50% to 80% of predicted value
- *Stage 3*: Severe FEV$_1$ = 30% to 50% of predicted value
- *Stage 4*: Very severe FEV$_1$ ≤30% to 50% of predicted value with hypoxia

Differential Diagnosis

- *CV*: Cardiac mass, cardiomyopathy, CHF, pulmonary embolism
- *GI*: GERD
- *HEENT*: Sinus disease
- *HEM*: Hodgkin's lymphoma
- *PULM*: Acute bronchitis, bronchiectasis, bronchiolitis, chronic cough, foreign body aspiration, lung cancer, pulmonary fibrosis, pulmonary migraine, TB
- *Other*: Sarcoidosis

 ALERT

AMS, cyanosis, peak flow <50%, pulse oximetry <90% or 88% in CO_2-retaining COPD requires SABA, oxygen, and immediate referral to the ED.

Diagnosis

Labs
- *CBC*:
  - Eosinophilia in allergen-triggered exacerbations
  - Polycythemia in advanced COPD
- *BMP*:
  - Hyperglycemia with oral steroids
  - Hypokalemia, hypocalcemia, and hypomagnesemia with SABA and LABA use
  - Bicarbonate elevated in CO_2-retaining COPD
- AAT testing in COPD presenting in age <40 years
- BNP level to distinguish CHF from COPD exacerbation
- Sputum c/s in persistent cough
- Arterial blood gases are performed in emergent situations
  - CO_2-retaining COPD patient is in fully compensated respiratory acidosis with hypoxemia

 CLINICAL PEARL

Acid–Base Disturbance in Acute Respiratory Distress
- *Asthma/non-CO_2 retaining COPD*: Respiratory alkalosis with PaO$_2$ <60 to 75 progressing to respiratory acidosis without intervention
- *CO_2-retaining COPD*: Partially compensated respiratory acidosis with PAO$_2$ <60 to 75 from fully compensated respiratory acidosis

Additional Diagnostic Testing

- PFTs for staging and managing asthma/COPD (gold standard)
- PEFR to identify airflow limitation
  - PEFR is the gold standard for measuring airflow limitation at POC
- Pulse oximetry to identify hypoxia
  - A normal pulse oximetry reading in asthma should not be interpreted as stable; must be compared to PEFR
  - Ambulatory pulse oximetry in advanced disease to prescribe home oxygen therapy
- Chest x-ray and chest CT
- Allergy testing to identify triggers
- 12-lead EKG may reveal atrial fibrillation and right-sided chamber enlargement in advanced disease
- Echocardiogram to identify right-sided HF in progressive disease

Treatment and Management

Treatment Goals

- Improve airflow limitation, control triggers, maximize gas exchange, and prevent complications.

Drug Treatment

- Asthma/COPD individualized action plans include symptomatic and maintenance plans
- Symptomatic therapy
- SABA prn PEFR <80% PV for symptoms
  - Low-dose budesonide–formoterol or low-dose ICS with SABA for patients with symptoms in step 1 asthma
- Consider adding SAMA to SABA for COPD or ACOS
- Consider short-term oral corticosteroids during exacerbations.

ALERT

Black Box Warning for Leukotriene Receptor Antagonists
- Increased risk of suicidality for adults and adolescents
- Behavior problems and nightmares in children

ASTHMA MAINTENANCE THERAPY

- Do not treat asthma in adults and adolescents with SABA alone. Prescribe according to step based on the frequency of symptoms.
  - *Step 1*: Symptoms <2×/month: Prescribe low-dose ICS whenever SABA is taken or low-dose budesonide–formoterol.
  - *Step 2*: Prescribe low-dose ICS whenever SABA is taken or low-dose budesonide–formoterol in addition to LTRA maintenance therapy.
  - *Step 3*: Prescribe daily low-dose ICS/LABA, medium-dose ICS, or low-dose ICS plus LTRA.
  - *Step 4*: Prescribe daily medium-dose ICS/LABA; add-on LAMA or LTRA.
  - *Step 5*: Prescribe daily high-dose ICS/LABA, add-on a low-dose ICS and refer for MAB.
- Consider nonsedating antihistamine; mast cell stabilizers for allergy-induced asthma/COPD.

CLINICAL PEARL

Add ICS to LAMA and/or LABA with ACOS or COPD exacerbations and hospitalizations.

COPD MAINTENANCE THERAPY

- Combination ICS, LAMA, LABA according to patient needs using monotherapy, dual, or triple therapy. LAMA has a more significant effect than LABA.
- Consider mucolytics and antioxidants such as *N*-acetylcysteine daily.
- Prescribe statins for COPD patients that meet criteria to improve outcomes.
- Alpha1-antitrypsin therapy can be considered for select patients.

(continued)

COPD MAINTENANCE THERAPY (*CONTINUED*)

- Collaborate with pulmonologist on phosphodiesterase inhibitors and long-term azithromycin in select cases.
  - Maintain theophylline level at 8 to 13 mcg/mL.
- Use home oxygen therapy for activity-induced hypoxemia.
- Update immunizations to reduce infections.

Interventions
- Instruct patient to monitor day-to-day variations in asthma/COPD journal and periodic PFTs and evaluate during follow-up visits.
- Evaluate the patient's understanding of medications, inhalers, and action plans.
- Provide nutritional referral for asthma (weight loss with obesity)/COPD (weigh gain in advanced disease).
- Refer patients to pulmonary rehabilitation after hospitalization.

Patient Education
- Instruct patient in tobacco cessation and irritant/allergen avoidance.
- Review individualized action plan.
- Discuss s/s of complications and adverse medications effects to report.

Patient Population Considerations

Women (conception/pregnancy/lactation)
- Most asthma medications are safe to use during pregnancy.

Geriatric
- Assess the inhaler technique regularly, especially if mild cognitive impairment develops. Discuss end-of-life planning and preferences for mechanical ventilation.

Pediatric
- Do not prescribe SABA-only treatment to children. Prescribe low-dose ICS with SABA for rescue in children ages 6 to 11 years old. Mepolizumab can be considered in children age ≥6 years old.

Referring Patients

- Pulmonology consult
- Allergy/immunology consult
- Cardiology consult
- Thoracic surgery consult

COMMUNITY-ACQUIRED BACTERIAL PNEUMONIA

Overview

- CAP is an infection of the lung parenchyma. Microbial invasion causes an inflammatory response in the alveoli that impairs gas exchange and can infiltrate bronchioles and pleura. Inflamed bronchioles produce excess mucous and become hyperresponsive. It can extend into the adjacent pleura causing painful irritation and effusion.
- Exclude all characteristics of hospital-acquired pneumonia to apply this diagnosis.

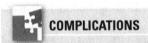

COMPLICATIONS

Acute: Bronchospasm, respiratory failure, sepsis, pleural effusion, pleurisy

Etiology

- *Exposure to bacteria*: Streptococcus pneumoniae, Haemophilus influenza, Moraxella Catarrhalis, Escherichia coli, Klebsiella (chronic alcoholism), and Staphylococcus (influenza); Pseudomonas aeruginosa in cystic fibrosis
- Alcohol use, tobacco use, obesity, recent travel, pollution, poor hand hygiene, substance abuse, tobacco, advancing age, residential facilities/crowded living conditions
- *Disease*: Alcoholism, aspiration, asthma, cancer, COPD, CVHD, cystic fibrosis, dementia, DM, GERD, HF, hiatal hernia, HIV, immunodeficiency neurodegenerative disorders, stroke

CLINICAL PEARL

Patients at risk for aspiration may have multiple bacteria. Screen patients for:

Aspiration: Alcoholism, drug intoxication, GERD, hiatal hernia, impaired consciousness, instrumentation, neurologic disorders

Dysphagia: Achalasia, advancing age, cleft palate, esophageal strictures, foreign bodies, hyposalivation, impaired dentition, neurologic disorders, radiation therapy, tumors/masses

Signs and Symptoms

- Dyspnea, cough, fever, malaise, pleuritic chest discomfort
- Nasal flaring, grunting, retractions in infants and children
- AMS or irritability may be present
- Tachypnea and use of accessory muscles
- Increased tactile fremitus
- Dullness to percussion
- Rales, crackles, wheeze on auscultation
- Egophony, whispered pectoriloquy, and bronchophony present
- Hypoactive bowel sounds
- Skin moist and warm; may be cyanotic, pale, or flushed

Differential Diagnosis

- *CV*: CHF, myocardial ischemia, myocarditis, pulmonary embolism
- *PULM*: Asthma, bronchitis, COPD, foreign body aspiration, alternative types of pneumonia (fungal, hospital-acquired, opportunistic, viral), lung cancer, pneumonitis, pertussis, TB

Diagnosis

Labs

- BMP to evaluate for hyperglycemia and rising azotemia and estimate GFR
- CBC with differential to assess for leukopenia, leukocytosis, bands, shift to the left
- Blood cultures to identify organisms
- Sputum c/s with gram stain
  - Do not wait for results to treat infections.
- *Infections*: HIV antibody test, QuantiFERON gold, legionella
- Determine treatment setting (outpatient or inpatient)—use CAP CDS alert or the pneumonia severity index tools

CLINICAL PEARL

Infections increased the risk for hyperglycemic emergencies. Obtain stat CBG in the primary care setting in the presence of suspected infection in a patient with diabetes.

Additional Diagnostic Testing

- Pulse oximetry to evaluate for hypoxia
- PEFR to evaluate for airflow limitation
- Chest x-ray

Treatment and Management

Treatment Goals
- Maintain airway, restore gas exchange, eradicate the infection, manage pain, and prevent complications.

Drug Treatment
- Prescribe antibiotics to eradicate infection.
  - Consider prescribing ampicillin, azithromycin, or doxycycline for a patient with no exposure to antibiotics for the past 3 months.
  - Otherwise, prescribe amoxicillin with clavulanic acid, cefpodoxime, cefuroxime, and a macrolide or doxycycline. If allergic, consider prescribing a fluoroquinolone.
- Treat symptoms of pneumonia.
- Prescribe inhaled SABA bronchodilator one to four puffs every 4 hr PRN wheezing.
- Consider inhaled corticosteroids or oral prednisone 6 to 20 mg daily to decrease inflammation.
- Offer guaifenesin to manage cough and thin secretions.
- Prescribe acetaminophen or NSAIDs for the pain to promote adherence to pulmonary hygiene.
- Update vaccinations to prevent respiratory infections.

Interventions
- Monitor results of cultures and adjust therapy as indicated.
- Assess the patient's pulmonary hygiene and provide assistive devices as indicated.
- Evaluate hydration and nutrition.

Patient Education
- Instruct the patient to avoid tobacco and alcohol and increase fluid intake.
- Discuss risk factor modifications to prevent infection transmission if indicated.
- Review s/s of complications and adverse medication effects to report.

Patient Population Considerations

Women (conception/pregnancy/lactation)
- Increased abdominal pressure can impede the function of the lower esophageal sphincter and diaphragm. These events increase the risk of reflux and reduce lung capacity. These factors can aggravate the risk of aspiration pneumonia in a pregnant woman. Encourage pregnant women with heartburn to sleep on the left side, with the head propped up with several pillows.

Geriatric
- Perform Mini-Cog© screening to identify patients at risk for neurocognitive disorders that are at increased risk for pneumonia. Examine the need for dental referral with poor dentition and denture fit. Assess for the presence of dysphagia and refer to speech pathology as indicated.

Pediatrics
- Cough is the most common symptom of pneumonia in infants, while younger children and adolescents report more constitutional symptoms.

Referring Patients

- Pulmonology consult
- Infectious disease consult

 ALERT

Refer patient with hypoxemia or two qSOFA signs to the ED immediately for evaluation for respiratory failure and sepsis.

 POP QUIZ 6.2

A 65-year-old male presents to the walk-in clinic for a persistent cough that started several days ago and is getting progressively worse. He has been taking dextromethorphan 30 mg 4 times a day with no relief. He reports sharp chest pain on inspiration, rated 4/10. He denies any history of chronic medical conditions, and he has smoked one pack of cigarettes per day for the past 50 years.

VS: RR 28, HR 92, BP: 106/58, T: 100.5°F (38.1°C). Tachypnea noted. Exertion dyspnea observed, increased accessory muscle use. Chest symmetric. AP diameter not increased. Lungs scattered wheeze with crackles at RLL. Dullness to percussion RLL with egophony present.

What is the patient experiencing and what are the next steps in care?

LUNG CANCER

Overview

- Lung cancer is the malignant transformation of the respiratory epithelium. *It can be divided into two groups*: SCLC and NSCLC (80%–95% of cases).
- Malignant lesions in the bronchi can block airflow leading to obstructive symptoms, atelectasis, and increase mucous production, causing cough and bronchospasm. Pressure from lesions can interfere with venous circulation causing SVC syndrome. Gas exchange is reduced by disruption to the parenchyma. Pleural and lung inflammation can produce exudates that accumulate and cause pleural effusion. Excess ACTH secreted by SCLC tumors causes ectopic Cushing's syndrome. ADH produced by SCLC causes SIADH.

Etiology

- Family history, genetic predisposition
- *Carcinogen exposure*: Arsenic, asbestos, chemicals, diesel exhaust, radiation, radon gas, second-hand smoke, tobacco use
- Pulmonary fibrosis

Signs and Symptoms

- Asymptomatic in early disease
- Wheezing, dyspnea, hemoptysis, decreased lung sounds, dullness to percussion
- Edema to face, neck, and arms, lymphadenopathy, digital clubbing
- Unexplained weight loss, hepatomegaly
- Bone pain, pathologic fracture
- S/s of Cushing's and SIADH

Differential Diagnosis

- *ENDO*: Cushing's syndrome, SIADH
- *HEM*: Hodgkin's lymphoma, metastasis from an alternative site of cancer, thymoma
- *PULM*: Acute bronchitis, atelectasis, asthma/COPD, benign tumor, bronchiectasis, foreign body aspiration, fungal infections, pneumonia, pulmonary fibrosis, pulmonary infarct, TB
- *Other*: Sarcoidosis

Diagnosis

Labs

- BMP to evaluate for adrenal metastasis and hormone-producing tumors of Cushing's syndrome and SIADH
- CBC with differential to assess for bone metastasis and infection
- PTT/PT/INR to assess for DIC
- Sputum for cytology
- LFTs and bilirubin to evaluate for liver metastasis

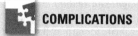

COMPLICATIONS

Acute: Tracheal obstruction, atelectasis, Cushing's syndrome, DIC, DVT, respiratory failure, malignant pleural effusion, respiratory infections, SIADH, SVC syndrome

Chronic: DIC, DVT/PE, dysphagia, metastasis to brain, liver bone, adrenal glands, protein-calorie malnutrition

CLINICAL PEARL

USPSTF Lung Cancer Screening Recommendations

Annual screening with low-dose CT in adults ages 50 to 80 who have a 20 pack/year smoking history and who currently smoke or have quit smoking within the past 15 years. (Recommendations are currently in revision as of November 2020).

ALERT

AMS, cyanosis, peak flow <50%, pulse oximetry <90% or 88% in CO_2-retaining COPD requires SABA, oxygen, and immediate referral to the ED.

Additional Diagnostic Testing
- Pulse oximetry to evaluate for hypoxia
- PEFR to evaluate for airflow limitation
- Chest x-ray
- Chest CT
- Refer to oncology for biopsy
  - Biopsy by bronchoscopy or percutaneous needle aspiration depending on location
  - Additional diagnostics to identify sites of distant metastasis following evaluation

Treatment and Management

Treatment Goals
- Identify complications and infection protection; make referrals as appropriate.
- Collaborate with the oncology team for palliation.

Drug Treatment
- Prescribe SABA without ICS PRN for wheezing to avoid an increased risk of respiratory infection.
- Collaborate with oncology in updating adult vaccinations.
  - If the patient is not scheduled for chemotherapy within 2 weeks, prescribe Tdap if not received in the past 10 years, influenza vaccine, and PPSV23 vaccine.
  - Evaluate for immunosuppression. Do not administer any live vaccines.

Interventions
- Monitor the patient's response to lung cancer treatment.
- Evaluate for the presence of complications of lung cancer and its treatment.
- Provide primary and secondary prevention for health conditions appropriate for age and health status.

Patient Education
- Encourage patients to avoid any nutraceuticals or OTC medications.
- Discuss strategies to prevent infection and bleeding.
- Teach patient s/s of complications and adverse medication effects to report.

Patient Population Considerations

Women (conception/pregnancy/lactation)
- Instruct women of childbearing age to avoid risk factors for lung cancer and initiate a tobacco cessation protocol.

Geriatric
- Refer patients for CT scan of the chest with smoking history as recommended by USPSTF.

Pediatric
- Teach caregivers and patients to monitor for s/s of lung cancer secondary to chest radiation for the treatment of hematologic cancer.

Referring Patients

- Pulmonology consult
- Oncology consult

PERTUSSIS

Overview

- Pertussis is a highly contagious bacterial disease known as whooping cough caused by *Bordetella pertussis* and *Bordetella parapertussis*.

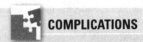

COMPLICATIONS

Acute: Coma, epistaxis, hernia, hypoxic encephalopathy, subdural hematomas, cerebral hemorrhage, pneumonia, seizures

- Gram-negative bacteria spread by aerosolized droplets are transmitted face to face by direct contact. Caregivers to infants are a common source. It incubates for 3 days, lasts for 1 to 2 weeks, and is transmissible for 3 weeks after the cough has started.
- *It progresses through three phases*: Catarrhal (URI symptoms), paroxysmal (whooping cough), and convalescent (chronic pertussis).
- The disease is more severe in infants <6 months and geriatric patients with comorbid conditions.
- Pneumonia can be a primary or secondary infection.

Etiology

- Contact with an infected person
- Unvaccinated patient
- Premature infants, infants with comorbid conditions
- Asthma, extremes of age, and obesity increase the risk of infection

Signs and Symptoms

- No complaints of fever
- Exhaustion, whooping sound, and vomiting
- Conjunctival hemorrhage, engorged neck veins, facial petechiae
- *Catarrhal phase*: URI symptoms (period of highest infectivity)
- *Paroxysmal phase*: Intense spasms of coughing followed by large whoop on inspiration and vomiting
- *Convalescent phase*: Chronic cough that lasts for weeks

Differential Diagnosis

- *CV*: Dehydration
- *HEENT*: Bronchiolitis, croup, cystic fibrosis, URI, RSV
- *NEURO*: Encephalitis, febrile seizures
- *PULM*: Afebrile pneumonia syndrome, asthma, foreign body aspiration, mycoplasma pneumonia

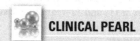

CLINICAL PEARL

Hospitalize patients who are at high risk for complication of severe disease.

Diagnosis

Labs

- *Serial CBC and differential*: Leukocytosis (15,000–50,000) with lymphocytosis
- BMP if fluid and electrolyte imbalance is suspected
- Nasopharyngeal swab and sputum culture
- PCR testing

Additional Diagnostic Testing

- Chest x-ray to rule out pneumonia
- Pulse oximetry to evaluate for hypoxemia

ALERT

CDC recommendations for testing

During an outbreak in a community, ensure that a sputum culture is obtained so that the pertussis outbreak can be confirmed. PCR testing varies in specificity.

Treatment and Management

Treatment Goals

- Prevent infection transmission, treat the infection, manage cough, and prevent complications.

Drug Treatment

- Prescribe azithromycin, clarithromycin, or erythromycin for treatment and chemoprevention of pertussis.
- Consider IV hydration and electrolyte replacement with dehydration and electrolyte losses.

Interventions

- Use droplet and contact precautions when examining the patient and report the infection to the health department.
- Encourage fluids to prevent dehydration.
- Evaluate response to therapy.
- Maintain transmission-based precautions for 5 full days of antibiotic treatment.

Patient Education

- Discuss supportive treatments to manage the infection.
- Teach s/s of complications and adverse medication effects to report.

Patient Population Considerations

Women (conception/pregnancy/lactation)

- Administer Tdap vaccine for each pregnancy at 27 to 36 weeks to reduce the risk of maternal transmission to infants.

Geriatric

- Older patients may require hospital admission and IV hydration and electrolytes.

Pediatric

- Adolescents and adults are sources of pertussis transmission to infants. Administer a Tdap vaccine as a booster at 11- and 12-year office visits.

Referring Patients

- Infectious disease consult
- Department of health

ALERT

Post Exposure Prophylaxis

Antimicrobial prophylaxis is prescribed for asymptomatic household contacts within 21 days of onset of cough in the index patient.

CLINICAL PEARL

Primary Prevention of Pertussis

All adults should receive a Tdap booster every 10 years, especially if they ever spend time with infants.

TUBERCULOSIS

Overview

- TB is a highly contagious infection caused by *Mycobacterium tuberculosis*. Infected droplets are inhaled and migrate to alveoli in the hilar region.
- In latent TB infection, T lymphocytes are sensitized and attempt to eliminate the bacillus. Any bacteria that remain are walled off by fibroblasts to form a granuloma. In this case, the patient will not have s/s of pulmonary TB but is experiencing latent TB infection.
- In TB disease, either the bacteria were not walled off effectively or the bacteria were unopposed and able proliferate to cause active pulmonary TB. This may occur over time when the patient's immune defense becomes compromised by advancing age, disease, or adverse effect of medications or treatments.

COMPLICATIONS

Latent TB infection: Active TB disease

Active TB disease: Acute respiratory failure, bronchospasm, dehydration, infection transmission, pain, protein calorie malnutrition, sepsis

Etiology

- Latent TB infection
  - Contact with an infected person or groups of infected people
  - Prolonged exposure to contaminated air
  - Increased incidence in alcoholism, DM, ESRD, HIV, immunosuppression by disease or treatment, IVDA, protein-calorie malnutrition, silicosis, smoking, young children
- Active TB disease
  - Close contact with a person with active TB disease whose immune system is ineffective in controlling the TB bacillus
  - A patient with latent TB infection whose immune system has become compromised by age, illness, medication, treatment or condition, tobacco smoke or alcoholism, DM, ESRD, HIV, IVDA, protein-calorie malnutrition, silicosis

CLINICAL PEARL

Considerations in TB Testing
- Perform IGRA testing for TB if patient has history of BCG vaccine, IVDA, is not likely to return for TST interpretation, and who are likely to be infected.
- Do not repeat skin testing in a person who has had a positive TST result in the past.
- Do not use IGRA and TST simultaneously.
- Measure induration, not erythema.

Signs and Symptoms

- Latent TB infection
  - No s/s of pulmonary TB
- Active TB disease
  - AMS, cough, fever, hemoptysis, lymphadenopathy, myalgia, night sweats
  - Crackles or rales on auscultation

Differential Diagnosis

- *HEM*: Neoplasm
- *PULM*: Actinomycosis, aspergillosis, aspiration pneumonia, blastomycosis, bronchiectasis, coccidioidomycosis, lung cancer

Diagnosis

Labs

- Latent TB infection
  - Diagnose latent TB infection with IGRA titer.
  - Diagnose latent TB infection with history taking and results of IGRA or TST. If TST or IGRA is inconclusive, but the risk for infection is high, repeat the test.
  - Obtain baseline blood work before starting antitubercular therapy: CBC, BMP, LFTs.
- TB disease
  - Sputum culture (the gold standard for diagnosis)
  - Sputum for acid-fast bacillus every morning for three consecutive mornings
    - ○ The sputum for AFB may be negative in a patient with active TB.
  - Drug susceptibility testing
  - CBC, BMP, LFTs
- See Table 6.1 for details on TB testing.

ALERT

TB in Primary Care Office

Patients with s/s of active TB disease who have had a recent close contact should be treated as a confirmed case of TB until proven otherwise.
- Apply personal PPE and N95 mask.
- Apply a simple face mask to the patient.
- Separate the patient from other people in the office.
- Call 911 for transfer to a hospital.
- Prepare to admit to a negative pressure room while undergoing workup for TB.

Table 6.1 Criteria for Classifying Reactions for TB Testing

Positive IGRA result or TST (PPD): ≥5 mm	Positive IGRA result or TST (PPD): ≥10 mm	Positive IGRA result or TST (PPD): ≥15 mm
• HIV-infected patient • Recent contacts of a patient with TB • Patient with fibrotic changes on x-ray • Organ transplant recipients • Immunosuppressed patients	• Recent immigrants (<5 years) from high-prevalence countries • IVDA • Residents and employees of high-risk congregate settings • Mycobacteriology laboratory personnel • Children <4 years of age, or children and adolescents exposed to adults in high-risk categories	• A person with no known risk factors

Congregate settings: Correctional facilities, shelters, assisted living, nursing homes, and other healthcare facilities.

Additional Diagnostic Testing
- A chest x-ray may reveal upper lobe involvement.

Treatment and Management

Treatment Goals
- *Latent TB infection*: Treat TB infection to prevent the development of active TB disease; promote adherence and tolerance.
- *Active TB disease*: Eradicate s/s of active disease and prevent the development of drug-resistant strains.

Drug Treatment
- *Latent TB infection*:
  - Twelve-dose once-weekly regimen of INH and RIF under direct observation
- *Active TB disease*:
  - Negative air pressure room, take a multidrug regimen of antitubercular agents according to susceptibility testing
  - Isolation until there is a clinical improvement of TB symptoms, and three sputum collections for AFB are negative.
  - Once clear of measurable infection, discharged to home with restrictions and receive directly observed treatment to complete their medication regimen

Interventions
- Use airborne transmission-based precautions when interacting with patients with active s/s of TB disease.
- Monitor the patient's response to therapy.
- Evaluate for the presence of adverse medication effects.
- Monitor CBC, BMP, and LFTs every 4 weeks, as indicated.

Patient Education
- Discuss the disease process and demonstrate infection protection strategies.
- Teach the patient to avoid any nutraceuticals or OTC medications that can contribute to hepatotoxicity.
- Review s/s of complications and adverse medication effects to report.

Patient Population Considerations

Women (conception/pregnancy/lactation)
- Treat pregnant women with active TB with EMB, INH, and RIF.

Geriatric
- Patients admitted to nursing homes and assisted living may be required to undergo TB testing.

Pediatric
- Children under age 5 who are close contacts of a patient with active TB disease may be tested with Mantoux skin testing.

Referring Patients

- Pulmonology consult
- Infectious disease consult
- Department of health

POP QUIZ 6.3

An asymptomatic 25-year-old male college student presents to student health services to have his TST test read 48 hr after insertion. On examination, the nurse practitioner notes a 12-mm induration with a 15-mm erythemic base.

What do these findings mean?

RESOURCES

Agency for Healthcare Research and Quality. (2018). *Community-acquired pneumonia in the primary care setting.* https://www.ahrq.gov/sites/default/files/wysiwyg/professionals/quality-patient-safety/quality-resources/tools/cap-toolkit/cap_pc-pamphlet.pdf

American Academy of Allergy, Asthma and Immunology. (n.d.). *AAAAI infographic: Work-related or occupational asthma.* https://www.aaaai.org/Aaaai/media/MediaLibrary/PDF%20Documents/Libraries/AsthmaInfo-Work.pdf

Baer, S. (2019). *Medscape: Community-acquired pneumonia.* https://emedicine.medscape.com/article/234240-overview

Bocka, J. (2019). *Medscape: Pertussis.* https://emedicine.medscape.com/article/967268-overview.

Carolan, P. (2019). *Medscape: Pediatric bronchitis.* https://emedicine.medscape.com/article/1001332-overview#

Cash, J. C., & Glass, C. A. (Eds.). (2019). *Adult-gerontology practice guidelines.* Springer Publishing Company.

Centers for Disease Control and Prevention. (2018). *Tuberculosis (TB).* https://www.cdc.gov/tb/default.htm

Centers for Disease Control and Prevention. (2019). *Pertussis (whooping cough).* https://www.cdc.gov/pertussis/index.html

Centers for Disease Control and Prevention. (2020). *Latent tuberculosis infection: A guide for primary health care providers.* https://www.cdc.gov/tb/publications/ltbi/pdf/LTBIbooklet508.pdf

Cochrane. (2017). *Antibiotic treatment for people with acute bronchitis.* https://www.cochrane.org/CD000245/ARI_antibiotic-treatment-people-acute-bronchitis

Codina Leik, M. T. (2018). *Family nurse practitioner certification: Intensive review.* Springer Publishing Company.

Fayyaz, J. (2019). *Medscape: Bronchitis.* https://emedicine.medscape.com/article/297108-overview

Gold. (2020). *Gold pocket guide.* https://goldcopd.org/wp-content/uploads/2020/03/GOLD-2020-POCKET-GUIDE-ver1.0_FINAL-WMV.pdf

Herchline, T. (2020). *Medscape: Tuberculosis.* https://emedicine.medscape.com/article/230802-overview.

Messenia, Z. (2020). *Medscape: COPD.* https://emedicine.medscape.com/article/297664-overview

Morris, M. (2019). *Medscape: Asthma.* https://emedicine.medscape.com/article/296301-overview

Rabe, K. F., Hurd, S., Anzueto, A., Barnes, P. J., Buist, S. A., Calverley, P., Fukuchi, Y., Jenkins C., Rodriguez-Roisin, R., van Weel, C., & Zielinski, J. (2007). Global strategy for the diagnosis, management, and prevention of chronic obstructive pulmonary disease: GOLD executive summary. *American Journal of Respiratory and Critical Care Medicine, 176*(6), 532–555. https://doi.org/10.1164/rccm.200703-456SO

Reddel, H. K., FitzGerald, J. M., Bateman, E. D., Bacharier, L. B., Becker, A., Brusselle, G., Buhl, R., Cruz, A. A., Fleming, L., Inoue, H., Wai-San Ko, F., Krishnan, J. A., Levy, M. L., Lin, J., Pedersen, S. E., Sheikh, A., Yorgancioglu, A., & Boulet, L. P. (2019). GINA 2019: A fundamental change in asthma management: treatment of asthma with short-acting bronchodilators alone is no longer recommended for adults and adolescents. *European Respiratory Journal, 53*(6), 1901046. https://doi.org/10.1183/13993003.01046-2019

Sethi, S. (2020). *Merck manual professional version: Acute bronchitis.* https://www.merckmanuals.com/professional/pulmonary-disorders/acute-bronchitis/acute-bronchitis

Sorenson, M., Quinn, L., & Klein, D. (2019). *Pathophysiology: Concepts of human disease* (1st ed.). Pearson Education.

Swerdel, J. N., Janevic, T. M., Kostis, W. J., Faiz, A., Cosgrove, N. M., Kostis, J. B., The Myocardial Infarction Data Acquisition System (MIDAS 27) Study Group. (2017). Association between dehydration and short-term risk of ischemic stroke in patients with atrial fibrillation. *Translational Stroke Research, 8*(2), 122–130. https://doi.org/10.1007/s12975-016-0471-9

United States Preventive Services Task Force. (2013). *Final recommendation statement: Lung cancer screening.* https://www.uspreventiveservicestaskforce.org/uspstf/recommendation/lung-cancer-screening

United States Preventive Services Task Force. (2020). *Lung cancer screening: An update in progress.* https://uspreventiveservicestaskforce.org/uspstf/draft-recommendation/lung-cancer-screening-2020

Waseem, M. (2020). *Medscape: Pediatric pneumonia.* https://emedicine.medscape.com/article/967822-overview

7

GASTROINTESTINAL SYSTEM

ACUTE APPENDICITIS

Overview

- Acute appendicitis is inflammation of the vermiform appendix. Lymphoid hyperplasia, fecalith, seeds, or parasites migrate into the appendix, and trigger obstruction, inflammation, and bacterial proliferation. Intraluminal pressure triggers tissue ischemia and necrosis that may result in perforation.

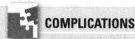

COMPLICATIONS

Acute: Perforated appendix/sepsis, AKI, electrolyte depletion, periappendicular abscess, obstruction, gangrene, peritonitis

Chronic: Chronic appendicitis

Etiology

- *Bacteroides, Escherichia coli, Peptostreptococcus,* and *Pseudomonas*
- Fecalith, chronic constipation, low fiber intake, calcified fecal matter
- Foreign body, swallowing small objects in children

Signs and Symptoms

- Periumbilical pain migrating to right lower quadrant pain
- Nausea and vomiting, anorexia, tachycardia, and fever
- Voluntary guarding, diarrhea, or constipation may be present
- Point tenderness present at McBurney point, rebound tenderness, rigidity
- *Accessory signs:* Rovsing sign, obturator sign, psoas sign, Dunphy sign, and Markle sign may be present

Differential Diagnosis

- *GI:* Adenitis, biliary colic, cancer, cholecystitis, colitis, Crohn's flare, diverticulitis, enteritis, gastroenteritis, pancreatitis, perforated duodenal ulcer
- *GU:* Obstructive uropathy, renal colic, UTI
- *REPRO:* Ectopic pregnancy, endometriosis, ovarian abscess or cyst, PID, uterine mass

ALERT

Patients with signs of acute appendicitis with severe pain, rebound tenderness or two qSOFA signs should be referred to the ED immediately for acute medical and surgical management.

Diagnosis

Labs

- UCG to exclude ectopic pregnancy
- Clean catch U/A and urine culture and specificity to exclude UTI and obstructive uropathy
- Serum amylase, lipase, and LFTs to exclude a hepatobiliary cause

(continued)

Labs (continued)

- CBC to evaluate for leukocytosis, shift to the left
- CRP level to evaluate for elevation early in evolution
- BMP to evaluate renal function and electrolytes
- Blood cultures with fever
- Stool c/s and gram stain

Additional Diagnostic Testing

- Abdominal flat and upright x-ray
- IV contrast CT recommended to exclude acute appendicitis
- *Pregnant patients*: Ultrasound is the initial imaging; consider MRI if ultrasound is not conclusive

Treatment and Management

Treatment Goals

- Manage pain, treat infection, and prevent perforation.

Drug Treatment

- Do not medicate for pain until evaluated for surgery. Ketorolac can be considered postsurgical evaluation.
- Prescribe antibiotic therapy (ampicillin, clindamycin, metronidazole, gentamicin) for gram-negative bacteria and anaerobes.
- Consider ondansetron for nausea/vomiting.

Interventions

- Assess hydration status, weight, and intake and output to evaluate for AKI.
- Initiate bowel rest and advance diet as tolerated after intervention.
- Monitor response to therapy.

Patient Education

- Instruct the patient to complete the entire course of antibiotics.
- Encourage oral fluids to replace losses and electrolytes from vomiting.
- Teach patient s/s of complications to report.

Patient Population Considerations

Women (conception/pregnancy/lactation)

- Ultrasound and MRI for diagnosis in pregnant patients. Avoid fluoroquinolones or aminoglycosides in pregnant patients.

Geriatric

- There is an increased risk of mortality from perforation in acute appendicitis in older adults. Early identification and observation are critical.

Pediatric

- Inflammatory bowel disease can contribute to obstructive stricture and requires further evaluation.

Referring Patients

- Surgery consult
- Gastroenterology consult
- Infectious disease consult for suspected sepsis

ACUTE CHOLECYSTITIS

Overview

- Acute cholecystitis is an inflammation of the gallbladder. Typically, gallstones block the cystic duct or trauma to the biliary tract occurs that triggers obstruction, while some cases are acalculous. Inflammation and bacterial proliferation develop, which can lead to perforation.

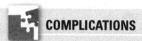

COMPLICATIONS

Acute: Perforated gallbladder/sepsis, AKI, electrolyte depletion, pneumonia, fistula formation

Chronic: Chronic cholecystitis

Etiology

- Adhesion, biliary lesion, gallstones, trauma from instrumentation
- Bariatric surgery, chemotherapy, contraceptives, estrogen replacement, family history, high-fat diet, liver transplant, obesity, opioid abuse, parenteral nutrition, pregnancy, rapid weight loss
- *Diseases*: Crohn's disease, DM, hepatic disease, pancreatitis

Signs and Symptoms

- RUQ pain radiating to the scapular following a fatty meal or fasting
- Chills, fever, nausea, vomiting
- Point tenderness present in RUQ with Murphy's sign
- Diaphoresis, pallor, tea-colored urine, clay-colored stools
- Rebound tenderness, rigidity with perforation

Differential Diagnosis

- *CV*: Aortic aneurysm
- *GI*: Biliary colic, gastroenteritis, cholangitis, gallbladder cancer or mass

ALERT

Patients with signs of acute cholecystitis with severe pain, rebound tenderness, or two qSOFA signs should be referred to the ED immediately for acute medical and surgical management.

Do not medicate for pain until evaluated for the surgeon.

Diagnosis

Labs
- UCG before x-ray for women
- BMP to evaluate renal function and electrolytes
- CBC to evaluate for leukocytosis, shift to the left, bands
- Bilirubin and LFTs to assess for elevated alkaline phosphatase
- Serum amylase, lipase to exclude pancreatitis
- U/A to exclude renal pathology
- Blood cultures with fever
- Stool c/s and gram stain

Additional Diagnostic Testing
- Abdominal flat and upright x-rays
- Gallbladder ultrasound, hepatobiliary scintigraphy
- CT is a secondary imaging tool to rule out perforation
- *Pregnant patients*: Ultrasound is the initial imaging; consider MRI if ultrasound is not conclusive
- ERCP

CLINICAL PEARL

Uncomplicated Cholecystitis

Gallbladder symptoms without fever, stable vital signs, no obstruction on imaging, who has no medical conditions, and not pregnant and has adequate pain relief

Treatment and Management

- Manage patients with uncomplicated cholecystitis conservatively as an outpatient.

Treatment Goals

- Manage nausea and pain, treat infection, and prevent perforation.

Drug Treatment

- Prescribe combination antibiotic therapy levofloxacin and metronidazole prophylactically.
- Consider promethazine or prochlorperazine for nausea/vomiting.
- Prescribe oxycodone with acetaminophen for moderate pain PRN.

Interventions

- Advance to a low-fat diet.
- Monitor response to antibiotic therapy.
- Evaluate the fluid balance.

Patient Education

- Instruct the patient to complete the entire course of antibiotics.
- Encourage oral fluids to replace losses and electrolytes from vomiting.
- Teach patient s/s of complications to report.

Patient Population Considerations

Women (conception/pregnancy/lactation)

- Cholecystitis is challenging to recognize in pregnant patients. Schedule planned surgery during the second trimester.

Geriatric

- Fever may be absent with nonspecific symptoms for cholecystitis in older adults.

Pediatric

- Pediatric cholecystitis is often associated with comorbid systemic diseases.

Referring Patients

- Gastroenterology consult
- Surgery consult
- Infectious disease consult for suspected sepsis

POP QUIZ 7.1

The nurse practitioner is precepting a student in an urgent care clinic who is preparing to assess a 30-year-old female with fever, abdominal pain, nausea, and vomiting. Before entering the room with the student, what would the preceptor expect the student to explain as the correct approach to the history taking and examination?

ACUTE PANCREATITIS

Overview

- Acute pancreatitis is an inflammation of the pancreas that can lead to autolytic destruction. Inflammation can extend to the structures of the biliary tract and sphincter of Oddi, contributing to hepatomegaly. Cases of pancreatitis range from mild to life-threatening.

Etiology

- *Environmental factors*: Alcohol abuse, surgical manipulation (ERCP), organophosphate poisoning, tobacco

COMPLICATIONS

Acute: ARDS, ATN, DIC, GI bleed, hemorrhage, hyperglycemia, hypocalcemia, AKI due to fluid shift

Chronic: Chronic pancreatitis, DM, malnutrition

- *Disease risk factors*: Cholelithiasis, biliary colic, infections (viral, bacteria, worms), tumors, immune-mediated vasculitis, and pancreatic cancer
- Family or personal history of hypertriglyceridemia, hereditary pancreatitis, hypercalcemia, congenital anomalies: pancreas divisum and annular pancreas
- Medications that can induce pancreatitis

Signs and Symptoms

- Sudden onset of upper abdominal pain described as severe, boring, with constant ache radiating through to the back
- Nausea, vomiting, diarrhea, anorexia
- Ascites, Cullen's sign, Turner's sign
- Abdominal rigidity, rebound tenderness
- Dyspnea, guarding, diminished breath sounds/crackles at bases
- Fever, tachycardia, and hypotension

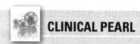 **CLINICAL PEARL**

Differentiating Chronic Pancreatitis

Chronic pancreatitis is characterized by intermittent attacks of pain, weight loss, steatorrhea, and possible elevation in amylase and lipase levels. Pancreatic calcification may be noted on abdominal films.

Differential Diagnosis

- *GI*: Adenitis, appendicitis, biliary colic, cancer, cholecystitis, colitis, Crohn's flare, diverticulitis, enteritis, gastroenteritis, perforated duodenal ulcer
- *GU*: Obstructive uropathy, renal colic, UTI
- *REPRO*: Ectopic pregnancy, endometriosis, ovarian abscess or cyst, PID, uterine mass

Diagnosis

Labs

- Serum amylase and lipase levels 3 times upper limit
- CMP reveals elevated LFTs, LDH, BUN and creatinine, BG, hypocalcemia, hyperglycemia
- Elevated CRP
- *CBC*: leukocytosis, hematocrit >47%, declining hemoglobin in hemorrhage
- ABGs may reveal hypoxia and mixed acidosis
- Blood cultures with fever

Additional Diagnostic Testing

- Abdominal flat and upright x-ray to identify perforation and free air
- Abdominal CT in the absence of clinical improvement
- Ultrasound or MRCP in pregnancy

Treatment and Management

Treatment Goals

- Manage pain, control risk factors, and prevent complications.

Drug Treatment

- Hold all medications associated with pancreatitis.
- *Pain management*: Acetaminophen in mild cases

Interventions

- Remove offending agents and manage contributing causes.
- Monitor for a decrease in serial amylase and lipase over time.
- Advance low-fat diet as tolerated.
- Initiate counseling for alcohol and tobacco cessation, if indicated.
- Monitor for chronic pancreatitis, DM, and malnutrition.

Patient Education

- Instruct the patient to limit fat to no more than 30 g daily.
- Explain the importance of alcohol and tobacco cessation.
- Teach the patient to report s/s of chronic pancreatitis and hyperglycemia.
- Encourage the patient to maintain BMI <25.
- Instruct patient in s/s of complications to report.

Patient Population Considerations

Women (conception, pregnancy, lactation)

- Consider acetaminophen for mild to moderate pain for pregnant patients, as opioids cross the placenta and cause fetal respiratory depression. Ultrasound, followed by MRI for diagnostic testing, is preferred to reduce radiation exposure.

Geriatric

- There is a higher incidence of organ failure in older adults. Gallstone pancreatitis can be managed with ERCP following acute pancreatitis at 6 weeks to improve survival outcomes at 1 year.

Pediatric

- Imaging in the early phase of acute pancreatitis is usually is not required to make a diagnosis.

Referring Patients

- Nutrition consult
- Endocrinology consult

COLORECTAL CANCER

Overview

- Colorectal cancer is a malignancy arising from a premalignant adenoma. The neoplasm grows slowly and sheds cells and blood in the stool in its early stage. As lesions enlarge and become circumferential, the bowel lumen narrows, and obstructive symptoms occur. Frank bleeding, fluid imbalance, electrolyte disturbance, and malnutrition follow. It is the third most common cancer and the second leading cause of death in the world.

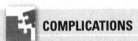 **COMPLICATIONS**

Acute: Bowel obstruction, lower GI bleed, AKI due to fluid shift

Chronic: Metastasis to lung, liver, bone, brain, and adrenal glands; anemia; protein calorie malnutrition

Etiology

- *Genetic predisposition*: HNPCC (Lynch syndrome) I or II, familial adenomatous polyposis, PJS, MAP
- Ethnicity: African American, Ashkenazi Jew
- Personal or family history of colorectal cancer, polyps
- Environmental; low fiber, low fruit, low vegetables, high animal fat, and processed meat diet, BMI >25, sedentary lifestyle, exposure to diagnostic or therapeutic radiation, alcohol consumption, tobacco
- Advancing age
- *Disease risk factors*: Crohn's disease, ulcerative colitis, type 2 DM
- Vitamin D deficiency

 CLINICAL PEARL

Colorectal Cancer Screening

Average risk: 45 to 76 years (age 76–85 based on personal preference):

- FIT or FOBT annually
- MT-sDNA every 3 years
- Virtual colonoscopy or sigmoidoscopy every 5 years
- Colonoscopy every 10 years
- Genetic testing offered according to criteria
- Epi proColon® blood test for people declining alternative testing

Signs and Symptoms

- Asymptomatic on screening
- Advanced disease
  - Rectal bleeding, change in the shape of stool or bowel pattern, leaking diarrhea, abdominal distention
  - Abdominal tenderness, palpable mass, ascites, hepatomegaly, s/s of metastasis
  - S/s of anemia and protein-calorie malnutrition

Differential Diagnosis

- *GU*: Obstructive uropathy, ascending UTI
- *REPRO*: Ectopic pregnancy, ovarian cyst, PID
- *Other*: Ileus, diverticulosis, inflammatory bowel disease, gastrointestinal lymphoma

Diagnosis

Lab

- U/A to evaluate for renal stones, infection
- BMP to evaluate renal function; LFTs to assess liver function
- CBC and PT/INR to evaluate for nutritional anemia, bleeding times, and bone marrow suppression
- Serum ferritin if microcytic anemia is present
- Baseline serum carcinoembryonic antigen CEA level and serum albumin for monitoring response to therapy
- Vitamin D level to identify deficiency
- Serum folate level if fluoropyrimidine is considered

Additional Diagnostic Testing

- Abdomen/pelvic CT
- Contrast ultrasound of abdomen and liver
- Diagnostic colonoscopy with biopsy
- *Staging*: Chest x-ray, PET scan, molecular testing to guide therapy selection:
  - RAS, BRAFV600, dMMR/MSI, KRAS

Treatment and Management

Treatment Goals

- Cure colorectal cancer, prevent/manage its risk for metastasis and recurrence, and manage acute and chronic complications: serum CEA and serum albumin at baseline.

Drug Treatment

- Secondary prevention
  - Prescribe daily low-dose aspirin to patients at higher risk for colon cancer.
- Tertiary prevention
  - Collaborate with oncology regarding chemotherapy and surgery for treatment according to the stage.
  - Prescribe duloxetine, gabapentin, or TCA for chemotherapy-induced neuropathy.
  - Prescribe iron supplementation with iron-deficient anemia.
  - Prescribe ondansetron for nausea (short term).
  - Prescribe vitamin D 5,000 IU weekly for vitamin D deficiency.
  - Prescribe enoxaparin 40 mg subcutaneous daily × 28 days after surgery.
  - Consult palliative care with refractory pain.

Interventions

- Order CEA level at each visit to monitor for cancer recurrence.
- *Monitor for chronic complications of cancer:* DVT, DIC, bowel obstruction, metastasis.
- Monitor serum albumin and weight loss and refer to a nutritionist if serum albumin <3.5.
- Monitor for leukopenia, thrombocytopenia, and anemia due to chemotherapy and radiation.
- Screen for depression and insomnia.
- *Monitor for complications following surgery:* Acute pain, ileus, SSI, pneumonia, GI bleeding, adhesions, hernia, CDAD, CAUTI, DVT.
- *Monitor for chronic complications of cancer:* DVT, DIC, bowel obstruction.

Patient Education

- Counsel patients for tobacco cessation and limit alcohol consumption.
- Discuss risks, signs, and prevention strategies of DVT, chronic DIC, neuropathy, pancytopenia, obstruction, malnutrition.
- Review guide for ERAS with the patient.
- *Follow dietary restrictions postoperatively:* Low residue, low fat.
- Discuss strategies to prevent infection, bleeding, and manage energy requirements.

Patient Population Considerations

Women (conception/pregnancy/lactation)

- Counsel women of childbearing age regarding colorectal cancer risks. If a genetic risk is present, discuss preconception counseling and referral for genetic testing.

Geriatric

- Do not screen patients older than age 75 years for colorectal cancer.

Pediatric

- Colorectal cancer in pediatric patients is rare but is rising. Most cancers are genetic syndromes. Symptoms of lower GI bleeding may be present. Careful screening of genetic risks is critical.

Referring Patients

- Surgery consult
- Hematology/oncology consult
- palliative care consult
- Enterostomal therapist, nutritionist, PT, if needed

 POP QUIZ 7.2

A 24-year-old male with HIV infection and bipolar I disorder presents to the primary care office following discharge from the ED for acute pancreatitis. He reports epigastric discomfort that is getting progressively worse. He drinks alcohol socially and denies substance abuse except for tobacco. The abdomen is soft and nontender, Normal BS throughout and no peritoneal signs. Medications include aripiprazole and single pill therapy for HIV (bictegravir/emtricitabine/tenofovir alafemanide).

What is the likely cause of his acute pancreatitis, and what are the appropriate next steps?

DIVERTICULITIS

Overview

- Diverticulitis is a disorder of inflamed diverticula that occur in pouches of diverticulosis in the sigmoid colon.
- Particles of undigested foods and fecaliths become trapped in diverticula in the sigmoid colon and become inflamed. As a result, bacteria proliferate, which increases the intraluminal pressure.
- The inflamed bowel is at risk for obstruction, bleeding, and perforation.

 COMPLICATIONS

Acute: Bowel abscess, bowel obstruction/ perforation, colovesical fistula, hemorrhage, AKI, electrolyte depletion

Chronic: Diverticulosis, colorectal cancer

Etiology

- Advancing age, constipation, high-fat diet, low-fiber diet, obesity, tobacco
- *Medications*: Corticosteroids, NSAIDs
- Diverticulosis by history

Signs and Symptoms

- LLQ abdominal pain, constipation alternating with diarrhea, fever, nausea, and vomiting

Differential Diagnosis

- *GI*: Appendicitis, biliary disease, cholecystitis, colon cancer, constipation, gastroenteritis, inflammatory bowel disease flare, intestinal perforation, mesenteric ischemia
- *GU*: Obstructive uropathy, renal colic, UTI
- *REPRO*: Endometriosis, ovarian abscess or cyst, PID, uterine mass

 ALERT

Patients with signs of acute diverticulitis with hemorrhage, severe pain, rebound tenderness, or two qSOFA signs should be referred to the ED immediately for acute medical and surgical management.

Diagnosis

Labs

- Clean catch U/A and urine culture and specificity to exclude UTI, obstructive uropathy
- Serum amylase, lipase, and LFTs to exclude a hepatobiliary cause
- CBC to evaluate for leukocytosis, shift to the left,
- BMP to evaluate renal function and electrolytes
- Blood cultures with fever
- Stool c/s and gram stain

Additional Diagnostic Testing

- Abdominal flat and upright x-ray to identify free air
- Abdominal and pelvic CT
- Colonoscopy during the nonacute phase to avoid accidental perforation
- Barium enema should be avoided with acute pain to prevent peritonitis

Treatment and Management

- Uncomplicated diverticulitis can be managed in the outpatient setting.

Treatment Goals

- Treat infection, prevent perforation, and modify risk factors.

Drug Treatment

- Prescribe a combination of metronidazole and either ciprofloxacin or TMP-SMX.

Interventions

- Prescribe a clear liquid diet for 2 to 3 days and then advance to low residue as tolerated.
- Monitor patient's response to antibiotics within 48 hr.
- Make follow-up appointment in 1 week to evaluate response.

Patient Education

- Instruct the patient to complete the entire course of antibiotics.
- Discuss modifiable risk factors to reduce events of inflammation.

(continued)

Patient Education (continued)
- Review fiber supplementation and high-fiber diet for diverticulosis after the resolution of inflammation.
- Discuss follow-up for colonoscopy and surgical evaluation.
- Teach patient s/s of complications to report.

Patient Population Considerations

Women (conception/pregnancy/lactation)
- Encourage a high-fiber diet to reduce the incidence of diverticulitis in women of childbearing age.

Geriatric
- There is an increased incidence of diverticulitis in geriatric populations.

Pediatric
- Meckel diverticulum is a congenital disease where a tube-like appendage at the distal ileum can develop complications of diverticulitis. It is managed with surgical resection.

Referring Patients

- Surgery consult
- Gastroenterology consult
- Infectious disease consult for suspected sepsis

GASTROESOPHAGEAL REFLUX DISEASE

Overview

- In GERD, gastric secretions into the esophagus triggering pain, inflammation, and erosion. It occurs in response to increased gastric volume, decreased lower esophageal sphincter tone, and recumbency shortly after eating. Hiatal hernia is a structural anomaly that causes GERD.

Etiology

- Truncal obesity, pregnancy, hiatal hernia
- Tobacco, alcohol, food, coffee, chocolate
- *Medications*: Bronchodilators, anticholinergics, CCB, TCAs, nitrates, progesterone

Signs and Symptoms

- Epigastric discomfort, heartburn, especially at night
- Water brash, hoarseness
- Coughing, wheezing
- Recurrent pharyngitis, dental erosions

Differential Diagnosis

- *CV*: ACS
- *GI*: Achalasia, cholelithiasis, cholecystitis, esophageal motility disorders, gastritis, intestinal motility disorders, PUD
- *PULM*: Aspiration pneumonia, nocturnal asthma

COMPLICATIONS

Acute: Aspiration pneumonia, asthma, pain, upper GI bleeding
Chronic: Barrett's esophagus, esophageal cancer

CLINICAL PEARL

Nocturnal asthma should trigger an evaluation of GERD as a likely cause because 50% of patients do experience heartburn with asthmatic symptoms.

Diagnosis

Labs
- CBC may reveal anemia
- Upper endoscopy
- FOBT

Additional Diagnostic Testing
- 24-hr pH testing
- Esophageal manometry
- Upper GI series
- Gastroesophageal reflux scintigraphy in infants and children

ALERT

GERD is the most common cause of noncardiac chest pain.

Patients with risk factors for CVHD require 12-lead EKG and exclusion of cardiac cause before ruling in GERD.

Treatment and Management

Treatment Goals
- Decrease episode of pain and nocturnal asthma and prevent complications of bleeding, Barrett's esophagus and cancer.

Drug Treatment
- Prescribe oral proton pump inhibitors daily for 6 to 12 weeks. May increase to twice daily in refractory GERD.
- Consider H2 antagonists with mild symptoms or in combination with PPI with more severe symptoms initially.
- Discuss the use of OTC antacids for symptomatic relief.

ALERT

Take H2 antagonist or PPI 30 min before dinner to minimize nocturnal asthma and GERD symptoms.

Interventions
- Monitor for upper GI bleeding, Barrett's esophagus, and esophageal cancer.
- Evaluate weight and lifestyle as a contributing cause.
- Review dietary factors that contribute to GERD.
- Refer for surgical intervention with refractory asthma or EENT manifestations.

Patient Education
- Counsel patient in tobacco and alcohol cessation, if needed.
- *Discuss lifestyle modifications*: BMI <25, frequent small feedings, avoiding foods that aggravate GERD, last meal 2 to 3 hr before bedtime, GERD pillow at bedtime. Do not take OTC H2 antagonist or PPI at the same time as other prescription medications.
- Caution patient to avoid OTC aspirin and NSAIDs.
- Reinforce dental hygiene and routine appointments.
- Teach complications of GERD and routine surveillance for complications.
- *Encourage the patient to seek consultation for dark, tarry stools and alarm symptoms*: Dysphagia, odynophagia, GI bleeding, anemia, and persistent vomiting.

Patient Population Considerations

Women (conception/pregnancy/lactation)
- Prescribe lifestyle modifications for GERD and reserve medications (antacids without salicylates, PPI, and H2 antagonists) for refractory disease.

Geriatric
- Older adults with GERD symptoms warrant prompt referral to the ED or cardiologist to rule out cardiac causes. Reduced gastroesophageal motility and prescribed medications may be at the root cause.

Pediatric
- Infants and small children cannot report typical symptoms. Parents of pediatric patients with GERD typically report crying, sleep disturbance, and decreased appetite. The constellation of symptoms should alert the provider to evaluate for GERD as part of the differential diagnosis.

Referring Patients

- Gastroenterology consult

HEPATITIS

Overview

- Hepatitis is an inflammation of the liver that can be caused by a viral infection, toxins, mechanical obstruction, and disease.
- Acute hepatitis leads to fulminant inflammation that interrupts liver function and hepatic circulation that may result in systemic complications
- In chronic hepatitis, fat infiltrates inflamed hepatocytes. When these inflamed hepatocytes die, collagen fibers replace cells causing fibrosis. Persistent fibrosis causes cirrhosis, and the tissue becomes vulnerable to malignant transformation to hepatocellular cancer.
- Hepatitis infections can be acute (A, B, C, E) co-infections (hepatitis D), or chronic (hepatitis B, C).
- In chronic hepatitis, the liver is subject to chronic inflammation that can lead to fatty infiltration, fibrotic changes, scarring, and malignant transformation.

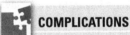 **COMPLICATIONS**

Acute: Hepatic encephalopathy, coagulopathy, hypoglycemia, ascites with or without SBP, esophageal varices, jaundice, hepatorenal syndrome

Chronic: Hepatocellular cancer (HCC)

Etiology

- *Viral infections*:
  - Hepatitis A, E (fecal-oral, sexual contamination)
  - Hepatitis B, C (parenteral, perinatal, blood and body fluids)
  - Hepatitis D (coinfection with hepatitis B)
    - Hepatitis A/B vaccine-naïve patients are at increases risk for hepatitis A or hepatitis B and D coinfection with adequate exposure to pathogen.
- *Toxins*: Alcohol, chemicals, hepatotoxic medications, and nutraceuticals
- *Mechanical obstruction*: Adhesions, cholangitis, common bile duct obstruction, biliary stricture, gallstone, gallbladder cancer, pancreatitis
- *Disease*: Auto-immune hepatitis, DM, hemochromatosis, hyperlipidemia, hypertriglyceridemia, metabolic syndrome, NAFL, NASH, Wilson disease
- High-refined carbohydrate diet, obesity

 ALERT

Average Incubation for Viral Hepatitis
Hepatitis A: 28 days (range 15–50)
Hepatitis B: 90 days (range 60–150)
Hepatitis C: 14–84 days (range 14–182)

Signs and Symptoms

- Abdominal and joint pain, anorexia, clay-colored stool, fatigue, fever, hepatomegaly, jaundice, nausea, tea-colored urine, vomiting
- S/s fulminant hepatitis

Differential Diagnosis

- *GI*: Cholangitis, bowel obstruction, pancreatitis, gastroenteritis, diverticulitis, Crohn's flare, enteritis, colitis, cancer, appendicitis, perforated duodenal ulcer, cholecystitis, biliary colic, adenitis
- *Other*: Acute HIV infection

Diagnosis

Labs
- Liver dysfunction
  - Elevated LFTs, bilirubin, elevated PT/INR
  - BMP, CBC, serum ammonia, serum albumin, blood, and urine cultures to identify complications

Additional Diagnostic Testing
- Abdominal ultrasound
- Liver biopsy
- *Toxicology screens for poisoning*: Alcohol, benzodiazepine, acetaminophen to identify contributing factors
- Positive ANA and anti-smooth muscle antibodies in immune-mediated hepatitis
- Evaluate hepatitis profile for susceptibility, incubation, active infection, and chronicity if indicated

Treatment and Management

Treatment Goals
- Provide supportive care during acute inflammatory events; protect from injury, infection, and hepatotoxins; vaccinate, maintain transmission-based precautions, malignant transformation, and identify and manage acute complications.

Drug Treatment
To protect the patient from further harm:
- Discontinue all hepatotoxins and provide hepatic dosing for prescribed medications.
- Administer antidotes for poisoning, as indicated by poison control.
- *Vaccinate as follows*:
  - Hepatitis A, B vaccination to prevent hepatitis from infectious etiology based on hepatitis profile
  - Influenza and pneumococcal vaccination
- *Infection management, if indicated*:
  - Interferons, antivirals, antiretrovirals according to hepatitis type
- *Immune protection*:
  - Corticosteroids for immune-mediated hepatitis
  - Immunoglobulin for passive immunity

Interventions
- Perform periodic evaluation of blood work to assess liver function and complications and hepatitis serology as indicated.
  - Prolonged PT, bilirubin >30 mg/dL, and hypoglycemia are suggestive of severe disease.
- Initiate counseling for alcohol and tobacco cessation, if indicated.

Patient Education
- Report viral infections to the health department for contact follow-up.
- Teach patient and household contacts to minimize infection transmission if indicated.
- Counsel in alcohol and tobacco cessation and avoiding OTC medications and nutraceuticals.
- Discuss s/s of complications to report and strategies to prevent complications.
- Discuss the risk of cirrhosis and hepatocellular cancer.

Patient Population Considerations

Women (conception/pregnancy/lactation)
- Discuss risk factors for hepatitis during preconception counseling and update hepatitis vaccinations, as necessary.

Geriatric
- Advancing age increases the risk of chronic hepatitis C–associated liver disease and related complications of cirrhosis and HCC. Many patients do not know they are infected.

Pediatric
- When hepatitis A is present, fulminant progression is rare.

Referring Patients

- Gastroenterology/hepatology consult

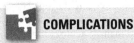

POP QUIZ 7.3

A 55-year-old female presents for evaluation of fatigue, jaundice, and anorexia that began 2 days ago. The patient has hypertension and hyperlipidemia and is taking HCTZ and simvastatin. Her BMI is 32. She denies recent travel and has never received hepatitis A or B vaccines. Her exam is unremarkable. What is the differential diagnosis?

PEPTIC ULCER DISEASE

Overview

- PUD is a disorder characterized by mucosal erosions in the stomach and duodenum that extend into the muscularis mucosa.
- *Helicobacter pylori* infection has been identified as a trigger for gastric mucosal inflammation and reduced duodenal bicarbonate secretion, causing dyspepsia triggered by food consumption (gastric ulcer) or relieved by food consumption (duodenal ulcer).

COMPLICATIONS

Acute: Pain, upper GI bleeding

Chronic: Refractory PUD, resistant *Helicobacter pylori*, gastric cancer

Etiology

- *Helicobacter pylori* infection (lower socioeconomic status, increased number of siblings, infected patent)
- NSAIDs, antiplatelets, anticoagulants, antithrombotics, thrombolytics
- Severe psychological or physical stress
- Genetic factors and hypersecretory states
- *Ethnicity*: African American, Hispanic, Native American, Alaska Native, and people born outside the United States

CLINICAL PEARL

Household contacts with preexisting *Helicobacter pylori*, crowded living conditions, and frequent gastroenteritis are risks for *Helicobacter pylori* infection.

Signs and Symptoms

- Epigastric discomfort, heartburn that is increased in recumbency
- Water brash, hoarseness
- Coughing, wheezing
- Recurrent pharyngitis, dental erosions

ALERT

PUD is a common cause of noncardiac chest pain.

Patients with risk factors for CVHD require 12-lead EKG and exclusion of cardiac cause before ruling in PUD.

Differential Diagnosis

- *CV*: ACS
- *GI*: Acute cholangitis, biliary colic, acute cholecystitis, esophagitis, GERD, esophageal motility disorders, variceal bleeding, gastroesophageal cancer, inflammatory bowel disease, diverticulitis

Diagnosis

Labs
- CBC may reveal anemia
- Upper endoscopy with biopsy
- Urea breath test, fecal antigen testing, or biopsy testing preferred
- Immunoassay for *Helicobacter pylori* less reliable
- FOBT

Additional Diagnostic Testing
- Serum gastrin level and secretin stimulation test in suspected hypersecretory disorders
- Chest x-ray to identify free air in perforation
- Angiography with massive bleeding

Treatment and Management

Treatment Goals
- Decrease episode of pain, eradicate *Helicobacter pylori* infection, and prevent/manage complications of bleeding gastric cancer.

Drug Treatment
- Prescribe empiric triple therapy antibiotics for *Helicobacter pylori* infection, if indicated.
- Consider pantoprazole 40 mg PO daily for maintenance therapy for at-risk patients.
- Oral antacids for symptomatic relief.

 ALERT

Repeat *Helicobacter pylori* testing should be performed 4 weeks after PPI has been withheld for 2 weeks to reduce chance of false-negative results.

Interventions
- Monitor for active upper GI bleeding and refer to ED if present.
- Evaluate medications and lifestyle factors as a contributing cause.
- Consider resistant *Helicobacter pylori* for recurrent symptoms after triple therapy.
- Discontinue NSAIDs for NSAID-induced ulcers. Switch to COX-2 inhibitor if NSAIDs must be continued and ensure cotherapy with PPI.
- Assess for the presence of alarms symptoms associated with gastric cancer.

Patient Education
- Counsel patient in tobacco and alcohol cessation, infection prevention to household contacts in *Helicobacter pylori*, if indicated.
- *Discuss lifestyle modifications*: Avoiding foods that aggravate symptoms. Do not combine OTC H2 antagonist and PPI with prescription medication.
- Caution patient to avoid OTC aspirin, NSAIDs.
- Teach complications of PUD and routine surveillance for complications.
- *Encourage patients to seek consultation for dark, tarry stools and alarm symptoms*: Dysphagia, odynophagia, GI bleeding, anemia, and persistent vomiting.

Patient Population Considerations

Women (conception/pregnancy/lactation)
- *Helicobacter pylori* infection is a risk factor for hyperemesis gravida. Consider *Helicobacter pylori* eradication to relieve symptoms in intractable cases.

Geriatric
- Older adults with PUD and comorbidities of CVHD, DM, HF, CKD, COPD, and HTN with polypharmacy have an increased risk for peptic ulcer perforation requiring emergency surgical management.

Pediatric
- Transabdominal ultrasound is a useful imaging tool in the diagnosis of PUD in children with low body weight.

Referring Patients

- Surgery consult for refractory PUD

RESOURCES

Abdalla, L. F., Chaudhry Ehsanullah, R., Karim, F., Oyewande, A. A., & Khan, S. (2020). Role of using nonsteroidal anti-inflammatory drugs in chemoprevention of colon cancer in patients with inflammatory bowel disease. *Cureus, 12*(5), e8240. https://doi.org/10.7759/cureus.8240

Abu-El-Haija, M., Kumar, S., Quiros, J. A., Balakrishnan, K., Barth, B., Bitton, S., Eisses, J. F., Foglio, E. J., Fox, V., Francis, D., Freeman, A. J., Gonska, T., Grover, A. S., Husain, S. Z., Kumar, R., Lapsia, S., Lin, T., Liu, Q. Y., Maqbool, A., Sellers, . . . Morinville, V. D. (2018). The management of acute pancreatitis in the pediatric population: A clinical report from the NASPGHAN Pancreas Committee. *Journal of Pediatric Gastroenterology and Nutrition, 66*(1), 159. https://doi.org/10.1097/MPG.0000000000001715

Alder, A. (2018). *Medscape: Pediatric appendicitis.* https://emedicine.medscape.com/article/926795-overview

Bath, M. F., Som, R., Curley, D., & Kerwat, R. (2020). Acute pancreatitis in the older patient: Is a new risk score required? *Journal of the Intensive Care Society,* 1751143720937877.

Bloom, A. (2019). *Medscape: Cholecystitis.* https://emedicine.medscape.com/article/171886-overview#a3

Cash, J. C., & Glass, C. A. (Eds.). (2019). *Adult-gerontology practice guidelines.* Springer Publishing Company.

Chan, S. L., Chan, A., Mo, F., Ma, B., Wong, K., Lam, D., Mok, F., Chan, A., Mok, T., & Chan, K. (2018). Association between serum folate level and toxicity of capecitabine during treatment for colorectal cancer. *The Oncologist, 23*(12), 1436–1445. https://doi.org/10.1634/theoncologist.2017-0637

Cheung, K. S., Chan, E. W., Seto, W. K., Wong, I. C., & Leung, W. K. (2020). ACE (angiotensin-converting enzyme) inhibitors/angiotensin receptor blockers are associated with lower colorectal cancer risk: A territory-wide study with propensity score analysis. *Hypertension, 76*(3), 968–975. https://doi.org/10.1161/HYPERTENSIONAHA.120.15317

Codina Leik, M. T. (2018). *Family nurse practitioner certification: Intensive review.* Springer Publishing Company.

Craig, S. (2018). *Medscape: Appendicitis.* https://emedicine.medscape.com/article/773895-overview

Dragonvich, T. (2020). *Medscape: Colon cancer.* https://emedicine.medscape.com/article/277496-overview#a5

Ghoulam, E. (2019). *Medscape: Diverticulitis.* https://emedicine.medscape.com/article/173388-overview

Gustafsson, U. O., Scott, M. J., Hubner, M., Nygren, J., Demartines, N., Francis, N., Rockall, T. A., Young-Fadok, T. M., Hill, A. G., Soop, M., de Boer, H. D., Urman, R. D., Chang, G. J., Fichera, A., Kessler, H., Grass, F., Whang, E. E., Fawcett, W. J., Carli, F., Lobo, D. N., . . . Ljungqvist, O. (2019). Guidelines for perioperative care in elective colorectal surgery: Enhanced recovery after surgery (ERAS) society recommendations: 2018. *World Journal of Surgery, 43,* 659–695. https://doi.org/10.1007/s00268-018-4844-y

Incensu, L. (2017). *Medscape: Appendicitis imaging.* https://emedicine.medscape.com/article/363818-overview

Matin, K. (2020). *Medscape: Colon cancer treatment protocols.* https://emedicine.medscape.com/article/2005487-overview

Moss, J. L., Roy, S., Shen, C., Cooper, J. D., Lennon, R. P., Lengerich, E. J., Adelman, A., Curry, W., & Ruffin, M. T. (2020). Geographic variation in overscreening for colorectal, cervical, and breast cancer among older adults. *JAMA Network Open, 3*(7), e2011645. https://doi.org/10.1001/jamanetworkopen.2020.11645

Nicholas, J. B. (2016). *Pediatric hepatitis A.* https://emedicine.medscape.com/article/964575-overview#a6

Omari, A. H., Khammash, M. R., Qasaimeh, G. R. (2014). Acute appendicitis in the elderly: Risk factors for perforation. *World Journal of Emergency Surgery, 9,* 6. https://doi.org/10.1186/1749-7922-9-6

Reid, M., Price, J. C., & Tien, P. C. (2017). Hepatitis C virus infection in the older patient. *Infectious Disease Clinics of North America, 31*(4), 827–838. https://doi.org/10.1016/j.idc.2017.07.014

Sangi, N. S. (2017). *Medscape: Viral hepatitis.* https://emedicine.medscape.com/article/775507-overview

Sayed, A. O., Zeidan, N. S., Fahmy, D. M., & Ibrahim, H. A. (2017). Diagnostic reliability of pediatric appendicitis score, ultrasound, and low-dose computed tomography scan in children with suspected acute appendicitis. *Therapeutics and Clinical Risk Management, 13*, 847–854. https://doi.org/10.2147/TCRM.S134153

Schwarz, S. (2017). *Medscape: Pediatric cholecystitis.* https://emedicine.medscape.com/article/927340-overview

Schwarz, S. (2019). *Medscape: Pediatric gastroesophageal reflux disease.* https://emedicine.medscape.com/article/930029-overview

Shalkow, J. (2020). *Medscape: Pediatric colorectal tumors.* https://emedicine.medscape.com/article/993370-overview#a7

Sorenson, M., Quinn, L., & Klein, D. (2019). *Pathophysiology: Concepts of human disease* (1st ed.). Pearson Education.

Tang, J. (2019). *Medscape: Acute pancreatitis.* https://emedicine.medscape.com/article/181364-overview

Tang, J. (2019). *Medscape: Gastroesophageal reflux disease.* https://emedicine.medscape.com/article/176595-overview

Wolf, D. (2019). *Medscape: Autoimmune hepatitis.* https://emedicine.medscape.com/article/172356-overview

GENITOURINARY AND RENAL SYSTEM

ACUTE KIDNEY INJURY

Overview

- AKI is an abrupt deterioration of kidney function due to prerenal, intrarenal, or postrenal causes. The events cause oliguria leading to uremia, acidosis, hyperkalemia, and fluid overload.
- Rapid intervention is needed to reverse AKI targeting its etiology. Otherwise, the patient will progress to uremic encephalopathy and congestive heart failure, and develop life-threatening arrhythmia. Reversible AKI can trigger ATN, irreversible necrosis due to hypoperfusion. Repeated episodes of AKI can contribute to cumulative damage and CKD.
- The role of the practitioner in primary care is to identify patients at risk, intervene promptly, and refer to specialists and ED as necessary.

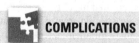 **COMPLICATIONS**

Acute: Ischemic ATN, fluid overload, atrial fibrillation, renal encephalopathy, anemia, hyperkalemia, metabolic acidosis, jaundice

Chronic: CKD

Etiology

Prerenal
- Hypovolemia, hypoperfusion due to HF, sepsis, HRS, shock, extrarenal losses, excessive diuresis

Intrarenal
- ATN due to sepsis, DM, hemolytic uremic syndrome, hydronephrosis, HTN, immune-mediated (SLE, TTP, Goodpasture syndrome, PSGN, interstitial nephritis), malignancy, pyelonephritis, renal thrombosis, rhabdomyolysis, tumor lysis syndrome, nephrotoxins (aminoglycosides, contrast, methanol, NSAIDs)

Postrenal
- Calculi, masses, obstructive uropathy due to strictures

Signs and Symptoms

- Oliguria, anuria
- AMS, anorexia, apathy, arrhythmia, nausea, vomiting secondary to uremia and electrolyte disturbance
- Dyspnea on exertion, rales, increased JVD, friction rub, S3, displaced PMI, tachycardia, HTN (intrarenal), hypotension (prerenal)
- Cool extremities, digital ischemia, prolonged cap refill, bilateral edema

 ALERT

Refer patient who are potentially unstable and require acute intervention to ED.

Differential Diagnosis

- *CV*: HF, hypertensive emergencies, pulmonary edema
- *GU*: ATN, CKD, hemolytic uremic syndrome, UTI, obstructive uropathy
- *HEM*: Sickle cell anemia, TTP
- *Other*: Goodpasture's syndrome postinfectious glomerulonephritis, SLE, vasculitis (immune); acidosis, DKA, hyperkalemia. hypermagnesemia, inborn errors of metabolism, rhabdomyolysis, tumor lysis syndrome (metabolic)

Diagnosis

Labs
- CMP
  - BUN and creatinine increased with decreased eGFR
  - Elevated K^+, Mg, phosphorus, and decreased HCO_3 and calcium
- ABGs
  - Uncompensated metabolic acidosis (uncompensated in AKI)
- U/A, urine for specific gravity, Na, osmolality to isolate the cause.
- CBC to evaluate for anemia, leukopenia, leukocytosis, eosinophilia, alterations in Hct, thrombocytopenia
- Serology tests for autoantibodies, serum complement
- Peripheral smear for hemolysis if immune-mediated event
- Antistreptolysin O for post-streptococcal glomerulonephritis
- Elevations in serum uric acid, CK, LDH to assess for TLS or rhabdomyolysis
- BNP level to evaluate for CHF

CLINICAL PEARL

Adults: Elevation in serum creatine 0.3 mg/dL (in 48 hr) or >50% (past 7 days) is diagnostic for AKI in adults.

Additional Diagnostic Testing
- Pulse oximetry to evaluate for hypoxia
- Chest x-ray and echocardiogram for patients with dyspnea and rales
- Bladder scan for urinary retention
- Noncontrast spiral CT or MRI to evaluate for obstruction, hydronephrosis/hydroureter
- Ultrasound for patients who are pregnant
- Renal biopsy to evaluate intrarenal causes

Treatment and Management

Treatment Goals
- Minimize progression to CKD and maintain eGFR >60. Maintain euglycemia, HbA1c <7%, and SBP <130 mmHg and promote kidney health.

Drug Treatment

PRERENAL
- For patients with mild HF with HTN, prescribe furosemide to achieve diuresis for >2 lb weight gain.
- Correct potassium level to minimize arrhythmia.
- Prescribe antiemetics and antidiarrheals judiciously in cases of gastrointestinal losses.
- Update vaccinations to prevent infection.

ALERT

Stop nephrotoxins and prescribe renal dose in all cases of AKI.

INTRARENAL
- Prescribe ACEIs or ARBs to maintain BP.
- Adjust antidiabetic therapy to achieve HbA1c <7%.
- Prescribe alpha blockers to improve urine outflow and 5-alpha-reductase inhibitors to reduce prostate size in male patients with BPH.

Interventions

- Monitor BP, HR, urine output, and fluid balance.
- Monitor BMI and electrolytes, especially sodium, potassium, phosphorus, calcium, and magnesium.
- *Control risk factors for AKI*: Avoid or manage infections and correct dehydration or fluid overload.
- Refer to urology for obstructive symptoms.
- Ensure tobacco cessation and modify ABCDE cardiovascular risk factors.
- Monitor diabetic risk factors, glycemic control, and adjust therapy as indicated.
- Treat according to the underlying source of AKI in consultation with nephrology and urology.

Patient Education

- Discuss the control of risk factors for AKI, such as dehydration, infections, BP, and BG.
- Avoid OTC, herbal, and nephrotoxins, especially OTC NSAIDs.
- Instruct in infection protection strategies.
- Avoid dehydration and maintain hydration.
- Teach s/s of complications to report.

Patient Population Considerations

Women (conception/pregnancy/lactation)

- Screen for preeclampsia with regular BP measurement throughout pregnancy.

Geriatric

- Older adults have an increased risk of AKI due to age-related decline in kidney function, decreased thirst response, comorbidities, and polypharmacology. Older males have added the burden of BPH and risk for advanced prostate cancer increasing risk for postrenal CKD.

Pediatric

- Infants are at particular risk for prerenal AKI since they are unable to communicate their need for hydration, have a higher ratio of surface area to volume and more significant fluid needs. Diarrhea is a frequent cause of prerenal AKI requiring intervention.
- All children with potential obstructive symptoms require urology consultation on the initial presentation.

Referring Patients

- Nephrology consult
- Urology consult
- Cardiology consult for ASCVD
- Rheumatology for immune-mediated disorders
- Infectious disease consult in suspected HAI or sepsis

ACUTE PYELONEPHRITIS

Overview

- Acute pyelonephritis is an upper UTI of the renal parenchyma. Bacteria, which are introduced by instrumentation, hematogenous spread, or increase in urine that is obstructed from emptying the kidney, ascend from the lower to the upper urinary tract. The microbes invade uroepithelium and trigger an inflammatory response leading to bacteremia. The inflammation, with or without obstruction, can cause hydronephrosis and renal damage. Fibrotic changes and atrophy can result from uncorrected obstruction and lead to chronic pyelonephritis.

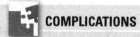

COMPLICATIONS

Acute: EPN, perinephric abscess, AKI, sepsis, hydronephrosis/hydroureter

Chronic: Chronic pyelonephritis, CKD

Etiology

- *Escherichia coli* are responsible for 70% to 90% of cases.
  - Consider *Enterobacter, Enterococci, Klebsiella, Proteus, Pseudomonas, Staphylococcus* as alternative
- UTI from sexual activity in women
- Obstructive uropathy
- Introduction of bacteria from instrumentation during procedures and surgery
- Bacteremia due to endocarditis, IVDA

 ALERT

Criteria for Referral to ED

Consider impending septic shock in patients with qSOFA score of ≥2 points
- SBP ≤100 mm Hg
- RR ≥22 breaths/min
- AMS (GCS score <15)

Signs and Symptoms

- Abdominal or flank pain, CVA tenderness, fever, nausea/vomiting
- *Recent or current UTI*: Dysuria, frequency, hematuria, pain, urgency
- Chronic constipation in children

Differential Diagnosis

- *GI*: Acute abdomen: appendicitis, diverticulitis
- *GU*: Acute and chronic prostatitis, cystitis, nephrolithiasis, retroperitoneal mass, urethritis
- *GYN*: Cervicitis, endometritis, PID

Diagnosis

Labs
- Clean catch U/A and urine c/s in ages 6 and older
  - Urinary catheterization if the patient is unable to perform collection.
  - *U/A*: Increased nitrites, LET >10 WBC, WBC >5 to 10, increased microscopic or gross RBCs, increased WBC casts, increased nitrites
- CBC to evaluate WBCs
- BMP to assess renal function and electrolytes

Additional Diagnostic Testing
- Contrast spiral CT is the gold standard if eGFR ≥30 mL/min
- MRI (pregnancy) or ultrasound (ultrasound does not exclude pyelonephritis)
- Tc-DMSA scintigraphy is preferred in children.
- CT and MR urography is replacing IV pyelogram.

Treatment and Management

Treatment Goals
- Prevention of recurrence, sepsis, and complications

Drug Treatment
Manage uncomplicated infection in the primary care setting.
- Prescribe ciprofloxacin 500 mg PO BID for 7 days.
- *Consider alternatives*: Amoxicillin and clavulanic acid, cefepime, TMP-SMX.
- Consider urinary analgesic phenazopyridine.
- Use caution with antipyretics that mask sepsis.

 ALERT

Fluoroquinolones Resistance

Consider single dose of parenteral antibiotics (ceftriaxone or an aminoglycoside) followed by oral therapy with TMP-SMX if suspected.

Interventions
- Assess hydration status, weight, I/O to evaluate for AKI.
- Follow up in 48 hr to adjust antibiotics with culture results.

Patient Education
- Instruct the patient to complete the entire course of antibiotics.
- Encourage oral fluids to replace losses and electrolytes from vomiting.
- Teach patient s/s of complications to report.
- Follow up with HCP within 48 hr.

Patient Population Considerations

Women (conception/pregnancy/lactation)
- It is essential to reinforce perineal hygiene throughout the pregnancy to prevent infection. Obtain a screening urine c/s at 16 weeks' gestation. Avoid fluoroquinolones or aminoglycosides in pregnant patients.

Geriatric
- Patients >80 years have an increased risk of septic shock.

Pediatric
- Refer pediatric patients for urologic evaluation with the first episode to rule out structural abnormalities.

Referring Patients
- Urology consult
- Infectious disease consult

NEPHROLITHIASIS

Overview
- Renal calculi coalesce from stone-forming crystals in the kidney that enlarge and lodge in the GU tract, causing an obstruction.
- Crystals identified in calculi include calcium (most common), oxalate, uric acid, phosphorus, cystine, xanthine, and drug precipitates.
- A high concentration of crystals in urine in the presence of dehydration favor aggregation and formation.

COMPLICATIONS

Acute: Acute pain, obstructive uropathy/nephropathy, postrenal AKI, ascending UTI, urosepsis

Chronic: Recurrent renal colic, chronic UTI, CKD

Etiology
- Dehydration, pregnancy, immobilization
- *Disease risks*: CKD, PKD, type 2 DM, hyperthyroidism, hyperparathyroidism, osteoporosis, malignancy, gout, IBD, obesity, chronic UTI/neurogenic bladder, sarcoidosis, Sjögren's syndrome, anorexia/bulimia
- Family or personal history
- High sodium, oxalate, animal protein diet based on stone type
- *Medications*: Sulfa agents, diuretics, calcium-based antacids, antiretrovirals, cephalosporins, quinolones, topiramate

CLINICAL PEARL

Factors most predictive of calculi follow **STONE criteria:**

S: Male sex

T: Short duration of pain

O: Of non-Black race

N: Nausea/vomiting

E: Erythrocytes (hematuria)

Signs and Symptoms

- Sudden onset severe flank pain radiating to the groin that is colicky
- Nausea/vomiting
- S/s of UTI may be present
- Microscopic/gross hematuria

Differential Diagnosis

- *GI*: Acute abdomen, appendicitis, bowel obstruction, cholecystitis, cholelithiasis diverticulitis, gastroenteritis, inflammatory bowel disease, pancreatitis
- *GU*: Acute glomerulonephritis, UTI, vesicoureteral reflux

Diagnosis

Labs

- U/A to assess for microscopic versus gross hematuria and evaluate urinary pH
  - Absence of RBCs does not exclude nephrolithiasis.
  - A pH >7 is associated with struvite; a pH <5 is seen with uric acid.
  - Indication of infection and AKI may be present based on the severity.
  - WBC >5 to 10 requires evaluation for hydronephrosis.
- Strain all urine for calculi and send to the lab to evaluate crystals.
- BMP to evaluate renal function and hydration
- Serum calcium, uric acid, PTH, and phosphorus
- CBC to evaluate for infection
  - Bands, WBC <4 or greater than 11 require ED referral
- Consider 24-hr urine collection

Additional Diagnostic Testing

- KUB x-ray to evaluate radiopaque stones
- Noncontrast spiral or plain CT of kidneys
- Ultrasound for patients who are pregnant or who have suspected hydronephrosis

Treatment and Management

Treatment Goals

- Manage pain, promote stone passage, hydration, encourage BMI <25, and adherence to dietary instruction according to type
- Prevention of recurrence and complications

Drug Treatment

- *Pain management*: Prescribed NSAIDs are the first choice, followed by opioids and desmopressin acetate.
- *Stone passage*: Prescribe terazosin, nifedipine, and tamsulosin to facilitate stone passage.
- *Additional therapy*:
  - Prescribe thiazide diuretics in the presence of high urine calcium and recurrent calcium stones.
  - Increase urinary pH with potassium citrate therapy to recurrent calcium, cystine, and uric acid stones.
  - Prescribe allopurinol to patients with calcium oxalate stones with hyperuricemia. Avoid in patients with uric acid stones.
  - Consider antiemetics for nausea/vomiting.

 CLINICAL PEARL

Pain Management

Best Practice to Minimize Opioid Abuse
- *Mild to moderate/tolerating PO*: Oral agents preferred. NSAIDs are first choice with opioid for breakthrough pain.
- *Moderate to severe/NPO*: Ketorolac IM/IV/intranasal if CrCl >30 mL/min. Parenteral opioid for breakthrough pain.
- **Consider DDAVP IV/intranasal** to reduce intraureteral pressure to relieve pain.

Interventions

- Strain all urine. Refer patients with large stones immediately to urology.
- Monitor response to pain management.
- Monitor for development of AKI and UTI.
- Prescribe hydration to achieve a urine output of 2.5 L.

Patient Education

- Teach the patient to increase fluid intake.
- Instruct the patient to maintain optimal body weight to reduce risk.
- Provide dietary instructions according to the type of stone.
- Instruct patient in s/s of complications to report.

Patient Population Considerations

Women (conception/pregnancy/lactation)

- Consider acetaminophen for mild to moderate pain with pregnancy as opioids cross the placenta and cause fetal respiratory depression.
- Ultrasound followed by MRI should be used for diagnostic testing in pregnant patients.

Geriatric

- The first event of renal colic is not likely in the older adult. Consider disease and medication risk factors as a possible cause. Be mindful that renal function declines with age.

Pediatric

- Ureteroscopy is the most common approach for children requiring nephrolithiasis treatment.

Referring Patients

- Urology consult

ALERT

Calcium: Limit Na and nondairy animal protein, consume 1 to 2 g of calcium daily and increase fruits and vegetables.

Calcium oxalate: Limit oxalate-rich foods (black tea, cocoa, nuts, Swiss chard, spinach, rhubarb, and beet greens), Na, and animal protein, and consume 1 to 2 g of calcium daily.

Uric acid stones: Limit intake of non-dairy animal proteins and lose weight if indicated.

POP QUIZ 8.1

A 25-year-old male presents to the walk-in clinic complaining of severe flank pain, nausea, and vomiting scaled at 10/10 that has gotten progressively worse over the past several days. The pain is described as continuous aching with intermittent stabbing pain radiating to his right groin. Patient denies chronic health conditions or medication use. *Vital signs*: HR 121; RR 20; T 101.1°F (38.4°C); BP 148/80. Pertinent exam findings include *CV*: No JVD, HT, S1, S2, no murmur, or S3. *Lungs*: CTA. *Abdomen*: last BM formed, brown. Abdomen round, BS normoactive, voluntary guarding, no rebound tenderness, and increased CVA tenderness.

What is the most likely diagnosis, and what is the next step in care?

URINARY INCONTINENCE

Overview

- Incontinence is an involuntary leakage of urine. The types are classified as follows:
  - *Stress*: Leakage due to increased abdominal pressure
  - *Urge*: Sudden urge to void
  - *Overflow*: Loss of urine when the bladder is full
  - *Functional*: Physical disability or barrier
  - *Reflex incontinence*: Nerve damage
  - *Mixed*: A combination of stress and urge
  - *Nocturnal enuresis*: Involuntary nighttime loss
- Incontinence can occur as a result of pelvic floor weakness, detrusor muscle dysfunction, urethral sphincter incompetence or impaired bladder contractility, barriers, instrumentation, or alternative pathology causing UAB or OAB.

COMPLICATIONS

Acute: Psychological stress, anxiety, acute urinary retention, autonomic dysreflexia in SCI

Chronic (Initial): Social isolation, alteration in intimacy and sexuality, increased sedentary lifestyle

Chronic (Refractory): Recurrent UTI, chronic urinary retention, pressure injury, CKD

Etiology

- *Increased abdominal pressure/pelvic floor weakness:* Pregnancy, obesity, multipara, increased age
- *Increased urine retention:* BOO (prostatic enlargement, surgical trauma, pelvic organ prolapses, tumor, neoplasm), medications (antihistamines, TCA, opioids, sympathomimetics, muscle relaxants, anticholinergics)
- *Neuropathic/detrusor muscle dysfunction (UAB):* Neurodegenerative disease, stroke, DM, SCI
- *OAB contractility:* Bladder irritants (caffeine, alcohol, tobacco), neuropathy, CNS disorders
- Patients with neurologic disorders may have a combination of UAB and OAB.

Signs and Symptoms

- Change in cognition, sensation, mobility, dexterity
- Continuous or spontaneous urine loss
- Increased nocturia, daytime frequency, hesitancy, or change in stream
- Palpable bladder, a sensation of incomplete emptying
- Urine loss while laughing, sneezing, lifting, or with an urge to urinate

 CLINICAL PEARL

Nocturnal polyuria in the adult is an early sign of CKD secondary to Na losses at the renal tubules.

Differential Diagnosis

- *ENDO:* Diabetes insipidus, SIADH
- *GU:* UTI, pyelonephritis
- *PSYCH:* Psychogenic polydipsia
- *Other:* Transient incontinence due to delirium, UTI, medications, immobility, fecal impaction
  - *Males:* BPH, prostate cancer, UTI, prostatitis, prostatectomy, priapism
  - *Females:* UTI in pregnancy, uterine prolapse, vesicovaginal fist

Diagnosis

Labs
- U/A, CBC to exclude infection
- BMP, eGFR to stage for CKD
- Elevated prostate-specific antigen with BPH
- Urine cytology with painless hematuria to evaluate for cancer, if needed

 ALERT

Transient incontinence due to delirium, UTI, medications, immobility, fecal impaction should be excluded in workup.

Additional Diagnostic Testing
- PVR >300 mL on two visits over 6 months defines chronic retention
- Urodynamic testing in complicated cases of OAB

Treatment and Management

Treatment Goals
- Correction or management of underlying causes and prevention of complications
- *OAB:* Target urination every 3 to 4 hr, *UAB:* target: UO 1 to 1.5 L/d
- A decrease in episodes of nocturia, PVR <300 mL, and no s/s of AKI/CKD

Drug Treatment
OAB
- Prescribe oral antimuscarinic (oxybutynin) or oral beta 3-adrenoceptor agonists (mirabegron) as second-line therapy, if not at goal.
- Consider intradetrusor onabotulinumtoxinA (100 U) injections for third-line therapy, if needed.

ALERT

Anticholinergic medications are contraindicated in patients with narrow angle-closure glaucoma.

UAB

- *Chronic urinary retention (male/female)*: Tamsulosin (an alpha-blocker) to relax sympathetic inhibition of urine flow; bethanechol (cholinergic) to improve bladder contraction and emptying.
- Consider 5-alpha-reductase inhibitors in males with BPH.

Interventions

GENERAL

- Correct underlying conditions and initiate behavioral therapy as first-line therapy.

STRESS INCONTINENCE

- Consider topical estrogens for atrophy and surgical consult to increase urethral outlet resistance if indicated.

UAB AND OVERFLOW INCONTINENCE

- Develop a catheterization regimen with patients who have neurodegenerative disorders and SCI.
- Consider a surgical consult for urinary diversion in addition to medications for chronic urinary retention.

ALERT

(First-Line Therapy)
- Schedule bathroom visits.
- Delay urination by 5 to 10 min to train bladder to hold more urine.
- Perform Kegel exercises.
- Manage fluid intake 6 to 8 glasses per day.

OAB

- Offer PTNS or sacral neuromodulation for third-line therapy if the patient is not a candidate for intradetrusor onabotulinumtoxinA injections and medication is ineffective.
- Monitor for PVR >300 mL.

FUNCTIONAL INCONTINENCE

- Collaborate with OT/PT to remove barriers to micturition and encourage home health services as needed to avoid skin breakdown.

Patient Education

- Instruct in use of absorbent products and barriers to protect skin integrity.
- Teach how to perform Kegel exercises to strengthen pelvic muscles.
- Explain risk factors for incontinence, such as avoiding constipation, smoking cessation, losing weight, and eliminating bladder irritants from the diet.
- Utilize bladder training to reduce and delay the urge to urinate.
- In neurogenic bladder, teach clean intermittent catheterization.
- Avoid using the Credé's maneuver in patients with neurogenic bladder.
- Report s/s of UTI, urinary retention, and adverse effects of medication immediately.

Patient Population Considerations

Women (conception/pregnancy/lactation)

- Instruct pregnant patients that incontinence is common. Review stress incontinence instructions and encourage patients to maintain appropriate weight gain for gestation.

Geriatric

- Monitor for impaired cognition closely to avoid dehydration.
- Collaborate with the physician as necessary according to state guidelines for home care evaluation.
- Provide instruction to family and caregivers on safety hazards that could increase the risk of falls in the event of nocturia.

Pediatric

- Evaluate constipation in all cases of pediatric incontinence.
- Reassure the family that most cases of enuresis abate with age.

Referring Patients

- Urology consult
- Infectious disease consult

URINARY TRACT INFECTION

Overview

- UTI is an infection of the bladder. Microbiol invasion and proliferation in epithelium trigger inflammation. Organisms can migrate into the systemic circulation, causing urosepsis. Ascension and reflux can cause pyelonephritis, hydronephrosis, and AKI. Host factors and functional and structural anomalies can cause recurrence.
- Immunosuppression, pregnancy, DM, and functional and structural anomalies can cause complicated UTI, which requires careful monitoring for CKD progression.

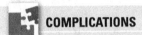 **COMPLICATIONS**

Acute: Pyelonephritis, AKI, sepsis, hydronephrosis/hydroureter
Chronic: Recurrent UTI and CKD

Etiology

- *Escherichia coli* is the most common causative organism; polymicrobiology may occur with instrumentation
- Advancing age, hygiene, pregnancy, sexual activity
- Structural or functional anomalies (urethral strictures, bladder stones, prolapse, prostatic enlargement, neurogenic bladder, estrogen loss)
- Instrumentation and surgery
- Cancer, DM, immunocompetence, immunosuppressive therapy, renal insufficiency, neurogenic bladder, SCI

CLINICAL PEARL

Prevalence of drug resistance to TMP-SMX, nitrofurantoin, fluoroquinolones, and first-generation cephalosporins requires careful monitoring of culture results and adjustment of therapy as indicated.

Signs and Symptoms

- Dysuria, frequency, urgency, bladder fullness, suprapubic tenderness
- Absent flank pain, nausea/vomiting, CVA tenderness
- No cervical motion tenderness, vaginal discharge in female, no scrotal enlargement mass in male
- Fever, chills, and malaise are more frequently seen in acute pyelonephritis than UTI.

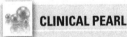 **CLINICAL PEARL**

DM, indwelling urinary catheters, and antibiotic use are risk factors for candiduria.

Differential Diagnosis

- *GU*: Acute and chronic prostatitis, acute urethritis, acute pyelonephritis, bladder irritants, epididymitis, interstitial bladder pain syndrome, masses, malignancy, OAB, orchitis, PKD, perinephric abscess, strictures, urethral syndrome
- *GYN*: Cervicitis, PID, vaginitis
- *REPRO*: Chlamydia, herpes simplex, gonorrhea

Diagnosis

Labs

- Clean catch U/A and urine c/s in ages 6 and older
  - Urinary catheterization if unable to perform collection
    - UCG in women of childbearing age
- *U/A*: WBC >10, increased nitrites, increased LET, increased microscopic or gross RBCs, increased low-grade protein, negative for WBC casts
  - If U/A is negative, await culture results before treating

 ALERT

UTI with 2 qSOFA signs should be referred to ED immediately.

Elevated PVR should be referred to urology.

Additional Diagnostic Testing

- Bladder scan to evaluate PVR

Treatment and Management

Treatment Goals

- Treat infection, manage symptoms, and prevent sepsis.

Drug Treatment

- *Do not treat asymptomatic bacteriuria. Asymptomatic bacteremia is colonization, not infection.*
- Prescribe acetaminophen for pain. If ineffective, consider urinary analgesic, phenazopyridine, for 1 to 2 days.
- *Nonpregnant female*:
  - *First-line therapy*:
    - Use nitrofurantoin, TMP-SMX, or fosfomycin 3 g as a single dose or equivalent.
  - *Second-line therapy*:
    - Prescribe amoxicillin–clavulanate or ciprofloxacin.
    - Consider topical estrogen therapy for women with vulvovaginal atrophy with recurrent UTI.
- *Complicated female and male patients*:
  - Prescribe a fluoroquinolone, TMP-SMX, minocycline, or nitrofurantoin.

Interventions

- Assess hydration status, weight, and I/O to evaluate for AKI; and encourage hydration.
- Follow up in 48 hr using culture results to adjust therapy.

Patient Education

- Instruct the patient to complete the entire course of antibiotics.
- Encourage patients to maintain hydration and avoid dehydration.
- Provide perineal hygiene recommendations for female patients.
- Take cranberry prophylaxis daily to reduce the incidence of recurrent UTI.
- Follow up with HCP within 48 to 72 hr.
- Teach patient s/s of complications to report.

Patient Population Considerations

Women (conception/pregnancy/lactation)

- Obtain a screening urine c/s at 16 weeks' gestation and treat for asymptomatic bacteriuria. Reinforce hygiene. Avoid fluoroquinolones or aminoglycosides in pregnant patients.

Geriatric

- Estrogen loss in female patients increases the risk of UTI, while prostatic enlargement increases the risk for recurrent UTI in male patients. Decreased host defenses in both genders increase the risk of urosepsis in the geriatric population.

Pediatric

- Admit patients who are septic, unable to tolerate anything by mouth, obstructive symptoms age less than 1 month. Febrile infants younger than 2 months should be evaluated for UTI and treated as acute pyelonephritis.

Referring Patients

- Urology consult for obstructive uropathy/ nephropathy
- Infectious disease consult in suspected HAI or sepsis

POP QUIZ 8.2

A 23-year-old female presents to primary care for multiple UTIs over the past 6 months, treated with amoxicillin at the walk-in clinic near her college. She has had no other diagnostic evaluation other than urine dipstick. She reports drinking diet green tea to try and "cure" it and increasing fluid intake with no relief. What details should be obtained in the history and what labs should be ordered?

RESOURCES

American Urological Association. (2016). *Non-neurogenic chronic urinary retention:* Consensus definition, management strategies, and future opportunities. https://www.auanet.org/guidelines/chronic-urinary-retention

American Urological Association. (2019a). *Diagnosis and treatment of overactive bladder (non-neurogenic) in adults: AUA/SUFU guideline.* https://www.auanet.org/guidelines/overactive-bladder-(oab)-guideline.

American Urological Association. (2019b). *Medical management of kidney stones: AUA guidelines.* Reviewed. 2019. https://www.auanet.org/documents/education/clinical-guidance/Medical-Management-of-Kidney-Stones.pdf

American Urological Association. (2019c). *Recurrent uncomplicated urinary tract infections in women: AUA/CUA/ SUFU guideline.* https://www.auanet.org/documents/Guidelines/PDF/rUTI-guideline.pdf

Brusch, J. (2020). *Medscape: Urinary tract infection and cystitis in females.* https://emedicine.medscape.com/ article/233101-overview

Brusch, J. (2020). *Medscape: Urinary tract infection (UTI) in males.* https://emedicine.medscape.com/ article/231574-overview

Cash, J. C., & Glass, C. A. (Eds.). (2019). *Adult-gerontology practice guidelines.* Springer Publishing Company.

Chaker, L., Bianco, A. C., Jonklaas, J., & Peeters, R. (2017). Hypothyroidism. *Lancet, 390,* 1550–1562. https://doi. org/10.1016/S0140-6736(17)30703-1

Codina Leik, M. T. (2018). *Family nurse practitioner certification: Intensive review.* Springer Publishing Company.

Dave, C. (2020). *Medscape: Nephrolithiasis.* https://emedicine.medscape.com/article/437096-overview

Drake, M. T. (2018). Hypothyroidism in clinical practice. *Mayo Clinic Proceedings, 93*(9), 1169–1172. https://doi. org/10.1016/j.mayocp.2018.07.015

Fischer, D. (2019). *Medscape: Pediatric urinary tract infection.* https://emedicine.medscape.com/ article/969643-overview

Fulop, T. (2019). *Medscape: Acute pyelonephritis.* https://emedicine.medscape.com/article/245559-overview

Gill, B. (2018). *Medscape: Neurogenic bladder.* https://emedicine.medscape.com/article/453539-overview#a7

Hsiao, C. Y., Chen, T. H., Lee, Y. C., Hsiao, M. C., Hung, P. H., & Wang, M. C. (2020). Risk factors for uroseptic shock in hospitalized patients aged over 80 years with urinary tract infection. *Annals of Translational Medicine, 8*(7), 477. https://doi.org/10.21037/atm.2020.03.95

Hughes, P. J. (2018). *Medscape: Classification systems for acute kidney injury.* https://emedicine.medscape.com/ article/233101-overview

Levy, M. M., Evans, L. E., & Rhodes, A. (2018). The surviving sepsis campaign bundle: 2018 update. *Intensive Care Medicine, 44,* 925–928. https://doi.org/10.1007/s00134-018-5085-0

Moore, D. (2018). Hypothyroidism and nursing care. *American Nurse Today, 13*(2), 44–46. https://www.auanet.org/ guidelines/chronic-urinary retention/

Sekido, N., Igawa, Y., Kakizaki, H., Kitta, T., Sengoku, A., Takahashi, S., Takahashi, R., Tanaka, K., Namima, T., Honda, M., Mitsui, T., Yamanish, T., & Watanabe, T. (2020). Clinical guidelines for the diagnosis and treatment of lower urinary tract dysfunction in patients with spinal cord injury. *International Journal of Urology, 27*(4), 276–288. https://doi.org/10.1111/iju.14186

Soler, Y. A., Nieves-Plaza, M., Prieto, M., García-De Jesús, R., & Suárez-Rivera, M. (2013). Pediatric risk, injury, failure, loss, end-stage renal disease score identifies acute kidney injury and predicts mortality in critically ill children: A prospective study. *Pediatric Critical Care Medicine: A Journal of the Society of Critical Care Medicine and the World Federation of Pediatric Intensive and Critical Care Societies, 14*(4), e189–e195. https://doi. org/10.1097/PCC.0b013e3182745675

Sorenson, M., Quinn, L., & Klein, D. (2019). *Pathophysiology: Concepts of human disease* (1st ed.). Pearson Education.

Stewart, J. G., & Dennert, N. L. (2017). *Family nurse practitioner: Certification review.* Jones & Bartlett Learning.

Vasavada, S. (2019). *Medscape: Urinary incontinence.* https://emedicine.medscape.com/article/453539-overview#a7

Ward, J. B., Feinstein, L., Pierce, C., Lim, J., Abbott, K. C., Bavendam, T., Kirkali, Z., Matlaga, B. R., & The NIDDK Urologic Diseases in America Project. (2019). Pediatric urinary stone disease in the United States: The Urologic Diseases in America Project. *Urology, 129*, 180–187. https://doi.org/10.1016/j.urology.2019.04.012

Washinger, K. (2017). Acute kidney injury in adults: An underdiagnosed condition. *The Journal for Nurse Practitioners, 13*(10), 667–671. https://doi.org/10.1016/j.nurpra.2017.08.005

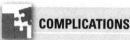

9

ENDOCRINE SYSTEM

DIABETES MELLITUS: TYPE 1

Overview

- Type 1 diabetes is a chronic, progressive, immune-mediated metabolic disorder.
- Destruction of beta cells in the pancreas leads to insulin deficiency resulting in hyperglycemia that compromises carbohydrate, fat, and protein metabolism and leads to acute and chronic complications. DKA may be the first manifestation of type 1 diabetes in children, adolescents, or LADA in early to mid-adulthood (30–40 years).

 COMPLICATIONS

Acute: DKA and hypoglycemia secondary to excess exogenous insulin

Chronic (microvascular): Retinopathy, angiopathy, nephropathy, and neuropathy

Chronic (macrovascular): ASCVHD, HTN, HF, CVD, PAD, stroke

Etiology

- Autoimmune in origin
- Genetic predisposition
- Environmental triggers; viral infection, exposure to cow milk in infancy

Signs and Symptoms

- *Classic symptoms*: Polyuria, polydipsia, and polyphagia
- Unintentional weight loss, anorexia, nausea, and vomiting
- Blurred vision
- Weakness, lack of energy, and fatigue
- Presence of an antecedent event that triggers hyperglycemia
- Acetone breath with DKA

ALERT

DKA can manifest with infection, MI, stroke, pancreatitis, insufficient insulin, or in the newly diagnosed.

Onset of DKA may be sudden in patients using insulin pumps due to absolute insulin deficiency.

Differential Diagnosis

- Type 2 diabetes
- Secondary hyperglycemia (medication-induced, adrenal/pituitary tumors, hypercortisolism, excess catecholamines, growth hormone, thyroid disorders)
- Chronic pancreatitis
- Cystic fibrosis

Diagnosis

Labs

- Must meet one of the following criteria *confirmed by repeat testing* on separate days unless there are signs and symptoms of a hyperglycemic crisis and the random plasma glucose ≥200 mg/dL
  - Elevated HbA1c >6.5%
  - Fasting plasma glucose ≥126 mg/dL
  - Two-hour postprandial plasma glucose ≥200 mg/dL during oral glucose tolerance test

Additional Diagnostic Testing

- *Lipid panel:* LDL-C >100 mg/dL
- Urinalysis for microscopic albumin
- Autoantibody testing may be considered
- Pertinent diagnostic testing for antecedent event, if suspected

Treatment and Management

Treatment Goals

- Self-management of glucose to maintain A1c <7% using nutrition, weight management, exercise, and insulin
- Premeal glucose level 80 to 130 mg/dL, random glucose <140 mg/dL

ALERT

During the honeymoon period following diagnosis of type 1 diabetes, insulin requirements may be decreased.

Drug Treatment

- Initiate intensive insulin therapy (basal/bolus) with SMBG:
  - Prescribe blood pressure control with ACEI/ARB to maintain BP <140/90 and lipid management with statins.
  - Prescribe SMBG using technology guided by patient preference and ability. (Real-time continuous monitoring [CGM] can improve glycemic control).
- Perform medication reconciliation at each visit to identify agents that can increase BG.

Interventions

- Initiate tobacco cessation protocol and diabetes education.
- Assess ASCVD risk assessment and CKD stage and examine feet.
- Provide for a follow-up to adjust therapy based on target HbA1c/BG.
- Provide immunizations based on age and health and instruction in infection protection.
- Admit to hospital for suspected DKA.
- If DKA is suspected, monitor for hypotension, unintentional weight loss, intake, and output. Correct fluid, electrolyte, and BG imbalances.

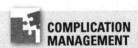

COMPLICATION MANAGEMENT

DKA requires administration of IV insulin, IV hydration, electrolyte replacements of K⁺, Mg⁺, Ca⁺, Phos⁺, and correction of precipitating event.

Patient Education

- Teach SMBG and insulin administration.
- Evaluate the ability to use prescribed devices to monitor BG and administer insulin.
- Instruct patient and family in hypoglycemia management for conscious and unconscious states.
  - Explain sick day guidelines to continue insulin, hydration, and criteria for consultation.
  - Provide instruction in medical nutrition therapy and optimal BMI.
  - *Teach exercise guidelines:* 150 min/wk for adults; 60 min/d for children <age 18.
  - Provide education and risks associated with alcohol consumption.
  - Teach foot care guidelines to reduce the risk of injury and complications.

Patient Population Considerations

Women (conception/pregnancy/lactation)
- Optimize HbA1c before conception.
- Perform medication reconciliation, including OTC and nutraceuticals to ensure safety.
- Increase the frequency of SMBG during pregnancy.

Geriatric
- Target HbA1c of <8%.
- Include caregivers in education.
- Screen older adults (aged >65 years) for cognitive impairment and depression.

Pediatric
- Target HbA1c of <7.5%.
  - Include parent/guardians in education.
  - Assess psychosocial issues and family stresses that could impact diabetes management.
  - Screen for disordered eating disorders beginning in children age 10 to 12.

Referring Patients

- Ophthalmology examination annually after 3 to 5 years from diagnosis
- Podiatry examination annually to evaluate for neuropathy
- Cardiology consult for hyperlipidemia, CVD, HTN, HF
- Nephrology consult for presence of microalbuminuria
- Mental health consult for stress and coping strategies if needed

DIABETES MELLITUS: TYPE 2

Overview

- Type 2 diabetes is a chronic metabolic disorder marked by increased insulin resistance and impaired insulin production, or excessive glucagon production resulting in hyperglycemia and hyperinsulinemia.
- The disorder affects the metabolism of carbohydrates, fats, and proteins and can lead to acute and chronic complications.
- Onset can begin in childhood, with the incidence increasing in the presence of elevated BMI.

COMPLICATIONS

Acute: HHS and hypoglycemia secondary to excess insulin secretagogues or insulin

Chronic (microvascular): Retinopathy, angiopathy, nephropathy, and neuropathy

Chronic (macrovascular: ASCVHD, HTN, HF, CVD, PAD, stroke

Etiology

- Interaction with genetics and environment
- Family history
- Obesity
- *Ethnicity*: Hispanic, Native American, African American, Asian American, Pacific Islander
- History of previously impaired glucose tolerance, gestational diabetes
- Acanthosis nigricans
- Medications that increase glucose
- Polycystic ovarian syndrome
- *Metabolic syndrome*: Impaired fasting glucose, hypertension, dyslipidemia, abdominal obesity
- Infections such as COVID-19

Signs and Symptoms

- May be asymptomatic
- *Classic symptoms*: Polyuria, polydipsia, and polyphagia
- Dehydration with sudden weight loss, anorexia, nausea, and vomiting
- Blurred vision
- Weakness, lack of energy, and fatigue
- Presence of an antecedent event that triggers hyperglycemia
- Numbness or tingling in the feet or hands

 CLINICAL PEARL

Newly diagnosed patients with type 2 DM are more likely to present with microvascular or macrovascular disorders as opposed to patients newly diagnosed with type 1 DM. Screen patients presenting with these disorders for hyperglycemia.

Differential Diagnosis

- Type 1 diabetes
- LADA
- Secondary hyperglycemia (medication-induced, adrenal/pituitary tumors, hypercortisolism, excess catecholamines, growth hormone, thyroid disorders)
- Chronic pancreatitis
- Cystic fibrosis

ALERT

HHS can manifest with infection, MI, stroke, pancreatitis, insufficient antidiabetic therapy or addition of agents that increase BG.

Diagnosis

Labs
- Initiate risk-based screening after age 10 or the onset of puberty. Must meet one of the following criteria confirmed by **repeat testing** on separate days unless there are signs and symptoms of a hyperglycemic crisis and the random plasma glucose ≥200 mg/dL:
  - Fasting plasma glucose ≥126 mg/dL
  - Elevated HbA1c >6.5%
  - Two-hour postprandial plasma glucose ≥200 mg/dL during oral glucose tolerance test

Additional Diagnostic Testing
- *Lipid panel*: LDL-C >100 mg/dL
- Urinalysis for microscopic albumin
- Pertinent diagnostic testing for antecedent event, if suspected

Treatment and Management

Treatment Goals
- Self-management of glucose to maintain HbA1c <7% using nutrition, weight management, exercise, and antidiabetic therapy
- Premeal glucose level 80 to −130 mg/dL

Drug Treatment
- Initiate metformin with SMBG using technology according to patient preference and ability.
- Prescribe dual-drug therapy with oral agents and/or insulin based on the presence of comorbidities if the patient is *not at HbA1c goal*.
- Control blood pressure with ACEIs/ARBs.
- Manage lipids with statins.
- Perform medication reconciliation at each visit to identify agents that can increase glucose.

Interventions
- Initiate tobacco cessation protocol and diabetes education.
- Assess 10-year ASCVD risk assessment, CKD stage, and examine feet.

- Encourage behavioral therapy in addition to diet and exercise in the presence of obesity, followed by pharmacotherapy and metabolic surgery. (*Note*: Insulin secretagogues, thiazolidinediones, and insulin can cause weight gain.)
- Provide for a follow-up to adjust therapy based on target HbA1c/BG.
- Provide immunizations based on age and health and instruction in infection protection.
- Admit to hospital for suspected HHS.
- *If HHS is suspected*: Monitor for hypotension, unintentional weight loss, intake and output, and correct fluid, electrolyte, and BG imbalances.

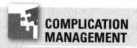

COMPLICATION MANAGEMENT

HHS has slower onset than DKA with higher plasma glucose. Like type 1 DM, it is triggered by an antecedent event. Prescribe IV insulin, IV hydration, and replace electrolytes K+, Mg+, Ca+, Phos+.

Correct precipitating event.

Patient Education

- Teach self-management of BG and lifestyle modifications.
- Instruct patients when making an appointment for any radiologic exam to notify the practice that they are on metformin, as they may need to withhold the medication prior to contrast studies.
- Instruct in hypoglycemia management for conscious and unconscious states once hypoglycemic agents are initiated.
- Explain sick day guidelines and provide criteria for consultation.
- Provide instruction in medical nutrition therapy.
- Evaluate the ability to use prescribed devices to SMBG and administer insulin, if needed.
- *Teach exercise guidelines*: 150 min/wk for adults; 60 min/d for children <age 18.
- Provide education and risks associated with alcohol consumption.
- Teach foot care guidelines to reduce the risk of injury and complications.

Patient Population Considerations

Women (conception/pregnancy/lactation)

- Optimize HbA1c prior to conception and refer to a multidisciplinary clinic with pregnancy.
- Switch to insulin during pregnancy since antidiabetics cross the placenta.
- Increase the frequency of SMBG during pregnancy.

Geriatric

- Target HbA1c of <8%.
- Include caregivers in education.
- Avoid crowds and people who are ill during influenza season.

Pediatric

- Target HbA1c of <7.5%.
- *Exercise*: 60 min daily for patients <18 years old.
- Include parent/guardians in education.
- Assess psychosocial issues and family stresses that could impact diabetes management.

Other

- The cut-off for treatment for patients of Asian descent is a BMI of 23 as opposed to 25.

Referring Patients

- Diabetes self-management program
- Bariatric surgery consult in patients who are morbidly obese
- Ophthalmology examination annually after 3 to 5 years from diagnosis

POP QUIZ 9.1

An adolescent patient with type 2 diabetes using an insulin pump and metformin is diagnosed with influenza and will be managed at home. What instructions regarding their diabetes management should be provided?

(continued)

Referring Patients (*continued*)

- Podiatry examination annually to evaluate for neuropathy
- Cardiology consult for hyperlipidemia, CVD, hypertension
- Nephrology consult for presence of microalbuminuria
- Mental health consult for ineffective stress and coping, if needed

HYPERTHYROIDISM (GRAVES' DISEASE)

Overview

- The most common causes of overactivity of the thyroid gland are Graves' disease, multinodular goiter, toxic adenoma, and painless thyroiditis.
- Graves' disease is a chronic, immune-mediated disorder of excess synthesis and secretion of thyroid hormone resulting in a hypermetabolic state, associated with exophthalmos and dermopathy.

> **COMPLICATIONS**
>
> *Acute*: Thyrotoxicosis/thyroid storm
> *Chronic*: Arrhythmia, CVD, cardiomyopathy, nephrolithiasis, osteoporosis, anxiety disorder, preeclampsia

Etiology

- Autoimmune in origin (Graves' disease)
- Family history (Graves' disease)
- Type 1 DM, primary adrenal insufficiency, and pernicious anemia
- Female gender
- Cigarette smoking
- *Ethnicity*: African American and Asian
- *Drug-induced*: Amiodarone, lithium, iodine contrast, excess thyroid hormone replacement
- High iodine intake

> **CLINICAL PEARL**
>
> The presence of Graves' disease has been associated with *polyglandular autoimmune syndrome Type 1* including pernicious anemia, vitiligo, Sjogren's syndrome, RA, SLE, systemic sclerosis, type 1 DM, Addison's disease, and myasthenia gravis.

Signs and Symptoms

- Unintentional weight loss
- Heat intolerance and diaphoresis
- Graves' triad of exophthalmos, pretibial myxedema, goiter
- *Cardio*: Tachycardia, hypertension, systolic murmurs, atrial fibrillation, palpitations
- *GI*: Increased frequency of bowel movements and diarrhea
- *Neuro*: Anxiety, nervousness, restlessness, tremors, hyperactive deep tendon reflexes, psychosis, fatigue from insomnia
- Palmar erythema, onycholysis, muscle wasting, and warm, moist skin
- *Women*: Menstrual irregularities, amenorrhea, and decreased fertility
- *Men*: Impotence, gynecomastia, and decreased libido

> **ALERT**
>
> Thyroid storm manifests with altered mental state, ineffective airway, pulmonary edema, tachycardia (atrial fibrillation), HF/cardiogenic shock, and fever.

Differential Diagnosis

- Factitious hyperthyroidism, subacute thyroiditis, toxic adenoma, multinodular goiter, pituitary tumor, drug-induced hyperthyroidism, iodine-induced hyperthyroidism, corticosteroid TSH suppression/euthyroid sick syndrome

Diagnosis

Labs

- TSH in range of 0 to 0.4 mIU/L
- Increase in free T4
- Positive thyrotropin antibodies and thyroid peroxidase antibody
- Hypercalcemia, hyperglycemia, and/or hypokalemia may be present
- Leukocytosis
- Decreased serum cortisol

Additional Diagnostic Testing

- The radioactive iodine uptake test shows increased uptake of iodine by the thyroid gland.
- Thyroid ultrasound is used to assess blood flow and the presence of masses or nodules.

Treatment and Management

Treatment Goals

- Increased TSH and decreased T4
- Symptomatic relief and prevention of acute/chronic complication

Drug Treatment

SYMPTOMATIC THERAPY

- Beta-adrenergic blockers for control of adrenergic symptoms of dysrhythmia, tachycardia, HTN
- Calcium channel blockers when beta-blockers are contraindicated to reduce blood pressure and heart rate

THYROID HORMONE INHIBITION

- Antithyroid thionamides to shrink the thyroid gland and decrease thyroid hormone secretion
- Iodine preparations to reduce the vascularity of the thyroid and minimize the release of the hormone
- Glucocorticoids to prevent additional thyroid hormone secretion and conversion of T4 to T3

Procedures

- RAI-131 for thyroid gland ablation
- Partial or total thyroidectomy

Interventions

- *Monitor for response to therapy*: Increase in TSH and decreased free T4.
- Assess for the presence of osteoporosis.
- Consider IGF-1 monoclonal antibody infusion in consultation with ophthalmology.

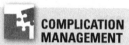

COMPLICATION MANAGEMENT

- Ensure adequate airway management and prescribe oxygen.
- Manage arrhythmias with IV beta-blockers or digitalis.
- Order external cooling and anti-pyretic.
- Initiate IV hydration and electrolyte management.
- Block thyroid hormone synthesis/release and circulation with thionamides, iodine, glucocorticoids, and cholestyramine.
- Initiate DVT prophylaxis.
- Obtain endocrine and surgical consults.

POST-THYROIDECTOMY

Monitor for airway obstruction, hemorrhage, laryngeal nerve damage, and thyroid storm.

Assess for Chvostek's or Trousseau's signs and prescribe IV calcium if present.

Patient Education

- Discuss with patients who received RAI to monitor for small increased risk for thyroid cancer.
- Explain that thionamides require 4 to 6 weeks to achieve a euthyroid state.
- Demonstrate to the patient how to protect eyes from injury with artificial tears and lubricants.
- Teach patients that weight gain may occur with treatment, reduced caloric intake, and a regular exercise program may help control weight.
- Instruction patients to avoid foods high in iodine.
- Instruct patients to report s/s of hypothyroidism.
- Instruct in lifelong thyroid replacement therapy and s/s of over- and undermedication.

Patient Population Considerations

Women (conception/pregnancy/lactation)
- RAI should never be used in a patient who is pregnant or nursing.
- Female patients requiring RAI should not breastfeed for at least 6 weeks before administration and should not be restarted after administration of RAI but can be safely done after future pregnancies.
- Female patients should wait at least 6 to 12 months to become pregnant following I-131 RAI treatment.

Geriatric
- Older patients with Graves' disease with underlying cardiac disease have an increased likelihood of decreased cardiac output. Concomitant atrial fibrillation can increase the risk of stroke.
- Due to the risk of malignancy among older adults, ultrasound and needle biopsy may be indicated.
- Create a safety plan in the presence of secondary osteoporosis from hyperthyroidism.

Pediatric
- Neonatal Graves' disease, caused by maternal IgG autoantibodies, is self-limited.
- Adolescents with hCG-secreting tumors can present with symptoms of hyperthyroidism.

Referring Patients

- Endocrine consult upon diagnosis
- Ophthalmology for exophthalmos
- Cardiology for arrhythmias, hypertension, and heart failure

HYPOTHYROIDISM (HASHIMOTO'S THYROIDITIS)

Overview

- Hashimoto's thyroiditis is a chronic, progressive immune-mediated metabolic disorder that is the most common cause of hypothyroidism.
- Autoimmune infiltration and destruction of the thyroid gland cause decreased synthesis of T3 and T4.
- Decreased circulation of thyroid hormones stimulates excess TSH resulting in a hypometabolic state with systemic effect (high TSH, low T3, T4).
- Onset may be insidious. Initially, the patient may be subclinical and may require periodic evaluation to determine the need for thyroid hormone replacement.
- Secondary hypothyroidism is the result of deficient TSH production by the pituitary gland or thyrotropin-releasing hormone from the hypothalamus (low TSH, T3, T4).

COMPLICATIONS

Acute: Myxedema coma

Chronic: Goiter, compressive symptoms leading to sleep apnea, atherosclerosis, heart failure, constipation, depression

Etiology

- Family history
- Presence of another autoimmune disorder, that is, rheumatoid arthritis, type 1 DM or lupus
- Vitamin D deficiency
- Female gender
- Middle age
- Radiation exposure
- Thyroidectomy with insufficient hormone replacement
- *Medication-induced*: Amiodarone, nitroprusside, sulfonylureas, thalidomide, interleukin, lithium, perchlorate, and interferon-alpha therapy

CLINICAL PEARL

Autoimmune polyglandular syndrome type 2 manifests with type 1 DM, Addison's disease, and autoimmune thyroid disease. In addition, primary hypogonadism, myasthenia gravis, and celiac disease may be present in people with hypothyroidism and should be further investigated.

Signs and Symptoms

- Fatigue, cognitive dysfunction, apathy
- Depression
- Daytime somnolence and sleep apnea
- Cold intolerance
- Constipation
- Goiter and hoarseness
- Menorrhagia, infertility, and loss of libido
- Dry skin, facial and eyelid edema
- Hair loss, brittle hair.
- Weight gain (modest)
- Erectile dysfunction and delayed ejaculation
- Hyperlipidemia, heart failure
- Impaired growth in children

 ALERT

Myxedema coma manifests as AMS, hypoventilation, pleural effusion, bradycardia, hypotension, pericardial effusion, and hypothermia caused by inadequate thyroid hormone that is life threatening.

Differential Diagnosis

- Autoimmune polyglandular syndromes, drug-induced hypothyroidism, factitious hypothyroidism, hypopituitarism, thyroid cancer, nontoxic goiter, diffuse toxic goiter, euthyroid sick syndrome, inadequate thyroid replacement post-RAI or thyroidectomy

Diagnosis

Labs

- Elevated TSH levels >4.5 to 10 mIU/L with low free T4
- TSH level 4.5 to 10 mIU/L with a normal T4 suggests subclinical hypothyroidism which should be monitored at regular intervals
- Anti-TPO and/or anti-Tg antibodies present
- Elevated LDL >130

Additional Diagnostic Testing

- Use thyroid ultrasound to examine shape, size, goiters, and nodules on the thyroid gland.
- Prescribe a sleep study in presence of compressive symptoms and goiter to detect apnea.

 CLINICAL PEARL

Instruct patient to avoid changing brands of levothyroxine and ensure that the pill color is not different after the prescription is filled. Concern regarding the FDA's methods for testing the equivalence of thyroxine preparations and the presence of subtle dose variations in pill brands has led most endocrinologists to recommend titrating with one brand.

Treatment and Management

Treatment Goals

- TSH level <5 mIU/L
- Absence of cognitive dysfunction and daytime somnolence
- Control of cardiovascular risk factors and no weight gain

Drug Treatment

- Prescribe levothyroxine 50 to 75 mcg daily and monitor the effect on TSH level in 6 to 8 weeks
- Titrate levothyroxine by 12 to 25 mcg until TSH is normalized, then monitor TSH level every 6 to 12 months.
- Treat hyperlipidemia and monitor for the development of the cardiac disease.

Interventions

- Assess for improving or worsening clinical manifestations.
- Assess for adverse effects of thyroid replacement therapy.
- Review other medications that the patient is taking for those that interfere with the absorption of thyroid hormone replacement.

Patient Education

- Instruct the patient to report s/s of under or over medication.
- Encourage patient to take thyroid hormone replacement in the morning, before breakfast, on an empty stomach with a full glass of water.
- Encourage physical activity and diet to reduce the risk of cardiovascular disease.
- Thyroid replacement therapy is required for life and should not be stopped without consulting a healthcare provider.

Patient Population Considerations

Women (conception/pregnancy/lactation)

- Untreated hypothyroidism can lead to birth defects and developmental problems in infants.
- Pregnant patients receiving thyroid replacement may require an increased dose to maintain a normal TSH and free T4.

Geriatric

- Monitor closely for the development of arrhythmias, atherosclerosis, and heart failure in the presence of hypothyroidism.
- Begin thyroid replacement at the lowest dose in older adults and patients with heart disease. Slowly increase the dose until TSH normalizes.

Pediatric

- Congenital hypothyroidism, cretinism, can occur because of an anatomic defect in the gland, an inborn error of thyroid metabolism, or iodine deficiency. It is characterized by hypotonia, coarse facial features, and umbilical hernia.
- Early diagnosis and treatment with levothyroxine are critical.
- Undiagnosed children with hypothyroidism may experience a slowed growth rate and intellectual disability.

Referring Patients

- Endocrine consult upon diagnosis
- Sleep specialist for daytime somnolence
- Nutritionist for weight gain
- Cardiology for dyslipidemia, hypertension, and heart failure

POP QUIZ 9.2

A patient with exophthalmos, weight loss, and heat intolerance has a very low serum TSH level and elevated serum free T4 and T3 levels. What test should be ordered next to complete the diagnostic workup?

RESOURCES

American Diabetes Association. (2019). Standards of medical care in diabetes-2019. *Diabetes Care, 42*(Suppl. 1). https://care.diabetesjournals.org/content/42/Supplement_1

American Diabetes Association. (2020). Standards of medical care in diabetes-2020 abridged for primary care providers. *Clinical Diabetes: A Publication of the American Diabetes Association, 38*(1), 10–38. https://doi.org/10.2337/cd20-as01

Cash, J. C., & Glass, C. A. (Eds.). (2019). *Adult-gerontology practice guidelines* (2nd ed.). Springer Publishing Company.

Chaker, L., Bianco, A. C., Jonklaas, J., & Peeters, R. (2017). Hypothyroidism. *Lancet, 390*, 1550–1562. https://doi.org/10.1016/S0140-6736(17)30703-1

Codina Leik, M. T. (2018). *Family nurse practitioner certification: Intensive review.* Springer Publishing Company.

Drake, M. T. (2018). Hypothyroidism in clinical practice. *Mayo Clinic Proceedings, 93*(9), 1169–1172. https://doi.org/10.1016/j.mayocp.2018.07.015

Joslin Clinic. (2017). *Joslin Diabetes Center & Joslin Clinic Clinical guideline for adults with diabetes.* https://joslin-prod.s3.amazonaws.com/www.joslin.org/assets/2019-08/Clinical-Guidelines-Adults-Diabetes-Rev-05-17-2017.pdf

Moore, D. (2018). Hypothyroidism and nursing care. *American Nurse Today, 13*(2), 44–46.

National Library of Medicine. (2020). *DailyMed. Tepezza—teprotumumab injection, powder, lyophilized, for solution.* https://dailymed.nlm.nih.gov/dailymed/lookup.cfm?setid=3e6c54a1-cefd-4a5b-a855-ab9f268b6cce

Ross, D. S., Burch, H. B., Cooper, D. S., Greenlee, M. C., Laurberg, P., Maia, A. L., Rivkees, S. A., Samuels, M., Sosa, J. A., Stan, M. N., & Walter, M. A. (2016). American Thyroid Association Guidelines for diagnosis and management of hyperthyroidism and other causes of thyrotoxicosis. *Thyroid, 26*(10), 1343–1421. https://doi.org/10.1089/thy.2016.0229

Rubino, F., Amiel, S. A., & Zimmet, P. (2020, June). New-onset diabetes in Covid-19. *The New England Journal of Medicine, 383*, 789–790. https://doi.org/10.1056/NEJMc2018688

Taylor, G. M., Pop, A., & McDowell, E. L. (2019). High-output congestive heart failure: A potentially deadly complication of thyroid storm. *Oxford Medical Case Reports, 2019*(6), omz045. https://doi.org/10.1093/omcr/omz045

REPRODUCTIVE SYSTEM

SEXUALLY TRANSMITTED INFECTIONS

Overview

- STIs are infections caused by bacteria, viruses, or parasites transmitted to partners during vaginal, anal, oral sexual contact, or with sharing of sex toys where there is contact with body secretions, mucous membranes, and abraded tissue.
- STIs can also be transmitted perinatally, causing congenital disease.
- Untreated STIs can cause acute infections that can lead to chronic complications and early mortality and morbidity.
- Since most people are unaware that they are infected, screening should be encouraged in sexually active patients.
- The presence of one STI presumes the risk for other STIs and coinfection with HIV and hepatitis B and C.
- The CDC provides guidance for screening for the presence of STIs to aid in early detection and treatment.

COMPLICATIONS

STIs can result in complications if left untreated:
- ***Chlamydia***: Fitz-Hugh–Curtis syndrome, infertility, PID, reactive arthritis, trachoma
- ***HSV 1 and 2***: Acute disseminated encephalomyelitis
- ***HPV***: Anal, cervical, penile, and oropharyngeal cancer
- ***HIV***: AIDS, malignancy, opportunistic infection
- ***Gonorrhea***: Gonococcemia, infertility, PID
- ***Syphilis***: Tertiary syphilis

Etiology

- Patient who has unprotected vaginal, anal, or oral sexual contact or does not use condoms correctly
- Contact with body fluids or objects contaminated with infected body fluids
- Patients who identify as MSM; patients with multiple sexual partners or aged 15 to 24 years
- Victim of a sexual assault or abuse
- Exposure to bacteria, viruses, or parasites during sexual contact (see select organisms in Table 10.1)
- Mother–baby transmission

Signs and Symptoms

- Patients with STIs may be asymptomatic and require screening for secondary detection.
- Patients may show acute presentation of pharyngitis, urethritis, vaginitis, cervicitis, epididymitis, genital or oral ulcer or lesion, or acute viral syndrome.
- Risk factors for STIs can be assessed using the "five P" history (see Tables 10.1 and 10.2).

CLINICAL PEARL

History Taking for STIs

Ask the five Ps: Partners, practices, prevention of pregnancy, protection from STDS, and past history

Table 10.1 STI Causes, Acute Presentation, and Screening

Etiological Agent	Acute Presentation	CDC 2015 Screening Recommendations
Chlamydia (*Chlamydia trachomatis*)	Pharyngitis, urethritis, cervicitis, epididymitis, vaginitis, genital ulcer known as lymphogranuloma venereum	• *Women*: Sexually active under age 25, age >25 years if an increased risk • *Pregnancy*: All women during first prenatal visit; retest in third trimester with increased risk of STIs • *Men*: Consider screening in high prevalence areas • *MSM*: Annually or every 3–6 months according to risk • Retest 3 months after treatment; 3 weeks in treated pregnant women
Herpes simplex 1 and 2 (HSV)	Genital or oral ulcers	• Consider HSV testing women, men, MSM, and HIV+ persons presenting for STI evaluation
HPV and genital warts (human papillomavirus)	Condyloma	• *Women 21–29 years*: Every 3 years with Pap test • *Women 30–65 years*: May consider Pap test alone every 3 years or Pap with HPV testing every 5 years
HIV infection	S/s of acute HIV infection (flu-like symptoms), s/s of AIDS-defining illness	• All patients age 13–64 offered HIV testing opt-out • All men and women seeking an evaluation of STIs • *Pregnancy*: Test at first prenatal visit • *MSM*: Annually with increased risk
Gonorrhea (*Neisseria gonorrhea*)	*Pharyngitis, urethritis, cervicitis*, epididymitis, *vaginitis; disseminated gonococcemia*: Classic joint pain in reactive arthritis rash, endocarditis, meningitis	• *Women*: Sexually active under age 25, age >25 years with increased risk • *Pregnancy*: First prenatal visit; retest third trimester with increased risk. • *MSM*: Annually or every 3–6 months, according to risk • Retest 3 months after treatment.
Syphilis (*Treponema pallidum*)	• Genital ulcer (primary) • Skin rashes, mucous membrane lesions, fever, myalgia, fatigue (secondary) • Multiorgan system disease (tertiary) • Asymptomatic (latent) • *Neurologic symptoms may be present at any stage*: Headache, motor-sensory deficit, dementia	• *Pregnancy*: First prenatal visit; high-risk patients should be screened in the third trimester and at delivery. • MSM who are sexually active annually or more frequently with higher risk • When initiating PrEP for HIV prevention

Note: MSM: Men who have sex with men
PEP, postexposure HIV antiretroviral prophylaxis; PrEP, preexposure HIV antiretroviral prophylaxis
Source: https://www.cdc.gov/std/tg2015/screening-recommendations.htm

Differential Diagnosis

- Chlamydia
  - *PULM*: RSV, congenital pneumonia in neonates
  - *GU*: Ectopic pregnancy, endometriosis, gonorrhea, orchitis, PID, trichomoniasis, urethritis, UTI, vaginosis
  - *HEENT*: Conjunctivitis, viral or bacterial pharyngitis
  - *INT*: Candidiasis, herpes simplex
  - *MSK*: Arthritis
  - *Other*: HIV
- Herpes simplex 1 and 2
  - *GU*: Chancroid, male urethritis, UTI
  - *HEENT*: Mouth ulcers, pharyngitis
  - *INT*: Herpes zoster, varicella-zoster virus
  - *MSK*: Arthritis
  - *NEURO*: Brain tumor/mass, CNS infection, seizures
  - *Other*: Drug eruptions, HIV, syphilis
- HPV and genital warts
  - *GU*: Benign or malignant vulvar or vaginal lesions, cervical polyp or cancer, chancroid
  - *HEM*: Nevi, skin cancer
  - *INT*: Condyloma lata, herpes simplex, lichen planus, molluscum contagiosum, psoriasis
  - *Other*: HIV, syphilis
- HIV infection
  - *CV*: Endocarditis, HF
  - *PULM*: pneumonia, tuberculosis
  - *GI*: Hepatitis
  - *GU*: Cervical cancer, chancroid, chlamydia, ectopic pregnancy, HPV, gonorrhea, orchitis, trichomoniasis, urethritis, UTI
  - *HEENT*: Frequent upper respiratory infection
  - *HEM*: Lymphoma, skin cancer
  - *INT*: Candidiasis, herpes simplex, herpes zoster, Kaposi's sarcoma, lichen planus, molluscum contagiosum
  - *NEURO*: Brain tumor/mass, CNS infection, seizures
  - *Other*: Cytomegalovirus, immune suppression from chemotherapy, syphilis, toxoplasmosis, valley fever
- Gonorrhea
  - *CV*: Endocarditis, HF secondary to rheumatic fever
  - *GI*: Hepatitis
  - *GU*: Chlamydia, endometriosis, orchitis, trichomoniasis, urethritis, UTI, vaginosis
  - *HEENT*: Conjunctivitis, viral or bacterial pharyngitis
  - *INT*: Herpes simplex, SLE rash
  - *NEURO*: Meningitis
  - *MSK*: Inflammatory, psoriatic, or septic arthritis
  - *Other*: HIV, syphilis
- Syphilis
  - *CV*: HF
  - *GI*: Hepatitis

- *GU*: Chancroid, chlamydia, ectopic pregnancy, endometriosis, epididymitis, genital warts, gonorrhea, orchitis, trichomoniasis, urethritis, UTI, vaginosis
- *HEENT*: Conjunctivitis, pharyngitis
- *HEM*: Cancer
- *INT*: Candidiasis, herpes simplex, herpes zoster, lichen planus, varicella-zoster virus
- *NEURO*: Brain tumor/mass, CNS infection, seizure, stroke
- *Other*: Drug eruptions, HIV, sarcoidosis

Diagnosis

Labs
- See Table 10.2.

Treatment and Management

Treatment Goals
- Prevent infection transmission, eradicate/manage infection, modify risk factors, and prevent complications.

Table 10.2 Labs and Treatment According to STI

Infection	Labs	Treatment and Management
Chlamydia	• U/A (mid-stream, first void) • NAAT endocervical (not pooled secretions); oropharyngeal, rectal, or urethral swab • Rapid PCR testing	***Drug Treatment*** • Azithromycin 1 g PO × one dose **OR** doxycycline 100 mg PO BID × 7 days • *Pregnancy*: Azithromycin 1 g PO × one dose ***Interventions*** • Report infection to public health and refer to partner notification services. • Retest pregnant women or women with PID with infection 3 weeks after treatment. • Retest all other patients treated for an infection in 3 months to identify reinfection. • Instruct patients that they can resume sex 7 days after their partner has been treated.

Herpes simplex 1 and 2	• HSV2 antibody test
	• Ulcer culture or PCR testing
		Drug Treatment
		• *First case of herpes*
		  • Valacyclovir 1 g PO q12h for 10 days; IV acyclovir in severe cases
		• *Recurrent case*
		  • Valacyclovir 500 mg PO q12h for 3 days
		• *Suppressive therapy for 1 year*
		  • Valacyclovir 1 g PO daily (immunocompetent) or 500 mg PO q12h with HIV infection
		Interventions
		• In known cases of HSV in pregnant women, refer to the obstetrician for suppressive therapy and planned cesarean section to prevent neonatal HSV infection transmission.
		• Consult with the obstetrician regarding prophylactic acyclovir or valacyclovir in infected women who are pregnant beginning at 36 weeks' gestation.

Infection	Labs	Treatment and Management
HPV and genital warts	• Acetic acid test whitens lesions • HPV PCR with Pap smear • Colposcopy and biopsy for suspicious lesions	**Drug Treatment** • Prevent infection through vaccination. • Vaccinate with recombinant human papillomavirus vaccine, two doses, 6 months apart for boys and girls age 9–12 years; or three doses 6 months apart, age 15–26 years. *Age 27–45 years*: Use a shared decision-making model. **Interventions** • Refer patients with suspected warts for biopsy and ablation. • Establish plan for long-term monitoring for cancer.

HIV infection	• Rapid HIV assay
	• Positive result must be confirmed by alternative HIV immunoassay for diagnosis.
		Drug Treatment
		• Prevent infection through PrEP for HIV-negative adolescents and adults.
		  • Prescribe daily combination antiretroviral therapy based on risk and sexual practices.
		• Refer patients to an HIV specialist to start antiretroviral therapy.
		• Refer patients to ED to evaluate accidental exposure to blood and body fluids for PEP within 96 hr of exposure.
		Interventions
		• Reevaluate patient taking PrEP every 3 months for adherence and tolerance of the medication. Teach the patient not to share medicine.
		  • Perform HIV rapid assay, CBC, BMP, HbA1c, LFTs, and lipid profile to monitor for adverse effects.
		  • If a second HIV test confirms HIV-positive rapid assay, refer to an HIV specialist.
		  • Report infection to public health.

Gonorrhea	• First catch urine • NAAT pharyngeal, endocervical, rectal, or urethral swab • Gram stain in symptomatic men • CBC, BMP, ESR with disseminated disease	**Drug Treatment** • *Uncomplicated*: Use azithromycin 1 g PO × 1 dose *AND* ceftriaxone 250 mg IM × 1 dose. • Refer complicated cases to infectious disease specialist. **Interventions** • Admit patients with disseminated disease to the hospital. • Report infection to public health and refer to partner notification services. • Retest in 2 weeks after treatment. • Retest all other patients treated for an infection in 3 months to identify reinfection. • Instruct patients that they can resume sex 7 days after their partner has been treated.

Syphilis	• Screening serology
	  • RPR, VDRL
	  • A treponemal test follows positive screens.
	• Lesion-based testing
	  • *Treponema pallidum* PCR testing and dark-field microscopic testing of the lesion
		Drug Treatment
		• Use benzathine penicillin G 2.4 million units IM in patients who have primary, secondary, or early latent syphilis.
		• Refer to infectious disease specialist for the management of latent syphilis which require increased PCN doses and frequency.
		Interventions
		• Refer patients with PCN allergy for skin test or oral challenge.
		• Report infections to public health and discuss partner notification services for partners within the past 90 days.
		• Consult an infectious disease specialist for long-term follow-up.

Patient Education
- Provide STI and HIV counseling to the patient and partner.
- Teach patient strategies to minimize the risk of infection transmission.

Patient Population Considerations

Women (conception/pregnancy/lactation)
- Provide conception counseling for the primary prevention of STIs to all women of childbearing age.
- Screen all women reporting symptoms of disorders that could be caused by an STI using the five Ps of history taking.
- Perform STI screening lab testing, including HIV rapid assay, HBsAg, RPR, VDRL, and additional testing for suspected STIs as clinically warranted.
- Screen all pregnant women for hepatitis C using anti-HCV antibody testing. All adult women should be screened at least once, depending on risks.

Geriatric
- Geriatric patients who are sexually active are at risk for STIs.
- Continue Pap testing after age 65 in women who have a history of abnormal cells, cervical cancer, or had a positive Pap smear within the past 10 years.

Pediatric
- Assess for the presence of STIs in prepubescent children who may be victims of sexual abuse. Do not presume the existence of STIs in an adolescent is from consensual acts. Provide privacy and gain trust to obtain an accurate history.
- Perinatal transmission can cause the following:
  - *Chlamydia*: Conjunctivitis, pneumonia
  - *HSV 1 and 2*: Disseminated neonatal herpes
  - *HPV*: Infection of unknown significance
  - *HIV*: AIDS, malignancy, opportunistic infection
  - *Gonorrhea*: Conjunctivitis, gonococcemia
  - *Syphilis*: Congenital syphilis

 POP QUIZ 10.1

A 15-year-old male presents to the primary care provider with dysuria. He is accompanied by his mother, who reports no personal or family medical history. She denies sexual activity on his behalf. He explains that he woke up this morning with dysuria. He denies frequency, urgency, or drainage. He also denies recent illness, injury, or insect bites. He reports recent overnight travel out of state on a school trip. What is the priority intervention?

Referring Patients
- Gynecology with reproductive anomalies and symptoms of pelvic inflammatory disease
- Infectious disease consult
- HIV specialist
- Neonatology with perinatal transmission of STI

MEN'S HEALTH

BENIGN PROSTATIC HYPERPLASIA

Overview
- BPH is a chronic progressive proliferation of prostate tissue that can lead to bladder outlet obstruction and urinary retention. The enzyme 5-alpha reductase converts testosterone into DHT, which binds with androgen receptors, increasing prostate size. The expanding gland impedes bladder outlet.
- Urinary retention can cause bladder calculi, hemorrhage, and UTI from urinary stasis.
- Progressive obstruction can cause postrenal failure that can progress to renal insufficiency over time.

 COMPLICATIONS

Acute: Bladder calculi, hemorrhage, obstructive uropathy, postrenal failure, UTI
Chronic: Renal insufficiency

Etiology

- Male gender; increases with age
- Testosterone supplementation
- Progression in African-American ethnicity is more severe

Signs and Symptoms

- LUTS with increased frequency, urgency, hesitancy; decreased force and intermittent stream
- Straining, dribbling
- Large, smooth, nontender prostate on DRE >two finger widths
- Increased PVR
- Palpable bladder, rising PSA, pain, frequent infections, hydroureter, and/or hydronephrosis, and associated neurological diseases require immediate referral to urology

Differential Diagnosis

- *GI*: Abdominal mass
- *GU*: Cystitis, bladder calculi, bladder cancer, overactive bladder, neurogenic bladder, pelvic floor dysfunction, prostate cancer, prostatitis, renal colic, urethral stricture

CLINICAL PEARL

AUA-SI Tool

Use this objective scale at each clinical encounter to measure course and severity of symptoms.

ALERT

Symptoms of acute urinary retention and oliguria should be referred to the ED immediately.

Diagnosis

Labs

- U/A to evaluate for leukocytes, nitrites, RBCs, protein, and casts
- Elevated PSA in response to hyperplasia
- BMP to evaluate for azotemia and estimate GFR
- CBC to evaluate for baseline Hgb, HcT, and platelets

Additional Diagnostic Testing

- Bladder scan to evaluate PVR
- Cystoscopy to evaluate for bladder malignancy
- Urodynamic study to distinguish detrusor underactivity
- Ultrasound of ureters and kidney to evaluate for hydroureter and or hydronephrosis
- Transurethral ultrasound and biopsy for suspicious prostatic lesions

Treatment and Management

Treatment Goals

- Manage LUTS, modify risk factors, and prevent complications.

Drug Treatment

- Prescribe terazosin or tamsulosin to promote bladder emptying.
- Do not prescribe tamsulosin with planned cataract surgery.
- Refer to urology for additional medications.
  - Drugs that inhibit 5-alpha reductase reduce prostate size but have higher sexual side effects.
  - Phosphodiesterase inhibitors cause smooth muscle relaxation and is preferred with concomitant erectile dysfunction.
  - Anticholinergics are prescribed by urology to reduce LUTS with irritation but aggravate urinary retention and should be managed by urology.

Interventions
- Monitor for UTI, calculi, and renal insufficiency.
- Evaluate AUA-SI score in response to therapy at periodic intervals.
- Monitor for increased risk of metabolic syndrome and manage it in order to promote euglycemia.
- *Monitor patients' use of nutraceuticals*: Examples include saw palmetto, pumpkin seeds, rye, African plum tree; compare to current medication profile for interactions or adverse effects.
- Monitor response to surgical interventions, suprapubic tube placement, and TURP. Monitor for complications.

Patient Education
- Counsel patient on strategies to manage LUTS.
- Review bladder irritants to avoid.
- Discuss risk for orthostatic hypotension with alpha blockers and encourage the patient to change positions slowly during nightly visits to urinate.

Patient Population Considerations

Women (conception/pregnancy/lactation)
- Drugs that inhibit 5-alpha reductase are teratogens and can be absorbed through the skin. Advise women of childbearing age or who are pregnant not to handle pills with bare hands to avoid harm to the fetus.

Geriatric
- Review a safety plan for managing nocturia in older patients at higher risk of falling to prevent accidental injury.

Pediatric
- Instruct patients to keep medication out of reach of children; 5-alpha-reductase inhibitors can be harmful to children if handled.

Referring Patients

- Urology consult

Overview

- Epididymitis is an infection of the epididymis from bacteria that may have been introduced from retrograde urine flow from the prostatic urethra through the vas deference.
- Inflammation from microbial proliferation can extend to testes, form abscesses, or cross over to systemic circulation. Excessive inflammation can produce ischemia in testes.
- Left untreated, testes may infarct, atrophy, and increase risk for infertility.

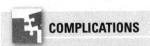

COMPLICATIONS

Acute: Abscess, orchitis, sepsis, testicular infarction

Chronic: Atrophy, infertility

Etiology

- Viral, bacterial, tuberculosis infection, environmental factors
- Urethral strictures
- STIs, urethritis, prostatitis, UTI
- Prolonged sitting, bicycling, motorcycle riding
- Unprotected sex, anal sex, instrumentation, indwelling catheters
- Increased incidence in males 18 to 50 years of age
- Coinfection with TB or recent BCG vaccine

Signs and Symptoms

- Scrotal pain and swelling that gets progressively worse, radiating to lower back and flank.
- Dysuria, frequency, or urgency; blood in semen; urethral discharge
- Fever, chills
- Scrotal edema, tenderness, urethral discharge, Prehn sign, normal cremaster reflex

ALERT

- Epididymitis must be distinguished from testicular torsion, which is an acute emergency that should be referred to the ED immediately.
- Refer patients with 2 qSOFA signs to ED immediately.

Differential Diagnosis

- *GI*: Inguinal hernia
- *GU*: Cyst, hydrocele, orchitis, scrotal hernia, STIs, spermatocele, testicular torsion, testicular tumor/mass/trauma, urethritis
- *Other*: Vasculitis

Diagnosis

Labs

- U/A shows pyuria; CBC reveals leukocytosis
- CRP may be elevated
- VDRL, RPR, HIV in possible sexual transmission
  - NAAT urethral swab for gonorrhea and chlamydia
- Urine culture and gram stain
- IGRA in suspected TB

Additional Diagnostic Testing

- Ultrasound to rule out testicular torsion and evaluate for presence of hydrocele
- Cystourethroscopy
- Chest x-ray in suspected TB

Treatment and Management

Treatment Goals

- Eradicate infection, promote comfort, and prevent complications.

Drug Treatment

- Treat infection
  - *STI*: Ceftriaxone 250 mg IM × one dose plus doxycycline 100 mg PO BID for 10 days
  - *Bacterial infection*: TMP-SMX for empiric treatment or levofloxacin as indicated
  - Infectious disease specialist consult if TB is suspected as cause
- Promote comfort
  - Acetaminophen and NSAIDs PRN for mild pain
    - Codeine with acetaminophen can be considered for breakthrough pain.

Interventions

- Apply ice and elevate using scrotal support.
- Sitz baths can be offered in addition to ice and scrotal support, as necessary.
- Monitor response to therapy and for the presence of complications.
- Adjust antibiotics according to culture results, if indicated.
- Report STIs to public health and discuss partner notification services if indicated.

Patient Education

- Discuss disease process, risk for recurrence, and chronic inflammation.
- Advise patient to limit activity; complete antibiotics and STI follow-up, if indicated.
- Teach s/s of complications and adverse medication effects to report.

Patient Population Considerations

Geriatric
- Older males with s/s of epididymitis should be evaluated for BPH.

Pediatric
- Development of this infection in infants and young children should alert the need for referral to urology to evaluate for urethral strictures. Reflux from Valsalva maneuvers during weight lifting with a full bladder may contribute to this infection. Teach males to empty their bladder before exercise.

Referring Patients

- Urology consult

ERECTILE DYSFUNCTION

Overview

- ED is a disorder of attaining and maintaining a penile erection that can be primary or secondary. It may or may not be associated with decreased libido.
- It can be caused by direct trauma to tissue, circulation, and nerve function of the penis or an early warning sign of other health conditions that affect tissue perfusion, nerve conduction, and smooth muscle relaxation.

 COMPLICATIONS

Acute: Anxiety, depression, interrupted family processes

Etiology

- Increased incidence with age, alcohol, drug use, malnutrition, obesity, tobacco, zinc deficiency
- Peyronie disease
- ASCVD, anxiety, BPH, cancer, CKD, COPD, dementia, depression, DM, epilepsy, hyperlipidemia, HTN, hyperthyroidism, hypogonadism, hypopituitarism, hypothyroidism, leukemias, neurodegenerative disease, PTSD, scleroderma, sickle cell anemia, sleep apnea, spinal cord injury, stroke, vasculitis
- Medications, surgery, radiation-induced vascular injury, anabolic steroid abuse

 ALERT

Medications That Can Induce Erectile Dysfunction

Anabolic steroids, antiandrogens, antihypertensives, antidepressants, antipsychotics, cimetidine, PPI, chemotherapy, cholesterol-lowering medications, opioids

Signs and Symptoms

- Report of difficult obtaining, maintaining a suitable erection
- Premature ejaculation
- Dissatisfaction with sex
- Deformity of penis, enlarged prostate, testicular atrophy
- Decreased secondary sex characteristics

CLINICAL PEARL

Standardized Instrument

Use of a questionnaire is useful to identify patients experiencing erectile dysfunction in preparation for a clinical encounter.

Differential Diagnosis

- *CV*: ASCVD, heart failure, hypertension, lipid disorders, peripheral arterial disease
- *ENDO*: DM, hyperthyroidism, hypogonadism, hypopituitarism, hypothyroidism
- *GI*: Abdominal vascular injury
- *GU*: BPH, Peyronie disease, prostate surgery, or radiation

- *HEM*: Cancer, chemotherapy, leukemia, sickle cell anemia
- *NEURO*: Anxiety, dementia, depression, neurodegenerative disorders, neuropathy, PTSD, sleep apnea, spinal cord injury
- *Other*: Alcohol or substance use, vasculitis, scleroderma

ALERT

Conduct a Mini-Cog® assessment and depression screen to identify early cognitive impairment and depression.

Diagnosis

Labs
- Serum testosterone levels < 11.1 nmol/L
- Serum prolactin and LH level low indicated pituitary origin, high levels indicate primary disorder
- TSH may be high or low
- BMP to evaluate for azotemia
- HbA1c to identify DM
- Lipid panel to identify hyperlipidemia or hypoalphalipoproteinemia
- CBC, serum albumin
- U/A

Additional Diagnostic Testing
- Ultrasound of vascular function of penis
- Angiography
- Urology for biothesiometry and prostaglandin E1 injection into the corpora cavernosa

ALERT

Appropriate Referral
- Patients with decreased secondary sex characteristics, low prolactin, and LH should be referred to endocrinology.
- Patients with deformity of the penis or enlarged prostate should be referred to urology.

Treatment and Management

Treatment Goals
- Correct erectile dysfunction, control contributing factors, and manage organic cause.

Drug Treatment
- Stop agents causing erectile dysfunction when possible and prescribe alternative agents.
- Prescribe agents to manage ASCVD, HTN, lipid disorders.
- Adjust antidiabetic therapy to maintain euglycemia.

Interventions
- Monitor response to oral medications and external vacuum devices.
- Monitor response to hormone replace therapy prescribed by endocrine and monitor for complications.
- Evaluate diabetes, heart disease, and hypertension at each clinical encounter.

Patient Education
- Provide alcohol and tobacco cessation counseling.
- Discuss the benefit of moderate-to-vigorous exercise on sexual dysfunction.
- Encourage a Mediterranean diet to achieve optimal BMI and improved sexual function.
- Discuss exercise and weight control strategies.
- Provide referrals for counseling and psychological care.

Patient Population Considerations

Geriatric
- Inform older patients with age-related low testosterone levels that the ACP suggests that testosterone replacement not be used for the purpose of improving energy, vitality, physical function, or cognition.

Referring Patients

- Urology consult
- Endocrine consult

PROSTATE CANCER

Overview

- Prostate cancer is an adenocarcinoma of the prostate that accounts for 10% of cancer deaths and affects males age >50 years.
- Circulating testosterone enhances cancer growth.
- Detected cancer cells are graded according to a Gleason score to determine their degree of differentiation and the cells' aggressiveness to guide therapeutic decisions. Higher Gleason scores are poorly differentiated and more likely to micro-metastasize.

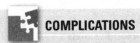

COMPLICATIONS

Acute: DVT, urinary retention, spinal cord compression, pathological fracture

Chronic: Infertility, metastasis to lungs, liver, adrenal, and bone; possible paraneoplastic syndrome

Etiology

- Increased incidence in age > 50 years
- Family history; African-American ethnicity is higher-grade with poorer prognosis

Signs and Symptoms

- Asymptomatic in early disease
- Palpable firm lesion on prostate by DRE
- Local growth and extension cause LUTS, hematuria, hematospermia, erectile dysfunction, and obstructive uropathy
- Advanced cancer demonstrates s/s of distant metastasis

CLINICAL PEARL

Prostate Cancer Screening

- First-degree relative of someone with prostate cancer should have PSA with or without DRE at age 45.
- Recommended beginning at age 40 with two first-degree relatives
  - *PSA ≥ 2.5 ng/mL*: Retest annually.
  - *PSA ≤ 2.5 ng/mL*: Retest every 2 years.
- The decision to undergo screening for prostate cancer in men age >50 years should be a shared decision between a patient and their provider.

Differential Diagnosis

- *GU*: BPH, bladder calculi, prostatitis, prostatic cysts, prostatic tuberculosis
- *HEM*: Secondary metastasis

Diagnosis

Labs

- Serum PSA used as tumor marker; is not diagnostic.
- *Serum PSA*: 4 to 10 ng/mL has 30% to 35% chance of prostate cancer; PSA >10 ng/mL has >67% chance of prostate cancer.
  - Elevates with cancer recurrence and approximates zero after prostate removal or irradiation.
- Elevations in serum acid phosphatase level is a poor prognostic indicator.
- Additional labs may be obtained by urology.
  - PCA3 testing following prostatic massage to determine if biopsy is indicated.
  - Epigenetic profiling can be performed in patients at high risk for occult cancer.
  - Cell cycle progression score for identifying recurrent cancer.
- Serum BMP, LFTs, Ca, Mg, Phos to evaluate electrolyte and hepatorenal function.
- CBC may reveal leukopenia, anemia, and thrombocytopenia in bone metastasis.

Additional Diagnostic Testing

- Transrectal ultrasound can be used to identify hypoechoic areas and biopsy can be performed.
- Endorectal MRI to localize cancer.
- CT of the abdomen, pelvis, and chest for metastasis.
- Bone scan for high Gleason score.

Treatment and Management

Treatment Goals

- Treat cancer according to type and stage.
- Manage complications of surgery, chemotherapy, and radiation.
- Prevent complications.

Drug Treatment

- Hormone therapy is used to deprive cancer cells of testosterone. *Medications used in addition to orchiectomy include LH–RH therapy, abiraterone acetate, antiandrogen therapy, estrogen therapy, antiadrenal therapy such as ketoconazole and aminoglutethimide.*
- Collaborate with hematology and palliative care in managing adverse effects.

Interventions

- Watchful waiting is used in addition to prostate removal with radical prostatectomy and radiation therapy (external beam vs. brachytherapy).
- Orchiectomy is considered in advanced cancer to reduce growth from testosterone and reduce symptoms.
- Monitor response to hormone therapy, radiation therapy, surgical interventions, and potential complications.
- Monitor for s/s of recurrence and advanced disease.
- *Monitor for adverse effects of androgen suppression when in use:* Anemia, gynecomastia, sexual side effects, osteoporosis, hot flashes, metabolic syndrome, and pulmonary edema.
  - Monitor HbA1c and lipid profiles and manage metabolic adverse effects.

Patient Education

- Initiate smoking cessation protocol, if indicated.
- Review postoperative instructions, radiation teaching as indicated.
- Teach s/s of complications and adverse medication effects to report.

Patient Population Considerations

Geriatric

- Men over 70 to 80 years should not consider the value of continued prostate cancer screening.

Referring Patients

- Urology consult
- Surgery consult
- Oncology consult

POP QUIZ 10.2

A 55-year-old male present to the primary care provider with dysuria. He is in a mutually monogamous relationship and uses condoms to prevent pregnancy. He explains that he woke up this morning with dysuria and has noticed increased frequency and urgency over the past month when traveling but finds his bladder is getting shy when he stops to use the bathroom. He denies urethral drainage, recent illness, and injury. He reports a recent long car trip across country. What is the likely cause of this patient's symptoms?

PROSTATITIS

Overview

- Prostatitis is an inflammation of the prostate gland that can be acute or chronic and can lead to LUTS and bladder outlet obstruction.
- Organisms spread to the prostate from ascending urethritis, reflux of infected urine into the prostatic ducts, or lymphatic spread from the rectum. Alternatively, it can be from viral pathogens, mycobacterium, or an idiopathic inflammatory process.
- Acute bacterial prostatitis can evolve into chronic bacterial prostatitis in patients with *Escherichia coli* or HIV infection. Alterations in bladder outlet can cause chronic bacterial prostatitis or chronic prostatitis without bacterial involvement.

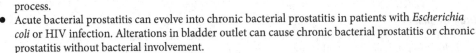

COMPLICATIONS

Acute: Abscess, acute urinary retention, AKI, pyelonephritis, sepsis

Chronic: Chronic, recurrent cystitis; CKD chronic pelvic pain syndrome; infertility

Etiology

- *Escherichia coli, enterobacter, serratia, enterococcus, pseudomonas,* and *proteus*
- *Neisseria gonorrhea* and *Chlamydia trachomatis* in younger males with LUTS
- CMV in patients with HIV
- *Mycobacterium tuberculosis* and candida have been observed
- STIs, UTI
- Increased age, decreased sexual activity, or trauma
- Sarcoidosis
- BPH or urethral strictures

ALERT

Risk of Urosepsis

Do not vigorously massage a prostate in suspected bacterial infection.

Signs and Symptoms

- Obstructive urinary tract symptoms, urethral discharge
- Pain to lower perineum, back, abdomen
- Pain with ejaculation, erectile dysfunction
- Tender enlarged boggy prostate by digital rectal exam
- Suprapubic abdominal tenderness
- Bladder is dull to percussion
- Fever, chills, malaise, myalgia in acute bacterial prostatitis

ALERT

Refer patients with s/s acute urinary retention, AKI, or sepsis to the ED immediately.

Differential Diagnosis

- *GI:* Anal fissures, inflammatory bowel disease
- *GU:* BPH, epididymitis, obstructive uropathy, prostate cancer, rectal foreign body, urethral stricture or calculi, urethritis, UTI
- *Other:* Sarcoidosis

Diagnosis

Labs

- U/A shows elevated WBC
- Urine culture and gram stain

- Urine for cytology in older males with no infectious symptoms
- CBC may reveal leukocytosis
- BMP may review azotemia
- VDRL, RPR, HIV in possible sexual transmission and males <50 years
  - NAAT urethral swab for gonorrhea and chlamydia
- IGRA in suspected TB
- Do not collect serum PSA level because elevated values do not assist in *diagnosis*

Additional Diagnostic Testing
- Bladder scan to evaluate PVR
- CT or ultrasound abdomen and pelvis to evaluate for hydroureter, hydronephrosis, strictures, calculi
- Cystoscopy with significant urinary retention
- Transrectal ultrasound to evaluate prostate size in acute inflammatory prostatitis but not in bacterial prostatitis because it can increase risk for sepsis
- Chest x-ray in suspected TB

Treatment and Management

Treatment Goals
- Treat infection/inflammation, reduce modifiable risk factors, and prevent complications.

Drug Treatment
- Reduce risk factors for complications.
- Stop all anticholinergics, imipramine α1 receptor agonists, and antihistamines that can contribute to bladder retention. Consult psychiatry if stopping TCAs.
- Prescribe stool softeners in presence of constipation and straining.
- Prescribe terazosin 5 mg PO daily to improve bladder outlet.
  - Consider tamsulosin if no planned cataract surgery.

TREAT INFECTION
- *STI*: Ceftriaxone 250 mg IM × 1 dose plus doxycycline 100 mg PO BID for 10 days
- *Acute bacterial infection*: TMP-SMX DS BID for 14 days if quinolone resistance is suspected
- When chronic bacterial infection is suspected, refer to urology for management; TMP-SMX DS may be continued for 60 to 90 days according to culture or levofloxacin 500 mg PO for 28 days
- Infectious disease specialist consult if TB is suspected as cause

PROMOTE COMFORT
- Acetaminophen and NSAIDs PRN for mild pain. Use caution with NSAIDs to protect kidney from harm.

Interventions
- Use a straight catheter (gently) to obtain urine if patient is unable to provide sample or retention is suspected. Refer to ED if straight catheter is unsuccessful in outpatient setting.
  - Monitor postoperative recovery following suprapubic tube insertion or TURP.
- Monitor response to therapy and for the presence of complications.
- Adjust antibiotics according to culture results, if indicated.
- Report STIs to public health and discuss partner notification services if indicated.

Patient Education
- Discuss disease process, risk for recurrence, and chronic infection.
- Advise patient to increase fluids and avoid dehydration constipation, unprotected sex.
- Encourage sitz baths for comfort, pelvic floor exercises, complete antibiotics, and STI follow-up, if indicated.
- Teach s/s of complications and adverse medication effects to report.

Patient Population Considerations

Geriatric

- Older males experience prostatitis at greater frequency. Primary prevention of acute prostatitis focuses on reducing infection and retrograde urine flow.
- Instruct patients to use condoms for sexual activity, avoid OTC and prescription medications that cause urinary retention as a side effect, and avoid bladder irritants like spicy food, tea, and coffee.
- Eat fiber to avoid constipation, empty the bladder regularly especially before strenuous exercise, avoid sitting and inactivity to reduce pressure on prostate, and maintain a BMI <25.

Pediatric

- Prostatitis is not seen in adolescents as frequently as adult or older males. When it occurs, it has been observed most often in boys after puberty. Orchitis most often develops in 4 to 6 days after the mumps begins.

Referring Patients

- Urology consult
- Infectious disease consult

TESTICULAR CANCER

Overview

- Testicular cancer is seminoma (sperm producing) and nonseminoma (nonsperm producing) carcinoma of the testes that affects males ages 15 to 35 years.
- Early identification and treatment with orchiectomy offers a cure.

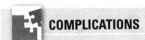 **COMPLICATIONS**

Acute: DVT, retroperitoneal adenopathy, obstructive uropathy

Chronic: Infertility, metastasis to lungs, liver, viscera, bone, and possibly brain

Etiology

- Exact etiology unknown
- Family history, European ancestry, maternal use of DES
- Caucasian cases outnumber cases in the African-American population, but African-American cases tend to be higher-grade with poorer prognosis.
- Cryptorchidism, mumps orchitis, HIV infection, testicular trauma, inguinal hernia as child

Signs and Symptoms

- Nontender, palpable testicular mass that does not transilluminate
- Enlarged scrotum with regional lymphadenopathy
- S/s of metastasis in advanced disease

Differential Diagnosis

- *GI*: Abdominal hernia
- *GU*: Epididymitis, hydrocele, orchitis, testicular torsion, varicocele
- *HEM*: Leukemia, lymphoma, retroperitoneal sarcoma, secondary metastasis

Diagnosis

Labs

- Serum alpha fetoprotein, beta hCG, and/or LDH may be elevated.
- Serum BMP, LFTs, Ca, Mg, Phos to evaluate electrolyte and hepatorenal function.
- CBC may reveal leukopenia, anemia, and thrombocytopenia in bone metastasis.

Additional Diagnostic Testing

- Testicular ultrasound is the best screening tool for complaint
- Biopsy for affected tests and contralateral testis
- CT of the abdomen and pelvis; CT of the chest for metastasis
- Brain MRI

Treatment and Management

Treatment Goals

- Treat cancer according to type and stage; manage complications of surgery, chemotherapy, and radiation; preserve fertility.

Drug Treatment

- Chemotherapy is done by oncology.
- Prescribe therapy to manage adverse effects in consult with hematology and palliative care.
  - Chemotherapy patients will receive analgesic, anxiolytic, antiemetic, SNRI, or anticonvulsant for peripheral neuropathy, topical treatment for oral mucous membranes, uricosurics for secondary gout, and stool softeners or antidiarrheals for bowel management. Prophylactic antibiotics and colony stimulating factors may also be needed, as indicated.

Interventions

- Surgical interventions include orchiectomy and retroperitoneal lymph node dissection, as indicated. Resection of thoracic metastasis or HSCT may be indicated in advanced disease.
- Monitor response to therapy and for potential complications from testicular cancer and its treatment.
- Monitor for the development of secondary malignancy and leukemia.
- Monitor for anxiety and depression, provide emotional support, and make referrals as necessary.

Patient Education

- Initiate smoking cessation protocol, if indicated.
- Discuss sperm banking before initiation of therapy.
- Review infection protection, bleeding precautions, and energy conservation, as well as skin care during chemotherapy and/or radiation.
- Explain routine testing for surveillance of cancer and demonstrate testicular self-examination in the remaining testis.

Patient Population Considerations

Geriatric

- It is rare for older patients to develop testicular cancer; however, the incidence rates of nonseminoma and seminoma have increased in patients over 50 years of age.

Pediatric

- Most cases of childhood testicular cancer can be treated with surgery alone.

Referring Patients

- Urology consult
- Surgery consult
- Oncology consult

TESTICULAR TORSION

Overview

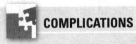

- In testicular torsion, the spermatic cord becomes twisted, obstructing perfusion to the ipsilateral testes, risking infarct. It can be further classified as intravaginal or extravaginal torsion.
  - Extravaginal torsion can occur in utero or in neonates where the testes freely rotate before fixation via the tunica vaginalis. Spermatic muscle contraction can trigger rotation.
  - Intravaginal torsion may be due to a congenital bell clapper deformity of the attachment of the tunica vaginalis to the testes. The deformity makes them vulnerable to torsion throughout the life span but it is more likely to occur in adolescence and young adulthood.
- Uncorrected, the testes will necrose and atrophy without surgical intervention.
- Its presentation can be confused with acute epididymitis, resulting in delayed treatment. Necrosis can occur after 6 hr of decreased perfusion.

> **COMPLICATIONS**
>
> ***Acute:*** Testicular infarction, orchitis, sepsis
> ***Chronic:*** Atrophy, infertility in late detorsion

Etiology

- Congenital anomaly, undescended testes
- Personal or family history of testicular torsion
- Vigorous exercise or sexual activity
- Trauma
- African American ethnicity, younger age, and lack of private insurance increase the risk of orchiectomy

Signs and Symptoms

- Scrotal pain of sudden onset followed by edema
- High riding testicle, hard testes
- Abdominal pain, fever, nausea, and vomiting may be present in ages >12
- History of recent sex, exercise, or trauma
- Unilateral scrotal edema, erythema, tenderness, loss of cremaster reflex
- Blue dot sign on upper pole of testes
- Hard scrotal mass in prenatal torsion

> **ALERT**
>
> Lightly stroke the inner part of the upper thigh and observe for contraction and elevation of the testes.
>
> Absence of response supports the likelihood testicular torsion in the absence of neurologic disease.

Differential Diagnosis

- *GI*: Appendicitis
- *GU*: Cyst, epididymitis, hydrocele, orchitis, scrotal hernia, STIs, spermatocele, testicular tumor/mass/ trauma, varicocele

Diagnosis

Labs

- U/A will be normal in most cases, but WBCs may be present
- CBC may be normal or reveals leukocytosis
- CRP may be elevated

Additional Diagnostic Testing

- TWIST score to evaluate risk for torsion
- Ultrasound to rule out testicular torsion
- MRI

> **CLINICAL PEARL**
>
> **TWIST Score Analysis**
>
> If there is testicular swelling or a hard mass in the testes in an afebrile patient, refer the patient to the ED for ultrasound.
>
> If there are two out of three of the following, refer the patient to the ED for ultrasound: nausea or vomiting, absent cremaster reflex, or high riding testing.

Treatment and Management

Treatment Goals
- Protect from harm, provide supportive care for surgical detorsion comfort, and prevent complications.

Drug Treatment
- The patient requires acute management by urology.
- Keep NPO; provide parenteral antiemetic. Parenteral analgesics can be provided after urology evaluation.

Interventions
- Following detorsion, monitor postoperative recovery for presence of complications.
- Discuss coping with altered body image.
- Reinforce that fertility function is preserved in salvaged testicles.

Patient Education
- Discuss complications to report following detorsion or orchiectomy.
- Reinforce postoperative instructions and follow-up with urologist within 2 weeks.

Patient Population Considerations

Geriatric
- Testicular torsion in older males is extremely rare but has been reported.

Pediatric
- Explore any history of sudden scrotal pain that resolves spontaneously in any patient's history taking. Intermittent torsion and spontaneous detorsion can occur and should be referred to urology for evaluation.

Referring Patients
- Urology consult

POP QUIZ 10.3

A 74-year-old male presents to the primary care office complaining of flank pain radiating to his groin, rated 10/1–10 scale, associated with urinary retention and constipation. He has a history of prostate cancer with a Gleason score of 8, for which he received brachytherapy 6 years earlier. His PSA level is 2 ng/mL. His bladder is palpable. He is able to void 30 mL dark cloudy urine, with a PVR of 800 mL. U/A reveals a large number of RBCs, WBCs, and casts. What is the priority intervention?

WOMEN'S HEALTH

BREAST AND CERVICAL CANCER SCREENING

Breast Cancer Screening
- Professional organizations, nonprofits, and governmental agencies do not proffer a unified breast cancer screening recommendation. Patients are encouraged to use a shared decision-making model with their HCP according to their preferences and examination of their personal and family risk.
- Breast cancer screening tools have been designed to calculate risk that can be completed by patients online.
- The American Cancer Society recommendations for breast cancer screening for the secondary detection of cancer include routine mammogram, MRI, and genetic counseling according to risk and condition. Ultrasound is an additional tool that is helpful in certain cases.
- The National Comprehensive Cancer Network recommends that all populations be assessed for personal and family risk factors for breast cancer no later than age 30 to early identify patients for supplemental screening.

Diagnostic Testing
- Genetic testing
- Mammogram or digital breast tomosynthesis
- Ultrasound
- MRI

General Recommendations Average Risk of Breast Cancer
- Women can choose to begin yearly mammograms by age 40 years or defer testing up until age 45 years, if they choose.
- All women should begin yearly mammograms by age 45 years.
- At age 55, women can schedule mammograms every 2 years but may continue with annual screening if that is their preference.
- Women should continue their screening if their life expectancy is 10 years or longer.
- Neither clinical breast examination nor breast self-examination are required as part of the screening recommendations. Women should know their breasts and report changes.

Recommendations in High-Risk Populations
- Genetic testing
  - Refer patients ≤age 30 years to genetic counseling for personal or family history of cancer on either side of the family with features suggestive of hereditary cancer.
- Breast MRI and mammogram
  - Refer high-risk patients for MRI and mammogram starting at age 30 years.
    - Examine personal and family history of cancer in first- and second-degree relatives to classify as high risk.
- Personal risk for breast cancer increases with a previous diagnosis of breast cancer or radiation therapy to the chest between the ages of 10 and 30 years.
- Inherited breast cancer is more likely in the following:
  - Ashkenazi Jewish heritage
  - Early age of onset <50 years
  - Bilateral breast cancers diagnosed at age 50 to 65 years
  - Breast cancer on both sides of the family
  - Multiple primary tumors (e.g., breast and ovarian)
  - Breast cancers in multiple first-degree relatives
  - Male breast cancers
  - BRAC1 or BRAC2 gene mutation in a first-degree relative
  - Li–Fraumeni syndrome, Cowden syndrome, or Bannayan–Riley–Ruvalcaba syndrome

Cervical Cancer Screening

- The American Cancer Society updated its recommendations for cervical cancer screening in July 2020. Clinicians can use either primary HPV testing, HPV DNA and Pap co-testing, or Pap testing alone for the secondary detection of cancer according to age and condition.
- Two HPV types, HPV 16 and HPV 18, are the high-risk HPV types that are associated with 70% of all cervical cancers. They can progress to low-grade cervical intraepithelial neoplasia within a few years of infection. The cure rate for cervical cancer if confined to the cervix can reach as high as 98%.
- ACS updated their screening recommendations with the development of more effective testing.
- Primary HPV testing is preferred because it increases the likelihood of detection of these high-risk types. HPV DNA and Pap co-testing can be used in its place. However, the testing can produce a false-positive test result for less high-risk HPV types. Pap testing alone does not test for the presence of HPV DNA; therefore, it may be less effective in the early detection of cancer. Pap testing alone is used when HPV testing is not available, but Pap testing frequency is increased to every 3 years.

Diagnostic Testing

- Perform primary HPV testing during cervical examination, every 5 years *OR*
- Perform HPV DNA with Pap co-testing every 5 years *OR*
- Perform Pap testing every 3 years.

Recommended Populations

- All women age 25 to 65 years
- Women who have had a hysterectomy for the treatment of cervical cancer or a serious precancer
- Women who have had a hysterectomy without removal of the cervix
- Women over 65 years who had been treated for a serious precancer (CIN ≥ 2) within the past 25 years or if they test negative over the past 10 years on all screens
- Women who were exposed to DES *in utero* or are immunosuppressed from HIV infection, long-term steroid use, or organ transplant may need to be screened more often and should follow their HCP's guidance

---

BREAST MASS (FIBROCYSTIC VS. BREAST CANCER)

Overview

Fibroadenoma, Fibrocystic Breast Change, Phyllodes Tumor

- Benign lesions are classified as fibroadenomas or fibrocystic changes and phyllode tumor.
  - Fibroadenoma is the most common breast mass of mixed fibrous and ductal tissue. They occur in adolescence and through reproductive years, sometimes resolving with menopause.
  - Fibrocystic changes are benign and describe discreet fluid-filled cysts with mastalgia that occur before menstruation. They can begin in adolescence or early adulthood and persist during reproductive years. Changes may or may not be associated with nipple discharge.
- Complicated cysts with debris in fibrocystic changes have a low rate of malignancy while complex cysts with a discreet solid component have a higher risk for malignant transformation.
- Phyllode tumors are fibroadenoma-like structures where fibrocystic changes and adenosis can occur. They can grow quickly and are complex in differentiation. Once removed they can locally recur. In rare cases, phyllode tumor can undergo malignant transformation.

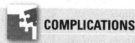

COMPLICATIONS

- Anxiety, malignant transformation of benign breast mass

Breast Cancer

- Breast cancer is a malignant transformation in breast cells in ducts (ductal), lobes (lobular), or parenchyma (infiltrative). It can be inflammatory and extend into overlying skin or circumscribed and discreet. Neoplasia can proliferate and extend into local structures and adjacent organs, micrometastasis, and travel by lymphatic spread.

COMPLICATIONS

Complications of Breast Cancer

Acute: DVT/PE, stroke, MI, renal colic, postoperative complications, adverse effect of chemotherapy, and radiation therapy

Chronic: Metastasis to bone, brain, liver, lung, breast cancer recurrence, secondary malignancy

Etiology

Fibroadenoma and Fibrocystic Breast Changes

- Exact etiology unknown
- Associated with estrogen and progesterone

Phyllode Tumor

- Exact etiology unknown
- Family history of Li–Fraumeni syndrome

Breast Cancer

- Increasing age
- Family history
- Genetic risk factors

(continued)

Etiology (*continued*)

- Benign breast disease
- Radiation exposure to chest
- Personal history of cancer (ovarian, endometrial, breast)
- Early menarche or late menopause
- Nulliparity or pregnancy after 30 years
- Sedentary lifestyle
- Tobacco, obesity, oral contraceptive, or hormone replacement use
- African-American women are more likely to get triple negative breast cancer

Signs and Symptoms

Fibroadenoma
- Solid breast lump
- Single or multiple
- Firm or rubbery
- Painless, mobile
- Can become uncomfortable if they enlarge

Fibrocystic Breast Changes
- Rubbery, tender masses
- Mastalgia
- With or without nipple discharge

Phyllodes Tumor
- Well demarcated mobile nontender mass
- May have overlying skin ulceration

Breast Cancer
- May be asymptomatic with risk factors
- Reports painless lump in breast that may be fixed
- Palpable axillary node
- *Skin changes*: Dimpling, inflammation, scaling, or ulceration
- Nipple discharge or retraction
- Lymphadenopathy

Differential Diagnosis

- *NEURO*: Neuropathy
- *ONC*: Breast cancer, Paget's disease
- *ENDO*: Pituitary tumor
- *Other*: Benign cyst or tumor, costochondritis, duct ectasia, fibroadenoma, mastitis

Diagnosis

Labs
- Diagnosis by clinical examination
- Elevated prolactin level with nipple discharge in pituitary tumor
- Genetic testing with high-risk family history

Additional Diagnostic Testing

- Ultrasound with or without fine needle aspiration or core needle biopsy
  - Palpable mass under age 30 years should be evaluated with ultrasound and MRI
- Diagnostic mammogram to detect microcalcifications with or without ultrasound

- MRI in age <30 years and/or presence of nipple discharge or skin changes
- Excisional biopsy
- Punch biopsy with skin ulceration

Treatment and Management

Treatment Goals

- *Benign mass*: Manage discomfort; modify risk factors for breast cancer.
- *Breast cancer*: Treat cancer according to stage, prevent micrometastasis and local extension, prevent recurrence and complications.
    - Breast cancer treatment may include chemotherapy adjuvant endocrine and targeted therapy with or without lumpectomy, mastectomy, and lymph node dissection, and oophorectomy according to stage and preference.

Drug Treatment

- *Benign mass*
    - Prescribe OTC acetaminophen or ibuprofen PRN for breast pain associated with fibrocystic changes.
- *Breast cancer*
    - Raloxifene or tamoxifen may be prescribed for the primary prevention of breast cancer.
        - Prescribe medication to prevent ASCVD according to risk profile.
    - Consult oncology for medication changes to avoid adverse event. Be mindful that polypharmacology in older patients can increase risks, reduce tolerance, and respond to cancer treatment.

Interventions

- *Benign mass*
    - Monitor for development of increased risks of breast cancer disease.
- *Breast cancer*
    - Adjuvant therapy can increase risk for thromboembolic events. Monitor BP and lipid profile and modify cardiovascular risk factors and hypertension.
    - Monitor fluid and electrolyte balance with vomiting and diarrhea with chemotherapy.
    - Monitor patient's response to therapy (chemotherapy, radiation, adjuvant therapy, and surgical interventions) and collaborate with oncology.
    - Monitor for secondary malignancy and complications.

CLINICAL PEARL

Interventions for Carcinoma In Situ
Stage 0 LCIS:
- Surveillance with raloxifene (postmenopausal) or tamoxifen (any)
- Elective bilateral prophylactic mastectomy if patient preference

Stage 0 DCIS:
- Lumpectomy versus mastectomy with or without radiation or sentinel node biopsy
- Tamoxifen can be considered for 5 years

Patient Education

- *Benign mass*
    - Discuss benign disease process, risk and screening for breast cancer, and s/s to report.
    - Instruct patient to wear a well-fitting bra and avoid caffeine if ingestion worsens symptoms.
- *Breast cancer*
    - Review primary prevention for breast cancer and risk factor modification.
    - Discuss cancer treatment according to type and stage and explain s/s of complications to report.
    - Review breast cancer surveillance following treatment.

Patient Population Considerations

Women (conception/pregnancy/lactation)

- Counsel women of childbearing age under 30 years to learn their personal and family risk for the development of breast cancer so that early testing and counseling can be performed.

Geriatric
- Breast cancer and comorbidities increase with age, as does cancer frequency. Cancer treatment tolerance is more difficult due to increased risk of adverse events and toxicities and requires more careful monitoring.

Pediatric
- Several inherited genetic syndromes (Ataxia-telangiectasia syndrome, Cowden syndrome, Li–Fraumeni syndrome, BRAC1, BRAC2) can cause pediatric breast disorders that require further inquiry to identify breast cancer.

Referring Patients
- Breast surgeon consult
- Oncology consult
- Genetic counseling

POP QUIZ 10.4

A 53-year-old female presents as a new patient to the primary care office for evaluation of a scaling lesion on her breast that is irritated by her bra strap.

What is the differential diagnosis?

CONTRACEPTION

Overview
- Contraception is a category of methods used to prevent pregnancy by either or both partners. Methods are mechanical, pharmacological, surgical, implanted, or a combination of more than one method. Contraceptive methods have been evaluated for their degree of efficacy when used properly (see Table 10.3).

Indications
- Desire to prevent pregnancy according to preference or necessity.
- Required prevention of pregnancy due to exposure to teratogens (medications, therapeutic or diagnostic radiation, environmental toxins)

Contraindications
- Current or suspected pregnancy for more than 120 hr is an absolute contraindication for hormonal, implanted, or inserted devices.
- In addition, there are many risk factors and health conditions that can cause complications when a method is used that may cause harm or outweigh the benefit.
- Refer to the CDC summary chart of medical eligibility for a detailed list and updated recommendations. Conduct further inquiry if a condition is present that correlates to the summary according to type

Table 10.3 Types of Contraceptives	
Classification	**Types**
Surgical	• Tubal ligation or vasectomy
Mechanical	• Abstinence, withdrawal, male and female condom, diaphragm, cervical cap, spermicidal agent
Hormonal	• *Combined hormonal contraceptives*: Estrogen and progesterone in pill, patch, or ring • Progestin-only pills and subdermal implants • Medroxyprogesterone acetate injection
Intrauterine	• Copper IUD, levonorgestrel-releasing (progestin) IUD

Relative or Absolute Contraindications According to Contraceptive Type

Combined Hormonal Contraceptive (Pill, Patch, or Ring)

Continued use of a contraceptive pill, patch, or ring may be contraindicated (relative or absolute) with the development of a specified disease or condition.

- *CV*: ASCVD (multiple risk), CVHD, DVT/PE (risk or active), PAD, hypertension, valvular disease (complicated), peripartum cardiomyopathy, HF, APLA syndrome
- *ENDO*: DM with microvascular or macrovascular disease, DM of ≥duration of 20 years
- *GI*: Severe cirrhosis, liver masses, history of bariatric surgery, gallbladder disease, past cholestasis, acute viral hepatitis, continuation in inflammatory bowel disease
- *REPRO*: Nonbreastfeeding <21 days postpartum, breastfeeding postpartum
- *HEM/ONC*: Current or past breast cancer in past 5 years, organ transplant
- *NEURO*: Migraines with aura, stroke, MS with prolonged immobility
- *Other*: Tobacco any age any amount, protease inhibitors, anticonvulsants, antitubercular agents

Progestin Only Pill

- *CV*: Continuation in CVHD
- *GI*: History of bariatric surgery, severe cirrhosis, liver mass
- *REPRO*: Breastfeeding postpartum
- *HEM/ONC*: Current or past breast cancer in past 5 years
- *NEURO*: Stroke
- *Other*: SLE, protease inhibitors, anticonvulsants, antitubercular agents

Progestin Implant

- *CV*: Continuation in CVHD
- *GI*: Severe cirrhosis, liver mass
- *REPRO*: Unexplained vaginal bleeding, breastfeeding postpartum
- *HEM/ONC*: Current or past breast cancer in past 5 years
- *NEURO*: Continuation in stroke
- *Other*: SLE

DPMA Injection

- *CV*: ASCVD (multiple risk), CVHD, hypertension
- *GI*: Severe cirrhosis, liver mass
- *ENDO*: DM with microvascular or microvascular disease, DM of ≥duration 20 years
- *REPRO*: Unexplained vaginal bleeding, breastfeeding postpartum
- *HEM/ONC*: Current or past breast cancer in past 5 years
- *NEURO*: Stroke
- *Other*: SLE, RA on immunosuppressants

Progestin IUD

- *CV*: Continuation with CVHD
- *GI*: Severe cirrhosis, liver mass
- *REPRO*: Distorted uterine cavity, unexplained vaginal bleeding or uterine disease, endometrial cancer, awaiting treatment for cervical cancer, insertion with current purulent cervicitis, current chlamydia or gonococcal infection, pelvic TB, postpartum puerperal disease, pregnancy, immediate postseptic abortion, postpartum sepsis
- *HEM/ONC*: Current or past breast cancer in past 5 years, insertion with organ transplant
- *Other*: SLE, antiretroviral therapy, initiation with AIDS

Copper IUD

- *REPRO*: Distorted uterine cavity, unexplained vaginal bleeding or uterine disease, endometrial cancer, awaiting treatment for cervical cancer, insertion with current purulent cervicitis, current chlamydia or gonococcal infection, pelvic TB, postpartum puerperal disease, pregnancy, immediate postseptic abortion, postpartum sepsis
- *HEM*: Insertion with organ transplant recipients
- *Other*: Wilson's disease

Treatment and Management

Contraception Counseling

- Use a comprehensive questionnaire and perform a history and physical when providing conception counseling.
- Obtain a health history to identify medical conditions and risk factors that increases the risk of certain contraindications or where the risk outweighs the benefits.
- Obtain an obstetrics, lactation, menstrual, and sexual history and perform urine pregnancy testing. Do not order exams and tests prior to initiation of contraception that could increase the likelihood that the patient will be lost to follow-up.
- Assess for the presence of medications and nutraceuticals that can interact with hormonal agents.
- Determine blood pressure to identify risk for hypertension if combined hormonal contraceptives are considered.
- Perform a physical exam to exclude medical conditions.
  - Do not require a pelvic exam before starting combined hormonal contraceptive. Bimanual examination and cervical inspection are required for cervical cap, diaphragm, and IUD insertion.
- Evaluate the patient's history, options, and preferences and prescribe or refer as indicated.
- Discuss initiation strategy and backup contraception, as necessary.
- Develop a plan for follow-up and STI prevention and notification.

Emergency Contraception

- Emergency postcoital contraception is medication or devices used to prevent implantation. The following options can be considered for emergency contraception:
  - Copper IUD
    - Refer overweight or obese patients for copper IUD since hormonal options are less likely to be effective.
  - Ulipristal (progesterone agonist) 300 mg PO taken in a single dose within 120 hr. Repeat dose if vomiting occurs within 3 hr.
    - Resume hormonal contraceptive methods no sooner than 5 days after ulipristal.
    - Use a backup method for contraception for 7 days.
  - Progestin-only pills 1.5 mg as a single dose **OR** 0.75 mg PO q12h for two doses within 72 hr.
    - Continue regular contraceptive methods immediately after emergency contraception.
    - Use a backup method for contraception for 7 days.
  - Combined estrogen/progestin oral contraceptives in two doses
    - Continue regular contraceptive methods immediately after emergency contraception.
    - Use a backup method for contraception for 7 days.

Referring Patients

- Gynecology consult

MENOPAUSE

Overview

- Amenorrhea for 12 consecutive months due to failure of ovarian follicular development and ovarian hormone depletion in a woman between age 45 to 55 with no alternative cause is referred to as menopause. Perimenopausal symptoms may precede amenorrhea for approximately 5 years.

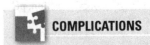

COMPLICATIONS

Acute: Anxiety, depression

Chronic: ASCVD, CVHD, osteoporosis, cancer

Etiology

- Natural maturational change
- Chemotherapy
- Primary ovarian failure
- Oophorectomy

Signs and Symptoms

- Hot flashes, night sweats
- Anxiety, depression, or mood swings
- Cognitive impairment
- Decreased libido
- Insomnia
- Vaginal dryness, atrophy, dyspareunia

> **CLINICAL PEARL**
>
> Variable patterns hormone sensitivity and release may contribute to irregular bleeding patterns resulting in testing for pelvic pathology.

Diagnosis

Labs

- FSH ≥ 40 IU/L

Differential Diagnosis

- *GU*: Pelvic TB
- *ENDO*: Cushing's syndrome, hypothyroidism, hyperthyroidism, pituitary disorder, PCOS
- *NEURO*: Brain mass, eating disorder, TBI
- *Other*: Sarcoidosis, chemotherapy, radiation

Treatment and Management

Treatment Goals

- Manage symptoms and prevent complications.

Drug Treatment

- Prescribe paroxetine 7.5 mg PO daily for vasomotor symptoms.
- Discuss risks and benefits of topical or oral hormone replacement therapy. Note that topical estrogen cream has reduced systemic adverse effects but does not eliminate risk for DVT, CVHD, stroke, and breast cancer.

Interventions

- Refer patients with dysfunctional uterine bleeding patterns to gynecology.
- Monitor and manage risk factors for development of CVHD, osteoporosis, or stroke.
- Monitor results of cervical, breast, and colon cancer screening results.

Patient Education

- Discuss risks and benefits of hormone therapy versus SSRI for the management of menopausal symptoms.
- Review modifiable risk factors for ASCVD, CVHD, and osteoporosis.
- Encourage vaginal lubricants for atrophic symptoms that interfere with sexual activity.

Patient Population Considerations

Women (conception/pregnancy/lactation)

- Encourage perimenopausal women to continue contraception to avoid pregnancy.

Geriatric

- Obtain a sexual health history using the "five Ps" assessment strategy (partners, practices, pregnancy, protection, and past history of STIs). Discuss the risk factors for STIs with unprotected sex. Continue primary HPV testing or HPV DNA and Pap co-testing every 5 years or Pap testing alone every 3 years in women over age 65 years. Stop testing if there are normal results in consecutive testing in the past 10 years and no history of CIN2 or more serious diagnosis within the past 25 years.

Referring Patients

- Gynecology consult

OVARIAN CANCER

Overview

- Ovarian cancer are predominantly epithelial tumors whose cells disseminate into the peritoneum and seed peritoneal surfaces of structures and organs such as the liver, diaphragm, bladder, mesenteric bowel, uterus, and lymph nodes.
- It is the most common cause of cancer death as compared to all other female reproductive cancers in women.

Etiology

- Personal history of breast cancer before age 40 years
- Family history of breast or ovarian cancer at any age
- Age over 50 years
- *Genetic factors*: BRAC1, BRAC2, Lynch II syndrome complex (HNCC)
- Ashkenazi Jewish ancestry
- Family history of premenopausal ovarian cancer
- Nulliparity
- Hormone replacement therapy in women age 50 to 79 years
- BMI > 25, use of talcum powder to vulva

Signs and Symptoms

- Asymptomatic in early disease.
- Report of bloating, distention, constipation or diarrhea, early satiety, urinary, or GERD symptoms should be further evaluated.
- Abdominal or pelvic mass, ascites bowel obstruction, and pleural effusion are associated with advanced disease.

Differential Diagnosis

- *GI*: Appendiceal mass, ascites, bowel adhesion, fecal impaction, GI cancer, irritable bowel syndrome, pancreatic cancer
- *GU*: Adnexal mass, cervicitis, ectopic pregnancy, hydrosalpinx, ovarian cysts, ovarian torsion, PID, urinary retention, uterine cancer, uterine fibroids

Diagnosis

Labs
- *Tumor markers*: CA-125 may be elevated in 50% of cases in stage 1 and is helpful in monitoring response to treatment.
- Carcinoembryonic antigen may also be measured.
- Check BMP, LFTs, Ca, Mg to evaluate electrolyte and hepatorenal function.
- Check CBC to evaluate for baseline Hgb, HcT, and platelets.

 COMPLICATIONS

Acute: Bowel obstruction, DVT, obstructive uropathy, pleural effusion

Chronic: Metastasis to liver, lungs, peritoneum, protein calorie malnutrition

CLINICAL PEARL

Risk for ovarian cancer is reduced with more full-term pregnancies, use of oral birth control, or tubal ligation.

ALERT

High-Risk Ovarian Cancer

Patients who are at high risk for genetic ovarian cancer should be referred to genetic counseling.

Patients with BRAC1 or BRAC2. HNPCC should be referred GYN-oncology for evaluation for salpingo-oophorectomy.

Additional Diagnostic Testing
- Transvaginal ultrasound is the most useful tool to evaluate a pelvic mass
- CT of the abdomen, pelvis, and chest to look for local and distant spread
- Coloscopy or barium enema
- Staging laparoscopy with biopsy

Treatment and Management

Treatment Goals
- Treat cancer according to stage (surgery, radiation, chemotherapy, targeted therapy), prevent micrometastasis and local extension, prevent recurrence and complications.

Drug Treatment
- Prescribe oral contraceptives to decrease the risk of developing ovarian cancer for average woman and BRCA mutation carriers.
- Consult oncology for medication changes to avoid adverse event. Be mindful that polypharmacology in older patients can increase risks, reduce tolerance, and respond to cancer treatment.

Interventions
- Monitor for development of risk factors that increase the risk of ovarian cancer.
- Targeted therapy can increase risk for myelodysplastic syndrome and gastrointestinal side effects. Monitor CBC for pancytopenia and BMP for fluid and electrolyte balance with vomiting and diarrhea with therapy.
- Monitor patient's response to therapy (chemotherapy, targeted therapy, and surgical interventions) and collaborate with oncology.
- Monitor for secondary malignancy and complications.

Patient Education
- Discuss disease process, risk, and genetic screening for high-risk patients.
- Review primary prevention for ovarian cancer and risk factor modification.
- Refer patients with genetic mutations for evaluation for bilateral salpingo-oophorectomy.
- Discuss cancer treatment according to type and stage and explain s/s of complications to report.
- Review ovarian cancer surveillance following treatment.

Patient Population Considerations

Women (conception/pregnancy/lactation)
- Assist patients in identifying their genetic risk for ovarian cancer before age 30 and refer for genetic counseling to reduce the mortality associated with ovarian and breast cancer.

Geriatric
- Older women are more likely to receive less aggressive interventions for ovarian cancer and suffer more death than younger patients. Standard of care chemotherapy treatment for older women may be feasible and tolerated. Age should not be a determining factor in selection of therapeutics.

Pediatric
- While most ovarian masses are not malignant in children, when malignancy occurs, it is most frequently found in females age 15 to 19 years. A recent study revealed that the rate for oophorectomy in benign ovarian disease is high. Refer pediatric patients to a pediatric oncologist who has experience in diagnosing ovarian cancer in children.

Referring Patients
- Gynecologic oncologist consult
- Pediatric and adolescent gynecology–oncologist consult

POLYCYSTIC OVARIAN SYNDROME

Overview

- PCOS is an endocrine disorder that is characterized by anovulation, hyperandrogenism, hyperinsulinemia, menstrual dysfunction, and multiple ovarian cysts.
- Increased gonadotropin-releasing hormone and insulin resistance causes an androgen excess that stops follicle development in the ovaries. Androgen excess further increases gonadotropin-releasing hormone which repeats the process and increases the LH:FSH ratio. Ovaries become polycystic.
- Resultant anovulation decreases fertility and regular menses and decreases progesterone release. Estrogen becomes unopposed due to decreased progesterone and endometrial hyperplasia follows.

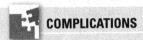

COMPLICATIONS

Acute: Acne, amenorrhea, hyperglycemia, anxiety, depression, NAFLD

Chronic: Dyslipidemia, insulin resistance, obesity, uterine cancer, gestational diabetes, preeclampsia

Etiology

- Genetics
- Obesity
- Sedentary lifestyle
- Intrauterine exposure to androgens

Signs and Symptoms

- Acanthosis nigricans
- Acne, alopecia, hirsutism
- Irregular menses
- Anovulation and miscarriage
- Anxiety or depression
- Elevated BP

Differential Diagnosis

- *CV*: Hyperlipidemia
- *GU*: Ovarian tumor, primary ovarian failure
- *ENDO*: Acromegaly, Addison disease, adrenal tumor, congenital adrenal hyperplasia (late onset), Cushing syndrome, hyperprolactinemia, metabolic syndrome, pituitary disease, thyroid dysfunction
- *Other*: Danazol, androgenic progestins, anabolic steroid abuse

Diagnosis

Labs
- Elevated serum androstenedione, luteinizing hormone, prolactin, testosterone level
- Low-serum FSH
- Elevated LDL, cholesterol, triglycerides, TSH
- Low HDL
- Elevated BG, HbA1c, OGTT > 140 mg/dL
- BMP, LFTs, Ca, Mg to evaluate electrolyte and hepatorenal function
- CBC to evaluate for increase platelet volume

Additional Diagnostic Testing
- Ovarian ultrasound
- Pelvic CT or MRI
- Ovarian biopsy

Treatment and Management

Treatment Goals
- Treat acute symptoms, regulate endocrine anomalies, and prevent complications of disease.

Drug Treatment
- Collaborate with gynecology, fertility specialist, endocrinology, and dermatology to manage disease.
- Prescribe statins, antidiabetics, and antihypertensives, as indicated.
- Patients will receive medications for PCOS as follows:
  - Metformin for acanthosis nigricans, anovulation, hyperglycemia
  - Spironolactone and oral contraceptives for acne, hirsutism, and irregular menses

Interventions
- Monitor effect of therapy and manage cardiovascular risk factors.
- Evaluate lab results for complications of disease and its treatment at periodic intervals.
- Make appropriate referrals as indicated.

Patient Education

- Discuss disease process and risk factor modification.
- Review importance of maintaining BMI at target, controlled carbohydrate diet, and regular exercise.
- Teach s/s of complications and adverse medication effects to report.

Patient Population Considerations

Women (conception/pregnancy/lactation)
- Clomiphene citrate may be considered by fertility specialists for anovulatory patients seeking to become pregnant.
- Patients with PCOS who are pregnant are at increased risk for miscarriage, gestational diabetes, hypertension, eclampsia, preterm birth, fetal demise, and stillbirth.

Geriatric
- Refer the patient for uterine ultrasound to monitor for hyperplasia secondary to the disease at periodic intervals.
- Instruct patients to report spotting or uterine bleeding when noted to identify uterine cancer.

Pediatric
- Refer adolescents with a family history of PCOS for endocrine evaluation if menstrual irregularities persist for 2 to 3 years past menarche. Early treatment with metformin and oral contraceptive is indicated in this population.

Referring Patients

- Gynecology consult
- Endocrine consult
- Dermatology consult
- Fertility specialist consult

PREGNANCY

Overview

Signs of Pregnancy

- Presumptive
  - Presumptive signs of pregnancy are the signs and symptoms that cause a person to think that they may be pregnant. It presumes recent sexual activity with or without consent. It may be intentional or accidental. Contraception may have failed or was used incorrectly.
    - Missed menstrual period
    - Fatigue, nausea, and vomiting
    - Nipple skin changes, change in vaginal mucosa
    - Frequent urination and breast tenderness
    - Report of quickening (16–22 weeks)
    - Positive home pregnancy test
- Probable
  - Probable signs of pregnancy support the presence of presumptive signs which may be caused by something other than pregnancy but do not exclude conditions other than pregnancy.
    - Enlarged abdomen
    - Elevation of basal body temperature
    - Chloasma, linea nigra
    - Positive serum beta hCG (elevated in ectopic)
    - Pelvic examination reveals:
      - Softening of cervix, softening of bottom of uterus, and bluish discoloration (CUB in sequence)
      - Goodell's sign (4–8 weeks), Hegar's sign (4–12 weeks), Chadwick's sign (6–8 weeks), Braxton Hicks contractions (16 weeks), ballottement (16 weeks)
- Positive
  - Positive signs of pregnancy confirm the presence of a fetus in utero.
    - Active fetal movement felt by practitioner
    - Transvaginal ultrasound to locate gestational sac at 4.5 to 5 weeks' gestation.
    - Abdominal ultrasound to detect the presence of the gestational sac at 6 weeks.

Naegele's Rules

- Naegele's rule is a calculation that is used to estimate the expected date of delivery for pregnancy. The EDD is compared to the first accurate ultrasound examination that determines gestational age. A final date is calculated. ACOG standards require accurate dating of pregnancy in the medical record. Suboptimal dating is presumed when a pregnancy confirms or revises the EDD before 22 weeks without ultrasound examination. Ultrasound measurement in the first trimester is considered more accurate. In case of *in vitro* fertilization, the EDD is assigned using the age of the embryo and the date of transfer.
  - Identify the first day of the last menstrual period.
  - Subtract 3 months from the month of last menses.
  - Add 7 days to the date of the LMP.
  - Add 1 year.

Drug Categories

- *The U.S. Food and Drug Administration Pregnancy and Lactation Labeling Rule replaces the traditional drug categories:* A, B, C, D, and X. *The PLLR also requires the label to be updated when information becomes outdated. Medications currently labeled for use are outlined in Table 10.4.*

Table 10.4 FDA PLLR Labels	
Label	**Description**
Pregnancy	List of approved drugs that can be prescribed to pregnant women throughout pregnancy and during labor and delivery includes subsections for risks, clinical considerations, and data.
Lactation	Provides information about using the drug while breastfeeding and the amount of drug in breast milk and potential effects on the breastfed infant.
Female and male reproductive potential	Specifies when pregnancy testing is indicated, contraception recommendation and information about fertility.

Complications

Gestational Diabetes

- GDM is a complication of hyperglycemia in pregnant women who have not been diagnosed with diabetes prior to pregnancy. It is believed that pancreatic beta cells become dysfunctional in combination with insulin resistance that is increased due to placental hormones and weight gain.
- Risk factors for GDM include family history of any diabetes, advanced maternal age, increased weight gain more than body requirements. Personal history of prior GDM; PCOS; African-American, Hispanic, Native American, or Asian American ethnicities; sedentary lifestyle, BMI > 25; previous baby weight >9 lb increases risk.
- Prevention and screening
  - See Table 10.5.
  - All women should receive preconception counseling to identify their personal risk for GDM, maintain BMI <25, eat a healthy diet, and exercise. Clinicians should explain risk factors for GDM, maternal and infant complications, and prevention.
    - All women should undergo risk assessment at the first prenatal visit. Any patient with a positive screen will be referred for additional testing.
    - Pregnant women may be asymptomatic and will be screened with an oral glucose tolerance test at 24 to 28 weeks. Diagnosis of GDM is made using the 2-hr OGTT. A result >153 to 199 mg/dL indicates gestational diabetes. A result >200 mg/dL is overt diabetes.
  - Treatment and Management
    - Controlled carbohydrate diet
    - SMBG 4 to 7 times daily
    - Weight control and increase exercise
    - Basal and bolus insulin injection if it is not controlled with dietary changes
    - Fundoscopic examination by ophthalmology
    - Cardiovascular risk management

Table 10.5 Complications of GDM	
Maternal Complications	**Infant Complications**
• Cesarean section	• Fetal demise
• Hyperglycemia	• Hyperbilirubinemia
• Preeclampsia	• Hypocalcemia
• Gestational hypertension	• Hypoglycemia
• Gestational diabetes in future pregnancy	• Hypothermia
	• Macrosomia (shoulder dystocia, fracture and nerve palsy)
	• Polycythemia vera
	• Premature birth
	• Respiratory distress syndrome

Preeclampsia

- A disorder of dysfunction of vascular endothelium and vasospasm that triggers hypertension, proteinuria, and edema. SBP >140 mmHg or DBP >90 mmHg on two separate occasions at least 4 hr apart in a person who was previously normotensive.
- Early preeclampsia may be asymptomatic, but the patient may report HA, dyspnea, and edema.
- Preeclampsia can progress to severe preeclampsia that is evident with SBP >160 mmHg or DBP >110 mmHg on two separate occasions at least 4 hr apart while the patient is on bed rest.
- Severe preeclampsia is associated with blurred vision and focal neurological deficits, seizure, worsening edema, pulmonary edema, and thrombocytopenia. It can lead to HELLP syndrome, a life-threatening disorder of hemolysis, elevations in hepatorenal function indicating liver damage, and low platelets causing bleeding.
- Risk factors for preeclampsia are nulliparity, multiple gestation, egg donation, *in vitro* fertilization, age >35 years, family history, African-American ethnicity, personal history of obesity, chronic hypertension, CKD, DM, RA, APLA, SLE. PCOS, MS, GDM, sickle cell disease, scleroderma, and migraines.
- Prevention and screening
  - All women should receive preconception counseling to identify their personal risk for preeclampsia, maintain BMI <25, eat a healthy diet, and exercise. Clinicians should explain risk factors for preeclampsia, maternal and infant complications and prevention.
  - All women should undergo risk assessment at the first prenatal visit, BP assessment, and urine checked for protein. Any patient with a positive screen will be referred for additional testing.
  - Pregnant women may be asymptomatic and will be screened with CBC, BMP, Mg, LFTs, LDH, uric acid, and 24-hr urine collection for protein.
- Treatment and management
  - Preeclampsia is managed with antihypertensives (intravenous labetalol, hydralazine, or oral nifedipine) and low-dose aspirin beginning at 12 weeks' gestation. Careful fetal monitoring and maternal observations for signs of eclampsia and HELLP syndrome. Labor will be induced at 37 weeks' gestation if preeclampsia is not severe.

Abruptio Placentae

- Abruptio placentae is a complication of premature separation of the placenta from the uterine wall causing bleeding at any time beginning at 20 weeks' gestation through the third trimester. Blood vessels in the placenta spontaneously rupture, if unable to repair or is aggravated by maternal hypertension, the blood can accumulate and shear the placenta partially or completely.
- Risk factors are prior abruptio placentae, hypertension, age <20 years or >35 years, and preeclampsia. Trauma, uterine anomalies, premature rupture of the membranes, fibroids, short umbilical cord, multiparity, smoking, substance abuse, lack of antenatal care, and disease risk factors of DM, APLA, SLE increase risk.
- May be asymptomatic, report decreased fetal movement or develop vaginal bleeding that can range from mild to severe and may be associated with back pain and contractions.
- Prevention and screening
  - All women should receive preconception counseling to identify their personal risk for abruptio placentae and receive counseling for tobacco, alcohol, and substance abuse cessation and primary prevention of HTN and DM.
  - All women should undergo risk assessment at the first prenatal visit. Any patient with a positive screen will be referred for additional testing.
- Treatment and management
  - A patient presenting with s/s of abruptio placentae should be referred to the obstetrician or ED based on the severity of their symptoms. Do not perform a pelvic examination which could worsen the patient's bleeding. A nonstress test will be performed and a biophysical profile score <6 suggests fetal compromise.

VAGINAL INFLAMMATION AND INFECTIONS

Overview

- Inflammation of vaginal tissue can be infectious or noninfectious.
- Common vaginal infections are bacterial vaginosis, candida vaginitis, and trichomonas vaginitis.
- Atrophic or inflammatory vaginitis occurs with genital atrophy from loss of collagen, inflammation from irritants, allergens, or possible autoimmunity.
- Bacterial vaginosis occurs when vaginal pH rises following a loss of healthy *Lactobacillus*, leading to bacterial proliferation.

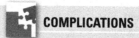

COMPLICATIONS

Acute: PID, postabortion and postpartum endometriosis, posthysterectomy vaginal cuff infection, chorioamnionitis, premature rupture of the membranes, preterm labor, and preterm birth

Etiology

- Cancer, diabetes, immunodeficiency, pregnancy
- Unprotected sexual activity, tight-fitting undergarments, soaps, vaginal deodorant, bubble baths, douching, spermicidal agents, excessive heat and moisture, smoking
- Antibiotics, corticosteroids, estrogen replacement therapy, immunosuppressants, IUD, oral contraceptives
- *Atrophic vaginitis*: Estrogen loss due to menopause, lactation, or ovarian failure from treatments or immune-mediated events
- *Bacterial vaginosis*: Gardnerella vaginalis, mobiluncus species, *mycoplasma hominis*, *prevotella* species, and *peptostreptococcus* species
- *Candidal vaginitis*: Candida albicans, Candida glabrata, Candida tropicalis, and *Candida krusei* overgrowth
- *Trichomonas vaginitis*: Trichomonas vaginalis parasite

Signs and Symptoms

- Vaginal pruritis, discharge, dysuria, dyspareunia, erythema, edema, and pain to vulva is seen in most inflammatory or infectious conditions.
- *Atrophic vaginitis*: Thinning, dry, and inflamed vaginal walls with loss of rugae, petechia, burning leukorrhea
- *Bacterial vaginosis*: Fish odor increased after sex and menses, white, gray, or green discharge
- *Candidal vaginitis*: Excoriation, thick cottage cheese-like discharge
- *Trichomonas vaginitis*: Fish odor, strawberry spots on vaginal walls and cervix, and copious, yellow-green, frothy vaginal discharge

Differential Diagnosis

- *GU*: Chlamydia vaginitis, gonococcal vaginitis, urethritis, UTI

Diagnosis

Labs

- *Atrophic vaginitis*: pH >5 parabasal cell on wet mount
- *Bacterial vaginosis*: Vaginal pH > 4.5, 20% clue cells on KOH wet mount, positive whiff test and leukorrhea (*Amsel criteria*: Homogenous discharge, positive whiff test, presence of clue cells, pH > 4.5; diagnosis requires three out of four criteria)
- *Candidal vaginitis*: Vaginal pH 4 to 4.5, pseudohyphae, budding yeast, or mycelia on KOH wet mount
- *Trichomonas vaginitis*: pH 5 to 6, trichomonads on saline wet mount, positive whiff test, direct microscopic examination of vaginal secretions, immunochromographic flow dipstick tests
- Bacterial or fungal cultures as indicated

Treatment and Management

Treatment Goals
- Treat infection, modify risk factors, and prevent complications.

Drug Treatment
- *Atrophic vaginitis*
  - *First-line treatment*: Offer vaginal moisturizers as needed to replace moisture.
  - Consider topical estrogen cream daily for 7 to 14 days if ineffective.
- *Bacterial vaginosis*
  - Metronidazole 2 g PO × one dose, *OR* 500 mg PO BID for 7 days, *OR* metronidazole 0.75% 5 g intravaginally daily for 7 days, *OR* 2% clindamycin vaginal cream daily for 7 days
  - Pregnant women in first trimester, use metronidazole gel
  - *Elective abortion*: Oral metronidazole prophylactically
- *Candidal vaginitis*
  - Fluconazole 150 mg PO for a single dose, especially after OTC topical ointment failure. Consider monthly suppression therapy for frequent reoccurrence.
- *Trichomonas vaginitis*
  - Tinidazole 2 g PO × one dose *OR* 500 mg PO BID for 7 days; treat sexual partner as well.

Interventions

- Monitor response to therapy in 1 to 2 weeks.
- Evaluate medication and health conditions contributing to inflammation.

Patient Education
- Discuss disease process and risk factor modification to reduce the likelihood for recurrence, hygiene practices, clothing, infection protection.
- Teach patient s/s of complications and adverse symptoms to report.

Patient Population Considerations

Women (conception/pregnancy/lactation)
- Refer pregnant patients to obstetrician. Consider HIV testing in women with frequent vaginal infections who have not been screened or have risk factors for HIV since their last test.

Geriatric
- Bacterial vaginosis, candidal vaginitis, and trichomonal vaginitis are uncommon among postmenopausal women. Evaluate for development of comorbid diabetes, cancer, immunodeficiency, unprotected sex, or medications that could be a contributing factor.

Pediatric
- Nonspecific vulvovaginitis can occur in children 2 to 6 years due to poor perineal and hand hygiene.

Referring Patients

- Gynecology consult
- Infectious disease specialist consult

RESOURCES

ACS. (2018). *Can ovarian cancer be prevented*. https://www.cancer.org/cancer/ovarian-cancer/causes-risks-prevention/prevention.html#:~:text=%20Can%20Ovarian%20Cancer%20Be%20Prevented%3F%20%20 1.may%20reduce%20the%20chance%20of%20developing…%20More%20

ACS. (2020a). *American Cancer Society recommendations for the early detection of breast cancer*. https://www.cancer.org/cancer/breast-cancer/screening-tests-and-early-detection/american-cancer-society-recommendations-for-the-early-detection-of-breast-cancer.html

ACS. (2020b). *The American Cancer Society guidelines for the prevention and early detection of cervical cancer.* https://www.cancer.org/cancer/cervical-cancer/detection-diagnosis-staging/cervical-cancer-screening-guidelines.html

American College of Obstetricians and Gynecologists. (2017). Methods for estimating the due date. Committee Opinion No. 700. *Obstetrics & Gynecology, 129*(5), e150–e154. https://doi.org/10.1097/aog.0000000000002046

Ayoade, F. (2018). *Medscape: Herpes simplex.* https://emedicine.medscape.com/article/218580-overview

Bevers, T. B., Helvie, M., Bonaccio, E., Calhoun, K. E., Daly, M. B., Farrar, W. B., Garber, J. E., Gray, R., Greenberg, C. C., Greenup, R., Hansen, N. M., Harris, R. E., Heerdt, A. S., Helsten, T., Hodgkiss, L., Hoyt, T. L., Huff, J. G., Jacobs, L., Lehman, C. D., & Kumar, R. (2018). Breast cancer screening and diagnosis, version 3.2018, NCCN Clinical practice guidelines in oncology. *Journal of the National Comprehensive Cancer Network, 16*(11), 1362–1389. https://jnccn.org/view/journals/jnccn/16/11/article-p1362.xml

Carroll, L. (2020). *Medscape: One in 10 gay and bisexual men may share HIV prep medications.* https://www.medscape.com/viewarticle/937296

Casey, F. (2020). *Medscape: Contraception.* https://emedicine.medscape.com/article/258507-overview#a6

Cash, J. C., & Glass, C. A. (Eds.). (2019). *Adult-gerontology practice guidelines.* Springer Publishing Company.

CDC. (2015a). *2015 Sexually transmitted diseases treatment guidelines.* https://www.cdc.gov/std/tg2015/default.htm

CDC. (2015b). *HPV-associated cancers and precancers.* https://www.cdc.gov/std/tg2015/hpv-cancer.htm#spec-con

CDC. (2020a). *Release of CDC vital signs report on newly reported cases of hepatitis C and updated hepatitis C screening recommendations.* https://www.hhs.gov/hepatitis/blog/2020/04/09/new-cdc-hepatitis-c-screening-recommendations-for-adults.html

CDC. (2020b). *Summary chart of U.S. medical eligibility criteria for contraceptive use.* https://www.cdc.gov/reproductivehealth/contraception/pdf/summary-chart-us-medical-eligibility-criteria_508tagged.pdf

Ching, C. (2020). *Medscape: Epididymitis.* https://emedicine.medscape.com/article/436154-overview

Codina Leik, M. T. (2018). *Family nurse practitioner certification: Intensive review.* Springer Publishing Company.

Croke, L. M. (2019). Gestational hypertension and preeclampsia: A practice bulletin from ACOG. *American Family Physician, 100*(10), 649–650.

Deem, S. (2018). *Medscape: Acute bacterial prostatitis.* https://emedicine.medscape.com/article/2002872-overview

Deters, P. (2019). *Medscape: Benign prostatic hypertrophy.* https://emedicine.medscape.com/article/437359-overview

Gearhart, P. (2020). *Medscape: Human papillomavirus (HPV).* https://emedicine.medscape.com/article/219110-overview

Ghazarian, A. A., Rusner, C., Trabert, B., Braunlin, M., McGlynn, K. A., & Stang, A. (2018). Testicular cancer among US men aged 50 years and older. *Cancer Epidemiology, 55*, 68–72. https://doi.org/10.1016/j.canep.2018.05.007

Gilroy, S. (2020). *Medscape: HIV infection and AIDS.* https://emedicine.medscape.com/article/211316-overview

Goje, O. (2019). *Merck manual: Overview of vaginitis.* https://www.merckmanuals.com/en-ca/professional/gynecology-and-obstetrics/vaginitis,-cervicitis,-and-pelvic-inflammatory-disease-pid/overview-of-vaginitis?query=Overview%20of%20Vaginal%20Infections

Gosain, R., Pollock, Y. Y., & Jain, D. (2016). Age-related disparity: Breast cancer in the elderly. *Current Oncology Reports, 18*(11), 1. https://doi.org/10.1007/s11912-016-0551-8

Green, A. (2020). *Medscape: Ovarian cancer.* https://emedicine.medscape.com/article/255771-overview

Grewal, H. (2019). *Medscape: Pediatric breast disorders.* https://emedicine.medscape.com/article/935410-overview#a7

Kim, E. (2018). *Medscape: Erectile dysfunction.* https://emedicine.medscape.com/article/444220-overview#a1

Krapf, J. (2018). *Medscape: Vulvovaginitis.* https://emedicine.medscape.com/article/2188931-overview#a6

Lannin, D. (2019). *Medscape4: Phyllodes tumor.* https://emedicine.medscape.com/article/188728-overview#a2

Lawrence, A. E., Gonzalez, D. O., Fallat, M. E., Aldrink, J. H., Hewitt, G. D., Hertweck, S. P., Onwuka, A., Bence, C., Burns, R. C., Dillon, P. A., Ehrlich, P. F., Fraser, J. S., Grabowski, J. E., Hirschl, R. B., Kabre, R., Kohler, J. E., Lal, D. R., Landman, M. P., Leys, C. M., . . . Mak, G. Z. (2019). Factors associated with management of pediatric ovarian neoplasms. *Pediatrics, 144*(1), e20182537. https://doi.org/10.1542/peds.2018-2537

Lu, Y., Chen, Y., Zhu, L., Cartwright, P., Song, E., Jacobs, L., & Chen, K. (2019). Local recurrence of benign, borderline, and malignant phyllodes tumors of the breast: A systematic review and meta-analysis. *Annals of Surgical Oncology, 26*(5), 1263–1275.

Lucidi, S. (2018). *Medscape: Menopause.* https://emedicine.medscape.com/article/264088-overview

Lucidi, S. (2019). *Medscape: Polycystic ovarian syndrome.* https://emedicine.medscape.com/article/256806-overview

Manohar, C. S., Gupta, A., Keshavamurthy, R., Shivalingaiah, M., Sharanbasappa, B. R., & Singh, V. K. (2018). Evaluation of testicular workup for ischemia and suspected torsion score in patients presenting with acute scrotum. *Urology Annals, 10*(1), 20–23. https://doi.org/10.4103/UA.UA_35_17

Miller, A. (2020). *Medscape: Breast abscesses and masses.* https://emedicine.medscape.com/article/781116-overview

NCI. (2019). *Childhood testicular cancer treatment (PDQ®)–health professional version.* https://www.cancer.gov/types/testicular/hp/child-testicular-treatment-pdq

NCI. (n.d.). *Online breast cancer risk assessment tool.* https://bcrisktool.cancer.gov/

Newton, E. (2020). *Medscape: Breast cancer screening.* https://emedicine.medscape.com/article/1945498-overview#a1

NHY DOH. (2019). *The diagnosis, management and prevention of syphilis an update and review.* https://www.nycptc.org/x/Syphilis_Monograph_2019_NYC_PTC_NYC_DOHMH.pdf

Ogunyemi, O. (2018). *Medscape: Testicular torsion.* https://emedicine.medscape.com/article/2036003-overview

Qaseem, A., Horwitch, C. A., Vijan, S., Etxeandia-Ikobaltzeta, I., & Kansagara, D. (2020). Testosterone treatment in adult men with age-related low testosterone: A clinical guideline from the American College of Physicians. *Annals of Internal Medicine, 172*(2), 126–133. https://doi.org/10.7326/m19-0882

Queshi, S. (2018). *Medscape: Chlamydia (chlamydia genitourinary infections).* https://emedicine.medscape.com/article/214823-overview

Rothstein, A., Ragini, S., & Wong, E. (2013). *Polycystic ovarian syndrome: Pathophysiology of PCOS.* McMaster Pathophysiology Review. http://www.pathophys.org/pcos/pcos-2/

Sachdeva, K. (2017). *Medscape: Nonseminoma testicular cancer treatment protocols.* https://emedicine.medscape.com/article/2006613-overview#a1

Sachdeva, K. (2019). *Medscape: Testicular cancer.* https://emedicine.medscape.com/article/279007-overview#a1

Shields, A. (2017). *Medscape: Pregnancy diagnosis.* https://emedicine.medscape.com/article/262591-overview

Sorenson, M., Quinn, L., & Klein, D. (2019). *Pathophysiology: Concepts of human disease* (1st ed.). Pearson Education.

Tew, W. P., & Fleming, G. F. (2014). Treatment of ovarian cancer in the older woman. *Gynecologic Oncology, 136*(1), 136–142. https://doi.org/10.1016/j.ygyno.2014.10.028

Trottier, H., Mayrand, M. H., Coutlée, F., Monnier, P., Laporte, L., Niyibizi, J., Carceller, A. M., Fraser, W. D., Brassard, P., Lacroix, J., Francoeur, D., Bédard, M. J., Girard, I., & Audibert, F. (2016). Human papillomavirus (HPV) perinatal transmission and risk of HPV persistence among children: Design, methods and preliminary results of the HERITAGE study. *Papillomavirus Research, 2,* 145–152.

Turek, P. (2019). *Medscape: Prostatitis.* https://emedicine.medscape.com/article/785418-overview#a3

Uthamalingam, M., & Periyasamy, K. (2016). Paget's disease of nipple in male breast with cancer. *Journal of Clinical and Diagnostic Research: JCDR, 10*(2), PD14–PD16. https://doi.org/10.7860/JCDR/2016/17778.7217

US Food and Drug Administration. (2015). *Pregnancy and lactation labeling final rule.* https://www.fda.gov/drugs/labeling-information-drug-products/pregnancy-and-lactation-labeling-drugs-final-rule

WedMD. (2019). *Prostatitis.* https://emedicine.medscape.com/article/785418-overview#a3

Zagaria, M. A. E. (2016). Ovarian cancer treatment considerations in older women. *US Pharmacist, 41*(9), 18–20. https://www.uspharmacist.com/article/ovarian-cancer-treatment-considerations-in-older-women

Zhou, Z. R., Wang, C. C., Yang, Z. Z., Yu, X. L., & Guo, X. M. (2016). Phyllodes tumors of the breast: Diagnosis, treatment and prognostic factors related to recurrence. *Journal of Thoracic Disease, 8*(11), 3361–3368. https://doi.org/10.21037/jtd.2016.11.03

11

HEMATOPOIETIC SYSTEM

ANEMIA OF CHRONIC DISEASE

Overview

- Anemia of chronic disease or inflammation results from decreased circulation RBCs due to reduced production, increased destruction, or chronic blood loss.
- Chronic inflammation of disease states impairs iron metabolism and suppresses erythropoiesis in combination with decreasing RBC life span.
- Cytokine TNF alfa facilitates the degradation of RBCs. IL-10 and INF gamma cause sequestration of iron in macrophages. Hepcidin released from the liver blocks some iron intake in the GI tract, further hampering RBC production.
- The patient may have concomitant IDA, functional iron deficiency in CKD or ESA, or mixed anemia (AI/IDA).

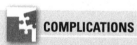

COMPLICATIONS

Acute: HF, ischemic CV events, exacerbation of HF, activity intolerance and fatigue
Chronic: Chronic HF, ASCVD

Etiology

- Anemia of critical illness, anemia of advanced age, obesity, concomitant bleeding, vitamin deficiencies (vitamins B_{12} and D, folic acid), hemolysis, radiation, renal dysfunction, infections, medications, hormones, dietary habits, genetics, and cancer
- *Disease risks:* Advanced liver disease cancer, CHF, CKD, collagen vascular disease, DM, immune-mediated disease, lymphoma, myeloproliferative disorders
- *Infections:* CMV EBV, *Helicobacter pylori*, hepatitis, HIV

ALERT

Medication-induced anemia
Anticonvulsants, aspirin, ACEIs/ARBs, antiplatelets, chemotherapy, DOAC, estrogen, heparin, NSAIDs, PPIs, and testosterone all can cause anemia.

Signs and Symptoms

- Fatigue, pallor, weakness, headache, cold intolerance
- Palpitations, dyspnea on exertion, activity intolerance
- Systolic murmur, hepatomegaly
- S/s of comorbid conditions

Differential Diagnosis

- *ENDO:* Hyperparathyroidism, hypoadrenalism, hypothyroidism, pituitary disorders
- *GI:* Inflammatory bowel disease, occult bleeding of GI cancers
- *HEM:* Aplastic anemia, iron deficiency anemia, hemolytic anemia, pernicious anemia
- *Other:* Medication-induced anemia

Diagnosis

Labs
- BMP and LFTs to evaluate renal and liver function
- PTT/PT/INR to identify coagulopathy
- TSH to assess thyroid function
- CRP to evaluate inflammation
- *CBC*: Normocytic normochromic early, may develop IDA
- Hgb <12 g/dL in women, <13 g/dL in men
- *MCV*: Normal (AI) or low MCV <80 fL (AI/IDA)
- *MCHC*: Normal (AI) or low (AI/IDA)
- Iron status
  - *Serum iron*: Low normal (AI) or low (AI/IDA)
  - *Serum ferritin*: AI has normal or increased >100 mcg/L while IDA <100
  - *Transferrin saturation*: >20% while IDA <20%
  - *TIBC and reticulocyte count*: Low indicates decreased production
- Renal status
  - Estimate to determine if GFR is normal or <60
- Vitamins
  - Vitamins B$_{12}$ and D; folic acid may be low
- Fecal occult blood test

> **CLINICAL PEARL**
>
> If serum ferritin is elevated >100, TSAT >20% check GFR.
> - If GFR <60, refer to **nephrology**.
> - If GFR >60, check B$_{12}$, D, and folic acid and refer to **hematology.**

Additional Diagnostic Testing
- Bone marrow aspiration may be considered, but not generally required.

Treatment and Management

Treatment Goals
- Treat the underlying cause, replace iron and vitamins if indicated, and increase RBC count and Hgb.

Drug Treatment
- Prescribe epoetin alfa SC for patients with CKD and nonmyeloid cancer if serum ferritin >100 and Hgb <7 g/dL.
- Prescribe ferrous sulfate with vitamin C to enhance absorption if IDA is present.
- Consider parenteral iron therapy if oral iron agents are ineffective, or the patient is symptomatic.
- Collaborate with hematology regarding PRBC transfusion with symptomatic anemia Hgb <7 to 8 and with CVHD, HF.
- Prescribe vitamins D and B$_{12}$, and/or folic acid if deficiencies are present to support RBC production.

Interventions
- Collaborate with gastroenterology, gynecology, hematology, rheumatology, and nephrology based on the cause.
- Discontinue any medications that increase bleeding, when indicated.
- Monitor for an increase in RBCs and Hgb with therapy. Stop epoetin alfa Hgb >11 g/dL.
- Monitor for complications of thromboembolic events and HF with ESA use.

Patient Education
- Teach patient energy management strategies based on comorbidities to avoid injury, ischemia, and decreased cardiac output.
- Provide dietary counseling to support nutritional therapy.
- Instruct the patient to monitor for hypertension and weight gain.

Patient Population Considerations

Women (conception/pregnancy/lactation)
- Pregnant women with true anemia of inflammation or chronic disease frequently are misdiagnosed with IDA.

Geriatric
- Evaluate microcytic anemia for an alternative cause in the older patient. Normocytic anemias of chronic inflammation may overlap.

Pediatric
- Evaluate for the presence of infection as a possible cause of anemia of inflammation in pediatric patients.

Referring Patients

- Hematology consult
- Nephrology consult
- Rheumatology consult
- Gastroenterology consult

APLASTIC ANEMIA

Overview

- Aplastic anemia occurs in the presence of bone marrow hypoplasia that causes decreased RBCs, WBCs, and platelet production. Hypoplasia causes symptoms of anemia, infection, and bleeding.
- It may be acquired, congenital, or secondary to disease states, and may occur in the presence of paroxysmal nocturnal hemoglobinuria.

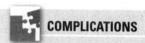

COMPLICATIONS

Acute: Hemorrhage, HF, ischemic CV events, myelodysplastic syndromes, opportunistic infections, sepsis

Chronic: Chronic transplant rejection

Etiology

- *Disease risks*: Bone cancer and metastasis, inherited bone marrow hypoplasia, Fanconi anemia, myeloproliferative disorders
- Idiopathic, no exact cause
- *Infectious*: Hepatitis, herpes virus, HIV
- *Other*: Benzene exposure, myelosuppressive medications, organ transplantation, radiation, TAGVHD

Signs and Symptoms

- *Anemia*: Fatigue, pallor, headache, cold intolerance, systolic murmur, tachypnea, tachycardia with effort, hypotension, hematuria, dark urine at night
- *Infection*: AMS, low-grade fever, hepatitis, s/s of opportunistic infection, frequent infections, candidiasis, ulcerations
- *Thrombocytopenia*: Occult or frank bleeding, petechial rashes, purpura

Differential Diagnosis

- *HEM*: Autoimmune hemolytic anemia, leukemia, lymphoma, megaloblastic anemia, multiple myeloma, myelodysplastic syndrome, myelofibrosis, myelophthisic anemia
- *Other*: Herpesvirus 6 (infection), medication-induced anemia, hemolytic anemia, pernicious anemia

Diagnosis

Labs
- *CBC*: Pancytopenia with low reticulocyte count
- Peripheral smear
- Hemoglobin electrophoresis
- Diepoxybutane test to exclude Fanconi anemia

Additional Diagnostic Testing
- Bone marrow aspiration with cytology, cytogenetics, and FISH

Treatment and Management

Treatment Goals
- Protect from further harm, transfuse PRBCs and platelets, and prepare for bone marrow transplantation.

Drug Treatment
- Stop all myelosuppressive medications or exposure to myelosuppressive environmental toxins.
- Hematologist will prescribe immunosuppressive therapy, colony-stimulating factors, and transfusions.

 ALERT

Hematology Consult
- Collaborate regarding immunosuppressive therapy, eltrombopag, and hematopoietic cell transplantation improve survival.
- Manage life-threatening bleeding with transfusion of single donor platelets.
- Treat symptomatic anemia with irradiated PRBCs.

Interventions
- Monitor response to immunosuppressive therapy and transfusion therapy.
- Evaluate response to eltrombopag (increased platelets) and filgrastim or sargramostim (increased WBCs).
- Employ bleeding precautions and infection protection.

Patient Education
- Teach patient energy management strategies and infection and bleeding prevention.

Patient Population Considerations

Women (conception/pregnancy/lactation)
- Provide conception counseling since pregnancy increases the risk of relapse.

Geriatric
- Obtain a home care consult for older adults who need assistance with ADLs secondary to aplastic anemia.

Pediatric
- Fanconi anemia is an inherited disorder that manifests with bone marrow failure. Distinguishing features of Fanconi anemia include café au lait spots, short stature, malformed hands and forearms, and organ defects in the kidney, heart, and GI tract.

Referring Patients

- Hematology consult

FOLIC ACID-DEFICIENCY ANEMIA

Overview

- FADA is macrocytic anemia caused by folate (folic acid) deficiency due to increased requirements, impaired absorption in the proximal jejunum, drug antagonism, or inadequate intake.

 COMPLICATIONS

Acute: Anemia, HF, ischemia, neural tube defects, depression, cognitive impairment

Chronic: Homocysteinemia, atherosclerosis, dementia

- Folic acid is essential in forming the heme component of hemoglobin and is a coenzyme for RBC DNA synthesis.
- Folic acid deficiency can lead to an accumulation of homocysteine that can contribute to cognitive decline, stroke, and CVHD.

Etiology

- *Decreased absorption*: Bariatric surgery, celiac disease, chronic alcoholism, Crohn's disease, folate (folic acid) antagonists, gastric resection, reduced gastric acid secretion due to gastritis, small bowel resection, zinc deficiency
- *Decreased intake*: Dietary restrictions due to chronic disease
- *Genetic*: Genetic disorders
- *Increased requirements*: Chronic hemolytic anemia, infection, malignancy, pregnancy, and breastfeeding
- *Increased loss*: Hemodialysis

 ALERT

- Women of childbearing age need adequate folic acid during the first month of pregnancy.
- Folic acid is responsible for closing the anterior and posterior neuropores at the 23rd and 26th day in fetal development respectively, preventing neural tube defects.

Signs and Symptoms

- S/s of anemia
- Cognitive impairment, depression, dementia
- Stomatitis and glossitis
- Hyperpigmentation of skin and mucous membranes
- Fever in the absence of infection

 CLINICAL PEARL

Medications That Reduce Folic Acid
Phenytoin, carbamazepine, primidone, phenobarbital, valproic acid, sulfasalazine, methotrexate, triamterene, pyrimethamine, trimethoprim–sulfamethoxazole

Differential Diagnosis

- Myeloproliferative disorder, pernicious anemia

Diagnosis

Labs
- *Serum folate*: <2.5 ng/mL
- Peripheral blood smear reveals large RBCs
- CBC reveals macrocytic, megaloblastic anemia
- MCV >100 fL
- Males Hgb <13.5 g/dL, females Hgb <12 g/dL
- Homocysteine level is elevated >16 mmol/L.
- Urine HCG to identify risk factor of pregnancy

Additional Diagnostic Testing
- Bone marrow aspiration if pancytopenia is present

Treatment and Management

Treatment Goals
- Treat the underlying cause, replace folic acid, increase RBC production, and avoid excess supplementation.

Drug Treatment
- Prescribe folic acid 400 to 1,000 mcg daily.
  - *Excess supplementation can slower brain development in children, increase cancer resurgence, and hasten cognitive decline among older adults.*

Interventions
- Stop offending agents.
- Provide alcohol and tobacco cessation counseling.
- Monitor for an increase in folic acid within range 2 to 10 ng/mL at regular intervals.

Patient Education
- Explain that folic acid replacement may take up to 4 months to demonstrate adequate replacement in severe disease.
- Review dietary measures to increase folic acid intake.
- Caution that excess folic acid has an inverse relationship with developing some cancers.

ALERT

- Folic acid supplementation can cause psychiatric adverse events in the presence of vitamin B_{12} deficiency since it masks the symptoms.
- Do not replace folate unless B_{12} anemia is ruled out.

Patient Population Considerations

Women (conception/pregnancy/lactation)
- Folic acid deficiency causes neural tube defects in the fetus during the first trimester. Instruct women of childbearing age to take daily prenatal vitamin with folic acid if planning to conceive.

Geriatric
- Evaluate older patients with cognitive impairment for unrecognized folic acid deficiency, especially when prescribed vitamin B_{12} replacement.

Pediatric
- Obtain a maternal history of folic acid supplementation when evaluating children with an autism spectrum disorder.

Referring Patients

- Hematology consult

IRON DEFICIENCY ANEMIA

Overview

- IDA results from decreased total iron stores, which causes the production of small, pale RBCs. Since iron functions as part of the oxygen transport mechanism of hemoglobin, symptomatic anemia can arise.
- In response to low iron stores, transferrin saturation increases to meet the body's demand for iron.

COMPLICATIONS

Acute: Tachycardia, premature or low-birth-weight neonates in women with anemia during pregnancy

Chronic: Cardiomegaly, heart failure, increased risk of infection, growth and development delays in children

Etiology

- *Decreased dietary iron intake:* Strict vegan diet, poor diet
- *Reduced iron absorption:* Gastric surgery, antacid consumption
- *Increased iron requirements:* Bleeding (chronic blood loss due to medication, menses, GI bleed) pregnancy

Signs and Symptoms

- Fatigue, palpitations, anorexia, s/s of anemia
- Systolic murmur
- Report of dark stools, heavy menses
- Cheilitis, glossitis, koilonychia in severe IDA

Differential Diagnosis

- *GI*: Inflammatory bowel disease, occult bleeding of GI cancers, gastrointestinal erosions
- *HEM*: Anemia of inflammation or chronic disease, aplastic anemia, cancer, hemolytic anemias, folic acid deficiency anemia, paroxysmal nocturnal hemoglobinuria, pernicious anemia
- *Other*: Lead poisoning

Diagnosis

Labs

- *CBC*: Microcytic hypochromic
- *Hgb* <12 g/dL in women, <13 g/dL in men
- *MCV*: Low MCV <80 fL
- *MCHC*: Low
- Iron status
  - *Serum iron*: Low
  - *Serum ferritin*: <30
  - Transferrin saturation <20%
  - *TIBC and reticulocyte count*: Low indicates decreased production
  - Perform BMP to determine if GFR is normal
  - Fecal occult blood test
  - U/A for gross hematuria
- Vitamins
  - If vitamins B_{12} and D, and folate (folic acid) are low concomitantly, this is considered mixed anemia

Additional Diagnostic Testing

- Endoscopy
- Ultrasound or CT if indicated
- Colposcopy

Treatment and Management

Treatment Goals

- Treat the underlying cause, replace iron and vitamins if indicated, and increase RBC count and Hgb.

Drug Treatment

- Hold agents that cause bleeding.
- Prescribe ferrous sulfate with vitamin C TID.
- Consider parenteral iron therapy if oral iron agents are ineffective or the patient is symptomatic.
- Prescribe vitamins D and B_{12}, and/or folic acid if deficiencies are present to support RBC production.

Interventions

- Monitor for an increase in RBC, Hgb, and serum ferritin at 4- to 8-week intervals.

Patient Education

- Teach the patient energy management strategies.
- Provide dietary counseling to support nutritional therapy.

Patient Population Considerations

Women (conception/pregnancy/lactation)
- Iron requirements rise steadily through pregnancy. Take iron with a daily vitamin.

Geriatric
- Offer parenteral iron preparations with symptomatic anemia in older adults who have malabsorption and cardiovascular comorbidities.

Pediatric
- IDA increases intestinal lead absorption. Primary prevention of lead poisoning includes the prevention of IDA.

Referring Patients

- Hematology consult

POP QUIZ 11.1

A 42-year-old Caucasian male with a history of DM type 1 and HTN, on basal/bolus insulin via pump and losartan 25 mg PO daily was evaluated in the office for worsening fatigue following the resolution of a respiratory infection. The following laboratory findings were reported the following morning:

BMP: K +4.9 mEq/L, BUN 36 mEq/L, and creatinine 1.8 mg/dL. GFR 45 mL/min/1.73m^2

CBC: WBC—4,200 cells/mcL, Hgb—8 g/dL, and HcT—32%. Platelets are 152,000/mcL. MCV 80 fL, Serum ferritin 104 mcg/L, and transferrin saturation 15%. How should these findings be interpreted? What is the next step in the plan of care?

PERNICIOUS ANEMIA

Overview

- Vitamin B$_{12}$ deficiency causes a megaloblastic, macrocytic, normochromic anemia because of impaired DNA synthesis. Adequate serum folic acid masks symptoms of B$_{12}$ deficiency.
- In some patients, autoimmune destruction of parietal cells decreases the available intrinsic factor responsible for its absorption. Also, chronic alcohol consumption, inflammation, or surgical resection may cause pernicious anemia. Inadequate intake and medication antagonists may be contributory.

Etiology

- *Disease risk*: Addison's disease, atrophic gastritis, chronic alcoholism, Crohn's disease, DM, Graves' disease, hypothyroidism, myasthenia gravis, pancreatic disorders
- *Decreased absorption*: Alcohol abuse, increased age, ileal resection, bariatric surgery, gastric resection
- *Reduced intake*: Dietary restrictions, vegan diet

Signs and Symptoms

- Traditional s/s of anemia
- Paresthesia, cognitive impairment, dementia, depression, diarrhea
- Glossitis and stomatitis

Differential Diagnosis

- *HEM*: Cancer, hemolytic anemia, hypothyroidism, iron deficiency anemia, immune thrombocytopenia, megaloblastic anemia, myelodysplastic syndrome
- *GI*: Celiac sprue, gastric cancer, liver disease, malabsorption, Zollinger–Ellison syndrome
- *Other*: Alcoholism

COMPLICATIONS

Acute: Anemia, peripheral neuropathy, depression, cognitive impairment, infection, bleeding

Chronic: Dementia

CLINICAL PEARL

Medications That Cause Vitamin B$_{12}$ Deficiency

Colchicine, H2 receptor antagonists, metformin, neomycin, PPIs

Diagnosis

Labs
- *CBC*: MCV >100 fL
- Serum vitamin B_{12} <150 to 200 ng/mL
- Males Hgb <13 g/dL, females Hgb <12 g/dL
- Folate (folic acid) normal between 2.5 and 20 ng/mL
- LDH and indirect bilirubin may be elevated
- Reticulocyte count may be low
- Peripheral smear reveals oval macrocytes with hypersegmented neutrophil
- Homocysteine level and serum methylmalonic acid is elevated in vitamin B_{12} deficiency
- Intrinsic factor antibodies
- Fecal occult blood test negative

Additional Diagnostic Testing
- Bone marrow aspiration in myeloid disorders and unexplained pancytopenia
- Gastric analysis
- Endoscopy

Treatment and Management

Treatment Goals
- Treat the underlying cause, replace vitamin B_{12} and folate (folic acid) and increase RBC production.

Drug Treatment
- Prescribe vitamin B_{12} injections 100 to 1,000 mcg IM daily for 7 days followed by 1,000 mcg IM monthly *OR*
- Intranasal cyanocobalamin spray in one nostril weekly

Interventions
- Stop all offending agents contributing to anemia.
- Monitor for an increase in reticulocytes, Hgb, and vitamin B_{12} in 2 weeks.
- Provide dietary counseling.

Patient Education
- Encourage alcohol and tobacco cessation.
- Teach patient energy management strategies based on comorbidities.
- Review dietary measures to increase vitamin B_{12} and folate (folic acid) intake.
- Review strategies for bleeding precautions infection protection.

Patient Population Considerations

Women (conception/pregnancy/lactation)
- Folate (Folic acid) deficiency is more common that vitamin B_{12} deficiency in pregnancy.

Geriatric
- An older patient with cognitive impairment and depression should be evaluated for B_{12} deficiency.

Pediatric
- Signs and symptoms of vitamin B_{12} deficiency mimic autism spectrum disorder.

Referring Patients
- Hematology consult

POP QUIZ 11.2

A 17-year-old female complains of palpitations and fatigue, daily headache, and decreased concentration in school. She reports that she was declined for blood donation at her high school blood drive. She has no chronic medication conditions by history. Menarche began 2 years ago with regular menses described as heavy.

What history taking and examination techniques should be prioritized?

SICKLE CELL ANEMIA

Overview

- Sickle cell anemia is an autosome-recessive hemolytic disease that is caused by the inheritance of a genetic mutation to hemoglobin. The beta chains in hemoglobin A are defective from a mutation in the HBB gene. It is replaced by hemoglobin S, which causes the RBC sickling with hypoxia triggering a vaso-occlusive crisis. RBCs are more fragile and hemolyze prematurely.
- Sickle cell trait occurs in the offspring of parents with sickle cell anemia or carriers of sickle cell trait. Parents with the defective gene must both pass the trait to their offspring for sickle cell anemia to develop. Patients with one copy of the mutation are not symptomatic unless exposed to a stressor. Extremely high altitude or dehydration can trigger a crisis in these patients.
- In a vaso-occlusive crisis, sickled RBCs trigger the clotting cascade in capillary beds, causing thrombosis, resulting in distal ischemia and pain.
- Patients with sickle cell anemia may also have sickle-beta thalassemia.

> **COMPLICATIONS**
>
> **Acute:** Acute chest syndrome, vaso-occlusive crisis, meningitis, stroke, cor pulmonale, renal failure, hepatic failure, splenic infarct, acute avascular necrosis, infection, CKD, priapism
>
> **Chronic:** Anemia, HF, ASCVD, retinopathy, nephropathy, PAD

Etiology

- Family history
- Parents with sickle cell trait or sickle cell anemia
- Common in patients of African Americans
- *Ethnicity*: Mediterranean descent, Middle Eastern, North African, Hispanic

> **CLINICAL PEARL**
>
> Screening for sickle cell anemia is part of the newborn screening in all 50 states.

Signs and Symptoms

- Symptoms of anemia after a few months of life
- Signs of vaso-occlusive crisis
    - *Presence of a precipitating stressor*: Acidosis, hypoxia, extreme physical activity, dehydration
    - Severe joint and bone pain; s/s of a thrombotic event
    - Fever, malaise, and leukocytosis
    - Hepatosplenomegaly
    - S/s of infections, leg ulcers, cor pulmonale, stroke, gallstones, priapism

Differential Diagnosis

- *CV*: Acute thrombotic events
- *HEM*: Hemolytic anemia, acute anemia, hemoglobin C disease, thalassemia
- *MSK*: Osteomyelitis, RA flare, septic arthritis

Diagnosis

Labs

- Hemoglobin electrophoresis demonstrates HbS (in HbSS) or HbSCBC
- CBC reveals microcytic, hypochromic anemia with leukocytosis and thrombocytosis
- ESR, LDH decreased
- Reticulocytes elevated
- *Peripheral smear*: Sickle cells, Howell–Jolly bodies
- BMP, LFTs, bilirubin to evaluate renal, hepatic function

Additional Diagnostic Testing

- Chest x-ray
- 12-lead EKG
- Ultrasound of abdomen
- Echocardiogram
- Bone scan or MRI
- Pulmonary function test

Treatment and Management

Treatment Goals

- Prevent vaso-occlusive crisis, manage chronic hemolytic anemia, promote adherence, and prevent complications.

Drug Treatment

- Collaborate with hematology for anemia management.
- Prescribe analgesics and TCAs for pain.
- Prescribe vasodilators to treat cor pulmonale.
- Provide immunizations to prevent infections.

 ALERT

Acute Crisis and Hematology Consult

Acute vaso-occlusive crises should be referred to the ED immediately.

Collaborate with hematology in use of hydroxyurea, monoclonal antibodies, and L-glutamine. Transfusions may be required, and stem cell transplantation may be considered.

Interventions

- Periodically evaluate CBC, BMP, LFTs, bilirubin, reticulocytes.
- Order pulmonary function tests and echocardiogram annually.
- Prescribe annual transcranial Doppler from ages 2 to 16 years.
- Target Hgb 10 g/dL before surgery.

Patient Education

- Initiate tobacco and alcohol cessation.
- Explain to patients with sickle cell trait about the genetic origin of the disease and encourage genetic counseling.
- Discuss strategies to prevent the vaso-occlusive crisis.
- Take folic acid and zinc as prescribed, and avoid cold weather, dehydration, and known triggers.
- Teach infection protection strategies and ensure vaccinations are up to date.

Patient Population Considerations

Women (conception/pregnancy/lactation)

- Counsel women of childbearing age that there is a high rate of fetal loss due to spontaneous abortion, placental infarction, abruption, and placenta previa.

Geriatric

- The median age of death for sickle cell anemia is 48 years for women and 42 years for men.

Pediatric

- Hand-foot syndrome in children <5 years, Hgb <7 g/dL, and leukocytosis in the absence of infection are poor prognostic indicators.

Referring Patients

- Hematology consult
- Nephrology consult
- Cardiology consult
- Pain management consult

THALASSEMIA MINOR

Overview

- Alpha thalassemia minor is an autosome-recessive hematologic disorder caused by inheritance of a genetic mutation or deletion of two of the four genes on chromosome 16 that decrease alpha-globin chain production hemoglobin. It causes mild symptoms of anemia.
- Beta thalassemia minor is an autosomal recessive hematological disorder caused by inheritance of one gene mutation of two genes that reduces the synthesis of the beta-globin chains of hemoglobin. Patients are clinically asymptomatic but may develop mild anemia.

Etiology

- Family history of thalassemia
- *Alpha*: Asian, Middle Eastern African descent
- *Beta*: Mediterranean (most often), Asian, African descent

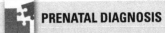

PRENATAL DIAGNOSIS

- Fetal cell analysis by fetoscopy can reveal imbalanced production of global chains.
- Chorionic villi sampling is used to evaluated DNA.

Signs and Symptoms

- Individuals with thalassemia minor are usually asymptomatic and have mild anemia
- Fatigue, pallor, weakness, headache, cold intolerance, palpitations, dyspnea on exertion, activity intolerance with anemia

Differential Diagnosis

- *HEM*: Iron-deficient anemia, anemia of chronic disease, sideroblastic anemia
- *Other*: Lead poisoning

Diagnosis

Labs
- CBC reveals microcytic and/or hypochromic anemia
- Males Hgb <13.5 g/dL, females Hgb <12 g/dL
- *Hemoglobin electrophoresis*: Carriers of beta-thalassemia trait demonstrate increased values of HbA_2 and HbF; carriers of alpha thalassemia trait will have Hb Bart
- Lead level <5 mcg/dL, exclude lead poisoning

Treatment and Management

Treatment Goals
- The patient understands increased genetic risk in offspring.

Drug Treatment
- No treatment is required.

Interventions
- Periodically evaluate CBC, especially in pregnancy.
- Refer to genetic counseling.

Patient Education

- Explain to patients with thalassemia minor about the genetic origin of the disease, to inform siblings, and seek genetic counseling in preconception counseling. Beta-thalassemia minor in both parents creates a 25% probability that a child will have thalassemia major.
- Teach patients with beta-thalassemia that iron replacement is not needed and will not improve their anemia.

Patient Population Considerations

Women (conception/pregnancy/lactation)

- Refer patients with a family history of thalassemia to preconception counseling to reduce the risk of incidence. Carriers of thalassemia should undergo chorionic villi sampling (11 weeks) and amniocentesis (16 weeks).

Pediatric

- It is essential to avoid misdiagnosis and treatment for iron deficiency anemia when thalassemia minor is present.

Referring Patients

- Hematology consult

POP QUIZ 11.3

A 22-year-old male presents to the urgent care clinical complaining of chest pain. He has a history of sickle cell anemia. What is the priority intervention?

RESOURCES

Advanci, P. (2019). *Medscape beta-thalassemia*. https://emedicine.medscape.com/article/206490-overview.

Amstad Bencaiova, G., Krafft, A., Zimmermann, R., & Burkhardt, T. (2017). Treatment of anemia of chronic disease with true iron deficiency in pregnancy. *Journal of Pregnancy, 2017*, 4265091. https://doi.org/10.1155/2017/4265091

Bacigalupo, A. (2017). How I treat acquired aplastic anemia. *Blood, 129*(11), 1428–1436. https://doi.org/10.1182/blood-2016-08-693481

Baker, R. D., & Greer, F. R. (2010). Diagnosis and prevention of iron deficiency and iron-deficiency anemia in infants and young children (0–3 years of age). *Pediatrics, 126*(5), 1040–1050. https://doi.org/10.1542/peds.2010-2576

Cash, J. C., & Glass, C. A. (Eds.). (2019). *Adult-gerontology practice guidelines*. Springer Publishing Company.

Codina Leik, M. T. (2018). *Family nurse practitioner certification: Intensive review*. Springer Publishing Company.

Harper, J. (2020). *Medscape: Iron deficiency anemia*. https://emedicine.medscape.com/article/202333-overview#a4

Herrin, V. (2018). *Medscape: Macrocytosis*. https://emedicine.medscape.com/article/203858-overview#a7.

Lanier, J. B., Park, J. J., & Callahan, R. C. (2018). Anemia in older adults. *American Family Physician, 98*(7), 437–442.

Maakaron, J. (2020). *Medscape: Sickle cell anemia*. https://emedicine.medscape.com/article/206490-overview.

Mayo Clinic. (2019). *Iron deficiency prevention in children: Tips for parents*. https://www.mayoclinic.org/healthy-lifestyle/childrens-health/in-depth/iron-deficiency/art-20045634.

National Institutes of Health. (2020). *Folate fact sheet for health professionals*. https://ods.od.nih.gov/factsheets/Folate-HealthProfessional/#h6

National Institutes of Health. (2020). *Medline plus: Thalassemia*. https://medlineplus.gov/ency/article/000587.htm

Petrakos, G., Andriopoulos, P., & Tsironi, M. (2016). Pregnancy in women with thalassemia: Challenges and solutions. *International Journal of Women's Health, 8*, 441–451. https://doi.org/10.2147/IJWH.S89308

Sorenson, M., Quinn, L., & Klein, D. (2019). *Pathophysiology: Concepts of human disease* (1st ed.). Pearson Education.

Weiss, G., Ganz, T., & Goodnough, L. T. (2019). Anemia of inflammation. *Blood, 133*(1), 40–50. https://doi.org/10.1182/blood-2018-06-856500

Yaisch, H. (2019). *Medscape: Pediatric thalassemia*. https://emedicine.medscape.com/article/958850-overview#:~:text=Pediatric%20Thalassemia%201%20Practice%20Essentials.%20Of%20genetic%20disorders,4%20Mortality%2FMorbidity.%20...%205%20Epidemiology.%20...%206%20Prognosis.

12

MUSCULOSKELETAL SYSTEM

ANKYLOSING SPONDYLITIS

Overview

- AS is a multisystem chronic inflammatory disorder that affects the axial skeleton and sacroiliac joints. Inflammation mediated by T lymphocytes, macrophages, cytokines, and TNF-alpha causes enthesitis, triggering fibrosis, and bone and joint changes that become arthritis and are vulnerable to fracture.
- AS is associated with reactive arthritis, psoriatic arthritis, and inflammatory bowel disease.
- It is similar to juvenile AS, with systemic signs of inflammation.

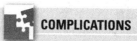

COMPLICATIONS

Acute: Pain, fractures, uveitis, arrythmia, cauda equina syndrome

Chronic: Arthritis, pulmonary fibrosis, aortic insufficiency

Etiology

- Exact etiology unknown
- Genetic predisposition
- Autoimmune in origin, family history of spondyloarthropathy

Signs and Symptoms

- Low back pain, insidious onset before age 40 years, morning stiffness
- Symptoms worse in the morning and improve with exercise
- Kyphosis, arthritis, inflammation of ligament and bone with point tenderness
- Decreased chest excursion
- *Extraarticular:* Uveitis, and CV, pulmonary, neurological, GI, renal, metabolic bone diseases
- *The following may be present:*
  - Painful red eye, tearing, blurred vision with photophobia
  - Abdominal pain and diarrhea of inflammatory bowel disease
  - AV block and aortic valve insufficiency
  - Atelectasis and pneumonia
  - Renal insufficiency
  - Pathological fracture

Differential Diagnosis

- Congenital degenerative disc disease, fractures, spinal deformity, kyphosis, lumbar spondylosis, OA, psoriatic arthritis, reactive arthritis

Diagnosis

Labs
- Increase in ESR and CRP
- BMP to evaluate renal function
- U/A to check for microscopic albumin

Additional Diagnostic Testing
- X-ray of spine (bamboo spine appearance in late disease)
- MRI and CT of spine
- Chest x-ray with pulmonary involvement
- 12-lead EKG may show heart block
- Bone mineral density

ALERT

Patients who experience degenerative changes and loss of function that interferes with activities of daily living should be referred to orthopedics.

Treatment and Management

Treatment Goals
- Relieve pain, promote mobility, protect from injury, and prevent complications.

Drug Treatment
- Prescribe NSAIDs or COX-2 inhibitors for pain and inflammation.
- Consider sulfasalazine daily to reduce inflammation.
- Consult with rheumatology on disease-modifying therapy with biologics, TNF inhibitors, and interleukin inhibitors.
- Consult with rheumatology for short-term corticosteroids for flares.
- Ensure immunizations are up to date for respiratory infections.

Interventions
- Evaluate for signs of systemic disease periodically and with symptoms.
- Encourage exercise, and prescribe ROM and spinal extension with PT.
- Monitor for the development of restrictive lung disease and vaccinate against respiratory infections

Patient Education
- Teach patients to participate in low-impact exercise on most days of the week.
- Explain to patients the importance of maintaining distance from people who are ill.
- Discuss nonpharmacologic interventions to promote comfort for arthritic pain.

Patient Population Considerations

Women (conception/pregnancy/lactation)
- Discuss the use of disease-modifying therapy in preconception counseling for women of childbearing age.

Geriatric
- Monitor blood pressure carefully and protect from infection with medications that place older patients at increased risk for complications.

Pediatric
- Juvenile spondylosis manifests in a similar pattern but is associated with systemic symptoms of fever.

Referring Patients

- Rheumatology consult for diagnostic workup and biologic therapy
- Orthopedic consult for degenerative changes or loss of function
- Ophthalmology consult for uveitis
- Pulmonary consult for pulmonary fibrosis
- GI consult for inflammatory bowel disease
- Cardiology consult for heart block

CARPAL TUNNEL SYNDROME

Overview

- Carpal tunnel syndrome is the compression of the median nerve in the wrist due to inflammation-causing paresthesia and weakness.
- It may occur from repetitive stress or malpositioning.

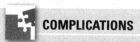

COMPLICATIONS

Acute: Pain, acute loss of function

Chronic: Local nerve damage, muscle wasting, permanent loss of function

Etiology

- Occupational exposure to repetitive stress, vibration, cold, extreme posture
- Use of manual wheelchair
- *Prior trauma to wrist:* Colles fracture
- Amyloidosis, DM, thyroid disorder

Signs and Symptoms

- Paresthesia to the palmar surface of first to fourth digits and palm
- Weakened grip on the affected side
- May be associated with autonomic symptoms of swelling, cooler temperature, and color changes
- *Weakness in motor function:* Adduction, abduction, flexion
- Positive Hoffman Tinel sign or Phalen sign
- Symptoms reproducible with carpal compression test

Differential Diagnosis

- *CV:* Raynaud's disease, compartment syndrome, thoracic outlet syndrome
- *ENDO:* Diabetic neuropathy, hypothyroidism, hypoparathyroidism, subtotal thyroidectomy
- *HEENT:* Myofascial pain
- *MSK:* Arthritis, cervical spondylosis, degenerative joint disease, epicondylitis, collagen vascular disease
- *NEURO:* Complex regional pain syndrome, GBS, mononeuropathy, MS, polyneuropathy, stroke, tumor
- *Other:* Lyme disease

Diagnosis

Labs
- No serology indicated.

Additional Diagnostic Testing
- Ultrasound or x-ray
- MRI
- Electromyography and nerve conductions studies

Treatment and Management

Treatment Goals
- Promote comfort, reduce risk factors, and prevent complications.

Drug Treatment
- NSAIDs may be considered for short-term pain and must be weighed against the risks.

Interventions
- Apply immobilizer for a minimum of 3 weeks.
- Provide periodic evaluation of response to therapy.
- Provide surgical referral for refractory symptoms interfering with function.

Patient Education

- Provide guidance for aerobic exercise if increased BMI is noted.
- Discuss workplace adaptations to reduce inflammation and refer to OT as indicated.

Patient Population Considerations

Women (conception/pregnancy/lactation)

- Women are more likely to get carpal tunnel syndrome. This has been explained by hormonal influences and smaller carpal tunnels than males.

Geriatric

- Perioperative positioning injury in older patients with OA may mimic symptoms of carpal tunnel syndrome after surgery or be confused with stroke signs.

Pediatric

- This disorder is rarely seen in the pediatric population.

Referring Patients

- Hand surgeon for surgical release of the transverse ligament

POP QUIZ 12.1

A 65-year-old male reports increased numbness to both of his hands. He reports that he types all the time at work and is concerned that it is work related. He received vaccinations for influenza 2 week ago. Extremities are symmetric on examination. Sensation to pinprick is decreased at the distribution of median, radial, and ulna nerves. Motor weakness is noted in bilateral extremities. What is the priority intervention?

DEGENERATIVE JOINT DISEASE/OSTEOARTHRITIS

Overview

- Degenerative joint disease is a "wear and tear" disease affecting joints, and a leading cause of chronic disability that affects the joints, subchondral bones, and synovia.

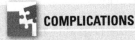

COMPLICATIONS

Acute: Joint effusion
Chronic: Fixed joint, disability

Etiology

- Family history
- Obesity
- Increasing age
- Repetitive stress or trauma

Signs and Symptoms

- Aching pain, morning stiffness, reduced ROM, edema, and crepitus
- History of repetitive stress or family history of OA

Differential Diagnosis

- *MSK*: AS, avascular necrosis, immune-mediated arthritis, septic arthritis, trauma
- *NEURO*: Fibromyalgia, neuropathic arthropathy
- *Other*: Gout and pseudogout, Lyme disease, RA, SLE

Diagnosis

Labs

- OA is more common in advanced age. Labs are not indicated for unilateral presentation in a younger patient with a history of repetitive stress; however, bilateral presentation in an adolescent or adult that cannot be explained by repetitive stress to both joints and requires an immune-mediated disease workup.
- ESR is usually normal in OA.

Additional Diagnostic Testing

- X-ray the affected joint to reveal loss of joint space and cysts.
- Arthrocentesis reveals an absence of crystals or infection.

Treatment and Management

Treatment Goals

- Promote comfort, prevent disease progression, and prevent complications.

Drug Treatment

- Hand OA
  - *Prescribe topical agents for pain*: Capsaicin or NSAIDs for pain.
  - Consider tramadol PRN for breakthrough pain.
- Knee OA
  - Prescribe acetaminophen alternating with oral NSAIDs for pain.
  - Consider tramadol PRN for breakthrough pain.
  - Refer to orthopedics for intraarticular corticosteroid injection.
- Chronic osteoarthritic pain
  - Prescribe duloxetine for chronic pain.

 ALERT

Referral to Orthopedic Surgeon
Fractures and decreased ROM interfering with ADLs for joint replacement or fusion

Interventions

- Review smoking cessation, weight loss, low-impact exercise, and footwear to cushion shock.
- Evaluate the effect of heat/cold application and encourage splints to hands when sleeping if hands are affected.
- Refer for functional exercise with PT/OT.

Patient Education

- Discuss the disease process and complication of chronically impaired mobility without intervention.
- Encourage smoking cessation, weight loss, and low-impact, closed-chain exercise.
- Review strategies for nonpharmacological therapy and s/s of adverse medication effects to report.

Patient Population Considerations

Women (conception/pregnancy/lactation)

- Women with arthritis who are pregnant should seek to achieve optimal body weight before conception and follow obstetrician guidelines for weight gain to minimize additional stress on joints.

Geriatric

- Avoid prescribing opioids to older adults due to the increased risk of falls.

Pediatric

- Pediatric OA is caused by congenital anomalies that affect joints and gait or could be a symptom of systemic disease and should be referred to a rheumatologist.

Referring Patients

- Orthopedics consult
- Rheumatology consult in symmetric presentation or features of autoimmunity

GOUT

Overview

- Gout is an inflammatory arthritis caused by a defect in purine metabolism that results in an inflammatory response to uric acid crystals formed in circulation triggering vascular injury, renal colic, and deposits in joints and tissue.
- Pseudogout is crystal formation other than urate.
- Secondary gout is caused by conditions that increase uric acid from another cause.

COMPLICATIONS

Acute: Acute pain, renal calculi, septic arthritis, infections
Chronic: Chronic gout, arthritis, ASCVD, CKD

Etiology

- Excessive alcohol, red meat, and seafood intake
- Diuretic use
- HTN
- Obesity
- Renal insufficiency

CLINICAL PEARL

Medications That Trigger Gout
Aspirin, chemotherapy, cyclosporine, niacin, thiazide diuretics, salicylates

Signs and Symptoms

- Erythema, edematous distal joint, warm to touch with limited ROM, especially great toe
- Tophi with skin erosion on outer ears, hands, and feet
- Degenerative joint disease

Differential Diagnosis

- *CV*: Hyperlipidemia, hypertension
- *ENDO*: Hypomagnesemia, hyperparathyroidism, hypoparathyroidism
- *GU*: Renal colic, renal failure
- *HEM*: Leukemia, multiple myeloma
- *INT*: Cellulitis, hyperproliferative skin disorders, skin cancer
- *MSK*: Charcot neuro-osteoarthropathy, septic arthritis
- *Other*: Lead poisoning, medication-induced gout, pseudogout, rhabdomyolysis, RA

Diagnosis

Labs
- Serum uric acid >6 in women and 6.8 in men
- Elevated ESR and WBC
- CMP with Ca Mg, Phos to evaluate renal function
- 24-hr urine for uric acid

Additional Diagnostic Testing
- X-ray of affected joint
- Arthrocentesis by orthopedics

Treatment and Management

Treatment Goals

- Treat acute attacks and prevent flares.

Drug Treatment

- Prescribe indomethacin or naproxen PO for pain in acute attacks.
- Prescribe allopurinol 100 to 300 mg PO daily to reduce serum uric acid.

Interventions

- Monitor electrolyte and uric acid levels. Do not treat asymptomatic hyperuricemia. Maintain uric acid <5 to 7.
- Monitor kidney function and pain.

Patient Education

- Teach patients to avoid alcohol, organ meat, red meat, and shellfish.
- Encourage patients to maintain BMI <25 and drink fluids during acute attacks.
- Discuss engaging in low-impact aerobic exercise such as swimming.

Patient Population Considerations

Women (conception/pregnancy/lactation)

- Women with gout who become pregnant may have flares of gout during pregnancy. Allopurinol has been given to women who are pregnant under the supervision of the obstetrician.

Geriatric

- Older patients with chronic gout should continue allopurinol during acute flares of disease.

Pediatric

- Gout is uncommon in pediatric patients.

Referring Patients

- Orthopedic consult
- Nephrology consult
- Rheumatology consult

> **ALERT**
>
> Colchicine is no longer the treatment of choice because of its narrow therapeutic window and risk for toxicity.
>
> If there's no response to NSAIDs, consider referral to orthopedics for intraarticular corticosteroid injections.

> **POP QUIZ 12.2**
>
> A 72-year-old male presents to primary care with a reddened toe that is painful and swollen. What is the differential diagnosis?

LOW BACK PAIN (STRAINS AND SPRAINS)

Overview

- Pain that can be acute (2–4 weeks) or chronic (>3 months) from acute or cumulative trauma to discs, ligaments, facet joints, muscles, and nerves that arise from the spine.
- Sprains result from overstretched ligaments whereas strains occur with overstretched muscle or tendon attached to the bone. About 70% of mechanical lower back pain is due to strains or sprains.
- Pain can become chronic as a result of the central processing of pain, patient perception of pain, deconditioning, and psychosocial barriers.

> 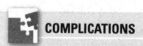 **COMPLICATIONS**
>
> **Acute:** Pain
> **Chronic:** Arthritis, neuropathy

Etiology

- Increasing age
- Occupation
- Anxiety, depression, obesity, sedentary lifestyle, smoking
- Congenital or acquired skeletal anomalies such as infections, inflammation, scoliosis, kyphosis, lordosis, spina bifida
- Mechanical stress such as trauma, sprains, and nerve compression

Signs and Symptoms

- Pain unrelieved or rest or repositioning
- Morning stiffness
- Decreased lumbar ROM (Schober test), step-off between vertebral bodies
- Motor impairment

Differential Diagnosis

- *CV*: Aortic aneurysm
- *GI*: Abdominal mass or tumor
- *GU*: Renal colic
- *HEM/ONC*: Primary or metastatic malignancy, multiple myeloma, sickle cell disease
- *MSK*: Degenerative disk disease, herniated disk, inflammatory arthropathy, metabolic bone disease, myelopathy, sacroiliitis, spinal fracture, synovial cyst
- *NEURO*: Cauda equina syndrome, CRPS, epidural abscess, fibromyalgia, sciatica
- *REPRO*: Endometriosis, ovarian cyst or cancer, pregnancy
- *Other*: Collagen vascular disease

Diagnosis

Labs

- ESR in suspected systemic or metabolic case

Additional Diagnostic Testing

- AP and lateral x-ray if age <20 years or >50 years, or suspected cancer, neurologic deficit, fever, or trauma is present in presentation <4 weeks; otherwise, defer x-rays and treat
- Bone scan in suspected systemic or metabolic case
- CT spine and MRI
- EMG and evoked potentials

Treatment and Management

Treatment Goals

- Treat pain, modify risk factors, and prevent injury.

Drug Treatment

- Prescribe acetaminophen PRN for acute pain. NSAIDs are acceptable for acute muscle pain but not for continued long-term use (increases CV, renal, bleeding complications).
  - Do not prescribe NSAIDs with suspected fractures due to delayed callus formation.

 CLINICAL PEARL

Assessing Motor Impairment

Function Test

- *L3*: Can squat and rise
- *L4*: Can walk in heels with ankle dorsiflexed
- *L5*: Can walk in heels with great toe dorsiflexed
- *S1*: Can walk or stand on toes

 ALERT

Labs are only indicated if the clinician suspects systemic infection or disease or if evaluation of renal or liver function is required for testing or therapeutic intervention.

 CLINICAL PEARL

Mackenzie Exercise

1. Lie prone with arms at side for 2 to 3 min. Add pillow under chest.
2. Lie prone and prop up on elbows and forearms with shoulders above elbows and feel for centralization of pain to spine.
3. Lie prone and prop up on hands with shoulders above them and press up and down for 10 reps.

- Prescribe duloxetine for chronic osteoarthritic pain.
- Consider a nonbenzodiazepine muscle relaxant or tizanidine to reduce muscle spasms short term.
- Consider anticonvulsant for neuropathic pain.
- Prescribe 5% lidocaine patch topical treatment for nociceptive and neuropathic pain.
- Correcting osteoporosis with bisphosphonates may help ease back pain.

Interventions
- Recommend weight loss, prevention of deconditioning, and heat/ice PRN for short-term improvement.
  - Bracing and traction are not recommended.
  - No conclusive evidence exists regarding the efficacy of TENS, acupressure, acupuncture, and massage; however, these therapies can be considered during shared decision-making.
- Monitor response to therapy and refer to orthopedics if patients do not improve in 4 weeks.

Patient Education
- Discuss disease processes, deconditioning, and evidence-based treatment protocols.
- Teach patient nonpharmacological strategies to manage pain; consider yoga as tolerated.
- Instruct in s/s of complications and adverse medication effects to report.

Patient Population Considerations

Women (conception/pregnancy/lactation)
- Weight gain can exacerbate low back pain in women who are pregnant. Obstructive uropathy should be excluded with complaints of low back pain. Review nonpharmacologic strategies to manage low back pain.

Geriatric
- Functional exercise and conditioning should be emphasized in older patients.

Pediatric
- Children and adolescents presenting with back pain should be evaluated for scoliosis.

Referring Patients

- Orthopedic consult
- PT/OT referral

OSTEOPOROSIS

Overview

- Osteoporosis is a primary or secondary metabolic bone disease that results in loss of bone density and increases the risk of pathological fracture.

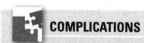

COMPLICATIONS

Acute: Compression fracture, pathological fractures, renal colic
Chronic: CKD

Etiology

- Advanced age, female gender, or Caucasian or Asian race
- Small body habitus, sedentary lifestyle, tobacco, excessive caffeine or alcohol, inadequate calcium, and vitamin D deficiency
- Bariatric surgery, bone metastasis, celiac disease, CKD, eating disorders, GERD, hypercortisolism, inflammatory bowel disease, hyperthyroidism, multiple myeloma, parathyroid disease, RA, seizures, SLE
- Medication-induced (levothyroxine, glucocorticoids, anticoagulant, anticonvulsants, immunosuppressant, PPIs, TZDs)

Signs and Symptoms

- Loss of height with advancing age
- Unexpected fracture

Differential Diagnosis

- *ENDO*: Cushing's syndrome, hypothyroidism, hyperparathyroidism
- *GU*: Renal osteodystrophy
- *HEM*: Bone cancer, homocysteinemia, leukemia, lymphoma, multiple myeloma, sickle cell anemia
- *MSK*: Osteogenesis imperfecta, osteomalacia, Paget disease
- *NEURO*: Seizures
- *Other*: Vitamin D deficiency, medications

Diagnosis

Labs

- CMP with serum Ca, Phos, Vitamin D, albumin LFTs, alk Phos
- Check testosterone level in men.
- CBC, ESR, and serum electrophoresis if hematology cause is suspected

Additional Diagnostic Testing

- BMD testing
    - T-score between −1.0 and −2.5 = low bone density or osteopenia
    - T-score of −2.5 or lower = osteoporosis
- X-ray in fractures

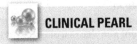

CLINICAL PEARL

USPSTF Screening for Osteoporosis
Prescribe BMD testing in:
- Women >65 years **OR**
- Postmenopausal women <65 years with increased risk for osteoporosis

Treatment and Management

Treatment Goals

- Preserve bone mass, modify risk factors, and prevent injury.

Drug Treatment

- Replace calcium and vitamin D as follows:
    - *9 to 18 years*: 1,300 mg of calcium, 600 IU of vitamin D
    - *19 to 50 years*: 1,000 mg of calcium, 600 IU of vitamin D
    - *51 to 70 years*: 1,200 mg of calcium, 600 IU of vitamin D
    - *>71 years*: 1,200 mg of calcium, 800 IU of vitamin D
- Prescribe bisphosphonates with normal serum calcium levels.
- Consider SERM in postmenopausal women.

Interventions

- Implement fall precautions and perform medication reconciliation for medications that increase the risk of falls and in weight-bearing exercise.
- Monitor response to therapy and for the presence of complications.
- Refer to endocrinology or rheumatology for refractory osteoporosis for additional therapy such as MAB and parathyroid hormone therapy.
- Refer to a spine specialist for percutaneous vertebroplasty and kyphoplasty in the presence of severe pain with vertebral compression fractures.

Patient Education

- Discuss the disease process and management.
- Review fall prevention strategies to improve home safety and OTC medications that increase the risk of falls.
- Instruct in s/s of complications and adverse medication effects to report.

Patient Population Considerations

Women (conception/pregnancy/lactation)
- Pregnancy-induced osteoporosis and bone loss with breastfeeding can be prevented with 1,000 to 1,300 mg of calcium per day based on age.

Geriatric
- Osteoporosis in men increases in ages >70 years and is often missed.

Pediatric
- Osteoporosis in children is genetic or secondary to medications or disease.

Referring Patients

- Endocrinology or rheumatology consult
- Spine specialist

POP QUIZ 12.3

A 72-year-old African American male presents to the primary care office for follow-up for a T11 fracture evaluated in the ED 2 days before. His medical history includes hypertension managed with chlorthalidone, epilepsy managed with topiramate, and BPH managed with finasteride. The x-ray reveals penciling of vertebrae with a compression fracture at T11. What is the likely cause of this finding and what should he be evaluated for?

RHEUMATOID ARTHRITIS

Overview

- RA is a systemic collagen vascular disease of articular and systemic inflammation. Autoimmune destruction of joints causes remodeling to elbows, shoulders, hips, knees, and hands.
- Systemic inflammation and vasculitis can cause strokes, scleritis, pleuritis, and pericarditis. Renal disease secondary to adverse effects of medications can occur. RA progresses through stages 1 to 4.

COMPLICATIONS

Acute: RA flare with joint effusion and arthritis, cervical subluxation, strokes, scleritis, pleuritis, pericarditis, avascular necrosis, infections

Chronic: Anemia, CKD, depression, complications of immobility, osteoporosis, cervical spine disease

Etiology

- Exact etiology unknown, autoimmune in origin
- Genetic factors, family history, female gender, ages 20 to 50

Signs and Symptoms

- Asymptomatic in stage 1
- Symmetric joint effusion, warmth, morning stiffness
- Extraarticular disease with impaired mobility
- Increase disease load and immobility
- Fatigue, low-grade fever, subcutaneous nodules
- *Joint deformities associated with RA:* Swan neck contractures with ulna deviation, Boutonniere's deformity (PIP joint)
- S/s of target organ inflammation

Differential Diagnosis

- *HEENT:* Sjögren's syndrome, keratoconjunctivitis
- *HEM:* Myeloid dysplastic syndrome
- *MSK:* OA, polymyalgia rheumatica, psoriatic arthritis, reactive arthritis, relapsing polychondritis
- *NEURO:* Fibromyalgia, paraneoplastic syndrome, polymyositis
- *Other:* Gout, sarcoidosis, SLE

Diagnosis

Labs
- ESR and C-reactive protein level is elevated
- CBC shows slight leukocytosis, anemia, and thrombocytopenia or thrombocytosis
- BMP to assess renal function
- ANA, ACCP, rheumatoid factor is positive
- PPD and hepatitis profile before biologic therapy

Additional Diagnostic Testing
- X-ray of affected joints as indicated
- MRI of cervical spine
- Arthrocentesis
- Ultrasonography of joints and tendons to evaluate synovial membrane, and even erosions
- Bone mineral density test

Treatment and Management

Treatment Goals
- Promote comfort, slow disease progression, and minimize/manage complications.

Drug Treatment
- Refer to rheumatology regarding corticosteroids and DMARD with biologic therapy (TNF).
  - *Note methotrexate may still be prescribed to select patients*: Monitor BMP, CBC, LFTs, and urine frequently.
- Prescribe acetaminophen alternating with NSAIDs PRN for pain. Monitor for liver and renal toxicity.
- Consider topical capsaicin and/or diclofenac epolamine as an adjunct for pain relief.
- Prescribe tramadol 25 to 100 mg PO PRN for breakthrough pain.
- Update vaccinations to prevent infection.

Interventions
- Augment pain management with hot/cold application, CBT, and mindfulness.
- *Prescribe devices and therapies for joint protection*: Orthotics, splints, adaptive equipment, OT, PT.
- Monitor response to therapy and modify risk factors for its systemic complications.

Patient Education
- Discuss joint protection strategies and DMARDs to protect joints from further harm.
- Explain the risk of systemic complications of vasculitis, infection, and strategies to avoid.
- Encourage mindfulness, nonpharmacologic management of pain, and refer to pain clinic.
- Teach s/s of adverse medications effects to report.

Patient Population Considerations

Women (conception/pregnancy/lactation)
- RA flares tend to remit during pregnancy and recur in the postpartum period.

Geriatric
- There is an increased risk for cardiovascular mortality and gastric bleeding in older patients with chronic NSAID use. Monitor carefully and use the lowest possible dose.

Pediatric
- Juvenile idiopathic arthritis describes a cluster of autoimmune and inflammatory arthritic conditions with systemic disease that can arise in children less than 16 years.

Referring Patients

- Rheumatology consult
- Orthopedic consult

SYSTEMIC LUPUS ERYTHEMATOSUS

Overview

- SLE is a relapsing, remitting systemic collagen vascular disease of type 3 hypersensitivity affecting the skin, joints, heart, lungs, kidneys, neurologic system, and blood vessels. Autoimmune activation following cell apoptosis produces antinuclear antibodies that form immune complexes. These immune complexes adhere to capillary bed walls causing injury and inflammation in the organ. This event occurs in response to a trigger and is characterized by increases in inflammatory markers and a decrease in serum complement.
- SLE vasculitis can cause inflammatory vascular events such as cerebritis, pneumonitis, myocarditis, and nephritis that lead to CKD.

COMPLICATIONS

Acute: SLE flare with joint effusion and arthritis, cerebritis, pneumonitis, myocarditis, nephritis, infections, DVT

Chronic: Anemia, CKD, depression, MI, stroke

Etiology

- Exact etiology unknown, autoimmune in origin
- Genetic factors, family history, female gender, ages 20 to 50
- *Environmental factors*: UV exposure, infection, medications, tobacco, low vitamin D

ALERT

Medications Causing Lupus-Like Reaction

INH, procainamide, estrogen, hydralazine, TMP-SMX, sulfa agents

Signs and Symptoms

- Asymptomatic in early stages
- Butterfly rash, discoid lesions with sun exposure
- Fatigue, low-grade fever, joint pain, and rash during flares
- *S/s of target organ inflammation*: Seizures delirium, oral ulcers, pleural or pericardial effusions
- Generalized petechial rash during flares

Differential Diagnosis

- *CV*: Endocarditis, myocarditis, pericarditis
- *GI*: Autoimmune hepatobiliary disease
- *HEENT*: Sjögren's syndrome
- *HEM*: Lymphoma, hemolytic anemia
- *MSK*: Mixed connective tissue disease, RA, scleroderma
- *NEURO*: Fibromyalgia, polymyositis
- *Other*: APLA syndrome, Lyme disease, mononucleosis

Diagnosis

Labs

- ESR and C-reactive protein level is elevated
- Serum complement is low flares
- CBC shows slight leukopenia, anemia, and thrombocytopenia
- ANA, anti-DNA, anti-Smith antibodies positive
- Anticardiolipin antibodies, lupus anticoagulant
- BMP, LFTs, and calculate GFR to stage CKD
- U/A reveal protein and casts
- Vitamin D level

Additional Diagnostic Testing
- X-ray of affected joints
- Renal biopsy
- Arthrocentesis
- *MRI*: Brain and lumbar puncture, if indicated

Treatment and Management

Treatment Goals
- Promote comfort, slow disease progression, and minimize/manage flares and complications.

Drug Treatment
- *Refer to rheumatology for DMARD with immunomodulators*: Hydroxychloroquine, cyclophosphamide, azathioprine, methotrexate, mycophenolate.
  - Monitor BMP, CBC, LFTs, and urine frequently.
- Prescribe low-dose corticosteroids for flares in consultation with rheumatology.
  - IVIG may be considered in place of corticosteroids.
- Prescribe acetaminophen alternating with NSAIDs PRN for pain and monitor for liver and renal toxicity.
- Prescribed vitamin D for deficiency to prevent disease progression.
- Update vaccinations to prevent infection.

Interventions
- Augment pain management with hot/cold application, CBT, and mindfulness
- Monitor response to therapy; modify risk factors for its systemic complications.
- Assess for renal dysfunction at each visit and control risk factors to maintain kidney function.

Patient Education
- Discuss the disease process and complications and develop a lupus action plan to handle flares.
- *Review protective factors*: Stress management, infection protection, vitamin D supplementation, nephroprotection, and sunscreen.
- Discuss avoiding activities and medications that can trigger lupus reactions.
- Teach s/s of adverse medications effects to report.

Patient Population Considerations

Women (conception/pregnancy/lactation)
- SLE flares tend to exacerbate during pregnancy due to rising hormones.

Geriatric
- There is an increased risk for cardiovascular mortality and gastric bleeding in older clients with chronic NSAID use. Monitor carefully and use the lowest possible dose.

Pediatric
- There is a higher percentage of pediatric SLE patients who are African American <20 years of age and who have an increased risk of death due to MI. Careful monitoring of cardiovascular risk factors is necessary to improve mortality and morbidity.

Referring Patients

- Rheumatology consult
- Nephrology consult

RESOURCES

Antoniou, T., Macdonald, E. M., Yao, Z., Gomes, T., Tadrous M., Ho, J. M.-W., Mamdani, M. M., Juurlink D. N., & Canadian Drug Safety and Effectiveness Research Network. (2018). A population-based study of the risk of osteoporosis and fracture with dutasteride and finasteride. *BMC Musculoskeletal Disorders, 19*(1), 160. https://doi.org/10.1186/s12891-018-2076-9

Ashworth, N. (2020). *Medscape: Carpal tunnel syndrome treatment & management.* https://emedicine.medscape.com/article/327330-treatment#d9

Bartels, C. (2020). *Medscape: Systemic lupus erythematosus.* https://emedicine.medscape.com/article/332244-overview

Bethel, M. (2020). *Medscape: Osteoporosis.* https://emedicine.medscape.com/article/330598-overview

Brent, L. (2019). *Medscape: Ankylosing spondylitis and undifferentiated spondyloarthropathy.* https://emedicine.medscape.com/article/332945-overview

Cash, J. C., & Glass, C. A. (Eds.). (2019). *Adult-gerontology practice guidelines.* Springer Publishing Company.

Chawla, J. (2018). *Medscape: Low back pain and sciatica.* https://emedicine.medscape.com/article/1144130-overview#a1

Codina Leik, M. T. (2018). *Family nurse practitioner certification: Intensive review.* Springer Publishing Company.

Hills, E. (2020). *Medscape: Mechanical low back pain.* https://emedicine.medscape.com/article/310353-overview

Klein-Gitelman, M. (2019). *Medscape: Pediatric systemic lupus erythematosus.* https://emedicine.medscape.com/article/1008066-overview

Kuhnow, A., Kuhnow, J., Ham, D., & Rosedale, R. (2020). The McKenzie Method and its association with psychosocial outcomes in low back pain: A systematic review. *Physiotherapy Theory and Practice,* 1–15. Advance online publication. https://doi.org/10.1080/09593985.2019.1710881

Lozado, C. (2020). *Medscape: Osteoarthritis.* https://emedicine.medscape.com/article/330487-overview#a1

National Institute of Neurological Disorders and Stroke. (2020). *Back pain fact sheet.* https://www.ninds.nih.gov/Disorders/Patient-Caregiver-Education/Fact-Sheets/Low-Back-Pain-Fact-Sheet#3102_3

North American Spine Society. (2020). *Evidence-based clinical guidelines for multidisciplinary spine care.* https://www.spine.org/Portals/0/assets/downloads/ResearchClinicalCare/Guidelines/LowBackPain.pdf.

Rothschild, B. (2020). *Medscape: Gout and pseudogout.* https://emedicine.medscape.com/article/329958-workup#c1

Smith, H. (2020). *Medscape: Rheumatoid arthritis.* https://emedicine.medscape.com/article/331715-overview

Sorenson, M., Quinn, L., & Klein, D. (2019). *Pathophysiology: Concepts of human disease* (1st ed.). Pearson Education.

US Preventive Services Task Force, Grossman, D. C., Curry, S. J., Owens, D. K., Barry, M. J., Davidson, K. W., Doubeni, C. A., Epling, J. W., Jr., Kemper, A. R., Krist, A. H., Kurth, A. E., Landefeld, C. S., Mangione, C. M., Phipps, M. G., Silverstein, M., Simon, M. A., & Tseng, C. W. (2018). Screening for adolescent idiopathic scoliosis: Us preventive services task force recommendation statement. *JAMA, 319*(2), 165–172. https://doi.org/10.1001/jama.2017.19342

13

INTEGUMENTARY SYSTEM

ACNE VULGARIS

Overview

- Acne vulgaris is a chronic skin disease characterized by blockage and inflammation of sebaceous glands distributed on the face, jawline, neck, back, chest, and shoulders.
- Androgen hormone stimulates hypertrophy of sebaceous glands and overproduction of sebum. Obstruction by hyperkeratinization of the epidermis forms a comedone that can be closed (whitehead) or partially open (blackhead). *Cutibacterium acnes* proliferates in trapped sebum-producing pro-inflammatory factors, increasing the lesion diagnosed size.
- Onset infancy through adult. Nodulocystic causes scarring.

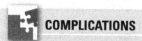

COMPLICATIONS

Acute: Pain, gram-negative folliculitis, anxiety, depression

Chronic: Acne scars

Etiology

- Family history
- *Environmental*: Cosmetics, skin, and hair products
- *Medications*: Steroids, lithium iodide, anticonvulsants
- *Conditions*: Pregnancy
- UV exposure may improve or worsen acne

ALERT

- PCOS is a common hormonal disorder in woman that can manifest with acne.
- Risk of long-term complications include metabolic syndrome, DM, and CVHD.

Signs and Symptoms

- Open and closed comedones
- Inflammatory papules; painful cysts
- Nodules greater than 5 mm
- Scars

Differential Diagnosis

- *ENDO*: Congenital adrenal hyperplasia, hypercortisolism, PCOS
- *INT*: Acneiform eruptions, acne maligna, acne conglobata, acne keloidalis nuchae, folliculitis, rosacea, seborrheic dermatitis, steroid-induced dermatitis
- *Other*: SLE, sarcoidosis

Diagnosis

Labs
- Diagnosed by clinical examination.

Additional Diagnostic Testing
- Urine HCG before and during the administration of retinoids
- Gram stain and culture for refractory acne resulting from long-term antibiotic use

Treatment and Management

Treatment Goals
- Reduce hyperkeratinization, treat inflammation and bacterial colonization, and minimize scarring.

Drug Treatment
- Consider a combination of benzoyl peroxide, retinoid, and topical antibiotic initially.
  - Prescribe tretinoin 0.02% to 0.1%; apply pea-size amount at bedtime.
    - *Pediatric*: <12 years—safety and efficacy not established
  - Prescribe topical antibiotics.
  - Prescribe clindamycin with benzoyl peroxide apply one amount daily.
    - Topical erythromycin, metronidazole can be considered
      - *Pediatric*: <12 years—safety and efficacy are not established
- If earlier combination therapy is ineffective, consider oral antibiotics and hormone therapy in females.
  - Prescribe doxycycline 50 to 200 mg PO daily
    - May consider oral erythromycin, minocycline, or TMP-SMX
  - Pediatric: <8 years; safety and efficacy are not established
  - Add hormone therapy
    - Spironolactone 50 to 200 mg PO daily in divided doses
    - Oral contraceptive to suppress androgens
- If persistent, collaborate with dermatology to prescribe oral retinoids.
  - Pediatric: <12 years—safety and efficacy are not established.

CLINICAL PEARL

Discontinue oral antibiotics if no improvement is noted after 3 months.

ALERT

- Oral isotretinoin agents have been associated with depression and suicidality.
- They are also associated with birth defects if taken when pregnant.
- Review the risks and benefits of therapy and discuss strategies to seek consultation.

Interventions
- Monitor adherence to skin regimen.
- Monitor BMP for hyperkalemia in spironolactone therapy.
- Prescribe systemic antibiotics for the shortest clinical course and reevaluate at 3 to 4 months.

Patient Education
- Review the environmental factors that trigger acne.
- Instruct the patient to avoid sunlight and apply liberal amounts of sunscreen with an SPF of 30 when prescribed retinoids or tetracyclines.
- Discuss the risk and benefits of oral retinoids in severe acne. Teach s/s of mood disorders and risk for self-harm.
- Discuss interventions to manage scarring to improve self-image.

Patient Population Considerations

Women (conception/pregnancy/lactation)
- Oral contraceptives and aldosterone antagonists are effective adjuncts for women with acne. Preconception planning is critical in women of childbearing age. Retinoids would be avoided.

POP QUIZ 13.1

A 30-year-old female develops adult-onset acne vulgaris, amenorrhea, and hirsutism associated with a 50-pound weight gain in the past year. She reports she has been using every topical agent in the drug store with no effect. She breaks down into tears stating, "I can't stand it anymore. I feel like my life is falling apart!" She is flushed and agitated. The patient does not have any chronic medical conditions or medications. Moderate to severe acne vulgaris is noted with several cysts described as painful. What are the possible causes of her acne, hirsutism, and weight gain?

Geriatric

- Acne vulgaris does not typically manifest in the geriatric population. Consider adrenal disorder as a likely cause.

Pediatric

- Neonatal acne occurs from maternal hormones and adolescence with the onset of puberty.

Referring Patients

- Dermatology consult
- Endocrine consult

ACTINIC KERATOSIS

Overview

- Actinic keratosis is a collection of atypical actinokeratocytes that overproduce keratin and are localized to a segment of the epidermis. UV light causes premalignant lesions.
- Bowen's disease tends to present in larger patches resembling eczema.

> **COMPLICATIONS**
>
> **Acute:** Anxiety
> **Chronic:** Squamous cell cancer

Etiology

- Cumulative exposure to UV light radiation
- Extensive exposure to radiation
- Some industrial chemicals
- Advancing age

Signs and Symptoms

- Small rough crusting area
- Red, dark tan, or pink lesion 3 to 10 mm in size
- Located in areas of sun exposure

> **CLINICAL PEARL**
>
> Almost everyone over 80 years of age will have some form of actinic keratosis.

Differential Diagnosis

- *HEM*: Bowen's disease, SCC, BCC, malignant melanoma
- *INT*: Seborrheic keratosis, porokeratosis, DLE

Diagnosis

Labs

- Clinical examination

Additional Diagnostic Testing

- Biopsy

Treatment and Management

Treatment Goals

- Eradicate premalignant lesions, prevent progression to SCC, and modify risk factors.

> **ALERT**
>
> Ten percent of cases will become SCC in 10 years.

Drug Treatment

- Managed by dermatology

Interventions
- Refer to dermatology for biopsy any suspicious lesion.
- Monitor response to therapy.
- Encourage risk factor modification.

Patient Education
- Discuss the likelihood of malignant transformation of premalignant lesions.
- Review risk factor modification of sun exposure, radiation, and certain chemicals.
- Instruct in a low-fat diet, which may help prevent progression.

Patient Population Considerations

Women (conception/pregnancy/lactation)
- Seborrheic keratosis is a common brown lesion due to increased hormone production in pregnancy. Do not confuse them with actinic keratosis.

Geriatric
- Using topical retinoids may reduce the incidence of skin cancer in this population.

Pediatric
- Actinic keratosis is not generally seen in this population. Instruct patients and caregivers in sun safety to protect against skin cancer development.

Referring Patients

- Dermatology consult

ATOPIC DERMATITIS

Overview

- Atopic dermatitis is a chronic pruritic inflammatory condition due to an IGE-mediated type I hypersensitivity reaction to allergens.
- It is referred to as eczema.

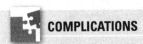

COMPLICATIONS

Acute: Anaphylaxis, secondary infection
Chronic: Chronic eczema, other atopic conditions

Etiology

- Family and/or personal history of an allergic reaction to irritants, seasonal or perennial, with onset in patients under age <20 years
- History of atopic asthma, allergic rhinitis, hay fever, food allergy

Signs and Symptoms

- Pruritus, erythema, eczema
- Xerosis
- Lichenification at skin margins

Differential Diagnosis

- *HEM*: Cutaneous lymphoma
- *INT*: Bacterial skin infection, fungal skin infection, seborrheic dermatitis, contact dermatitis, photosensitivity reaction
- *Other*: DLE, autoimmune vasculitis

Diagnosis

Labs
- Clinical examination; labs are not required

Additional Diagnostic Testing
- Biopsy if needed to rule out other conditions

Treatment and Management

Treatment Goals
- Relieve symptoms, protect skin from injury, implement environmental control measures, and avoid allergens.

Drug Treatment
- Prescribe OTC routine care.
  - Petrolatum healing ointment or equivalent topical as needed to maintain skin integrity
  - Hydrocortisone topical 1% to 2.5%, 2 to 3 times per day
    - More potent topical steroid if indicated or short-term oral prednisone in severe cases
- Prescribe oral antipruritic if indicated.
  - Hydroxyzine 25 mg PO q6h to q8h (decrease frequency on advanced age)
- Manage secondary skin infections.
  - Mupirocin 2% to affected area q8h × 10 days
    - Oral antibiotics if cellulitis present

Interventions
- Review environmental control measures and refer patients to the National Eczema Association for Science and Education.
- Monitor for secondary infection and progression in atopic march.
- Reevaluate in 1 to 2 weeks to determine response to therapy and adjust as needed.
- Collaborate with an allergist and dermatology for refractory moderate to severe disease.
- Monitor for acute food reactions (urticaria and anaphylaxis) in children.

Patient Education
- Provide counseling for tobacco cessation and avoidance.
- Teach patient to avoid triggers and foods that cause a reaction, and to use bedding and wear clothing made with cotton, bamboo, or silk. Maintain environmental humidification and avoid extremes of temperature. Use allergen-free detergents and household products. Apply moisturizer frequently and before entering the pool. Use mineral-based sunscreen.
- Discuss daily therapy to prevent acute events.
- Review steps for diluted bleach bath.
- Teach patient and family s/s of anaphylaxis to seek attention in the ED.
- Teach patients about medication adverse effects and symptoms to report.

Patient Population Considerations

Women (conception/pregnancy/lactation)
- Changes in eczema patterns and severity are not predictable during pregnancy. Mild to moderate steroids can continue to be used. Wash off steroids applied to nipples before breastfeeding.

Geriatric
- The use of antihistamines for pruritus increases the risk of falls in geriatric patients.

Pediatric
- Eczema manifests between the ages of 6 months and 5 years in children.

Referring Patients

- Dermatology consult
- Allergist referral

CANDIDIASIS

Overview

- Fungal infection of skin, scalp, nails, and mucous membranes caused *by Candida albicans, Candida guilliermondii, Candida glabrata, Candida parapsilosis, Candida tropicalis, Candida krusei, or Candida auris* found in warm, moist environments. Candida is part of the patient's normal flora of the skin and mucous membranes that can increase under conditions of immunosuppression due to disease, medication, and extremes of age.
- In cutaneous candidiasis, lesions are typically found in the groin/buttocks, skin folds, interdigital spaces, and nails. The skin and gastrointestinal tract from the mouth to anus can be colonized. Immunosuppression can lead to disseminated disease.

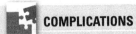 **COMPLICATIONS**

Acute: Sepsis, secondary infection
Chronic: Chronic mucocutaneous candidiasis

Etiology

- Family history of a hereditary immunodeficiency disorder
- *Disease*: HIV, IgA deficiency, congenital immunodeficiency, DM, Cushing's syndrome, hypothyroidism, hypoparathyroidism, polyendocrinopathy, autoimmune disorders, malignancy
- *Medications*: Immunosuppressants, chemotherapy, corticosteroids, immunomodulatory therapy
- Trauma, surgical implantation, hospital admission, nursing home residence, acquired in utero or during delivery
- Extremes of age, incontinence, protein-calorie malnutrition, immobility

 ALERT

Newly emerging pan-resistant *Candida auris* is a drug-resistant form that can survive on surfaces for weeks.

Signs and Symptoms

- Asymptomatic in colonization
- Erythematous maculopapular rash that may scale
- Associated maceration, erosion, and satellite lesions
- Pearly white lesions on mucous membranes with angular cheilitis in oropharyngeal presentation
- Edema, erythema, nail dystrophy and onycholysis in candida paronychia

Differential Diagnosis

- *ENDO*: DM, hypercortisolism
- *HEM/ONC*: Cancer, myelosuppression, leukemia
- *HEENT*: Leukoplakia, stomatitis
- *INT*: Allergic dermatitis, seborrheic dermatitis, contact dermatitis, psoriasis, lichen planus, leukoplakia, herpes, erythema multiforme, pemphigus
- *REPRO*: STI, vaginosis
- *Other*: Acquired or inherited immunodeficiency, incontinence, HIV, medication-induced

Diagnosis

Labs

- Clinical examination
- KOH scraping reveals spores and pseudomycelium
- CBG testing and HbA1c testing with recurrent infections
- STD screening

Additional Diagnostic Testing

- Suspected *Candida auris* requires sequencing or mass spectrometry.

Treatment and Management

Treatment Goals
- Prevent infection transmission in drug-resistant strains, control contributing factors, treat infection, and heal skin injury.

Drug Treatment
- The CDC does not recommend the treatment of *Candida auris* in skin colonization without symptoms of an infection; if an infection is present, refer immediately to an infectious disease specialist.
- Topical antifungal therapy
- Mycostatin powder to moist cutaneous lesions on skin and feet 3 times per day
- Nystatin ointment to the affected area twice daily
  - *Pediatric*: May be used as abovementioned in neonate and older
  - Nystatin oral suspension with oral candidiasis for 7 to 10 days

Interventions
- Review environmental control measures to prevent candida infection, contact precautions or enhanced barrier precautions and disinfection, moisture control, breathable coverings/clothing, judicious use of antibiotics, and antifungals.
- Reevaluate at periodic intervals to determine response to therapy and adjust as needed.

Patient Education
- Teach patient and family s/s of systemic infection to seek attention in the ED.
- Teach patients about medication adverse effects and symptoms to report.

Patient Population Considerations

Women (conception/pregnancy/lactation)
- Hormonal changes during pregnancy increase the risk or candida infections.

Geriatric
- Evaluate recurrent infections in geriatric patients for hyperglycemia.

Pediatric
- Congenital candidiasis can occur within 12 hr of delivery.

Referring Patients

- Dermatology consult
- Infectious disease consult

CELLULITIS

Overview
- Bacterial infection of the dermis and subcutaneous tissue that is non-necrotizing following a disruption in the integument. An abscess is a pocket of pus from a skin infection. See Figure 13.1.

 COMPLICATIONS

Acute: Sepsis, necrotizing fasciitis, acute compartment syndrome
Chronic: Chronic edema

Etiology

- *Causative organisms*: *Staphylococcus* species, especially CA-MRSA, or Group A *streptococcus*, *Streptococcus pneumoniae*, and *Vibrio vulnificus*
- Prior cellulitis or chronic skin disorder by history
- Recent trauma; insect, human, or animal bite

(*continued*)

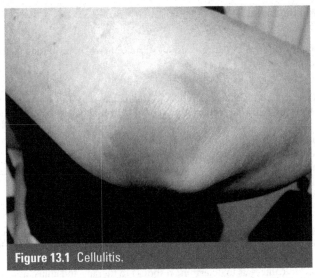

Figure 13.1 Cellulitis.

Source: Lyons, F., & Ousley, L. (2015). *Dermatology for the advanced practice nurse.* Springer Publishing Company.

Etiology (*continued*)

- Burn, surgical/invasive procedure, tattoo/body piercing
- *Disease*: HIV, DM, Cushing's syndrome, hypothyroidism, hypoparathyroidism, polyendocrinopathy, autoimmune disorders, malignancy, venous insufficiency, immunodeficiency, liver disease, CKD, chronic alcoholism, IVDA, PAD, COPD
- *Medications*: Immunosuppressants, chemotherapy, corticosteroids, immunomodulatory therapy
- Extremes of age

Signs and Symptoms

- Acute pain
- Edema, erythema, warmth to the site
- Violaceous color and bullae
- Wound opening with purulent drainage
- Red streak with lymphadenopathy may be present
- Systemic symptoms; fever chills myalgia

 ALERT

Violaceous color and bullae are signs of serious infection, especially within 24 hr of injury or event. Circumferential edema increases the risk for compartment syndrome.

Differential Diagnosis

- *HEM/ONC*: Leukemia cutis, cutaneous lymphoma, cutaneous metastasis of adenoma, inflammatory breast disease
- *INT*: Superficial cellulitis, dermatitis, abscess, erysipelas, necrotizing fasciitis
- *MSK*: Osteomyelitis
- *Other*: Medication-induced skin reaction

Diagnosis

Labs
- Wound culture
- X-ray if osteomyelitis is suspected

- Capillary blood glucose in DM
- Exclude systemic signs of infection especially in the presence of immunosuppression

Additional Diagnostic Testing
- Bone scan with periosteal lift if complications are suspected

Treatment and Management

Treatment Goals
- Eradicate infection, control contributing factors, and heal wounds when present.

Drug Treatment
Outpatient treatment if no signs of systemic illness (adult dosing provided):
- Prescribe cephalexin 500 PO q12h for uncomplicated mild cellulitis.
- May consider amoxicillin, dicloxacillin, or amoxicillin/clavulanate.
- Prescribe macrolides or clindamycin in PCN allergic patient.
  - Prescribe TMP-SMX, clindamycin, doxycycline, or linezolid in suspected CA-MRSA skin lesions.
- Refer moderate to severe infections for IV antibiotics.
- Adjust dosing for renal impairment.

> **ALERT**
>
> The presence of 2 qSOFA signs in a patient with s/s of cellulitis requires immediate referral to the ED.

Interventions
- Reassess and adjust antibiotic therapy with culture results accordingly at 48 to 72 hr.
- Perform wound cleaning and management and monitor effectiveness.
- Perform incision and drainage on an uncomplicated abscess.
- Implement strategies to protect from further injury and edema.
- Apply warm or cool compresses to cellulitis with intact skin 4 times daily.

Patient Education
- Instruct the patient to take the entire antibiotic prescription as ordered and to return for reevaluation in 48 to 72 hr.
- Remind patients to keep elevated and protect from injury. Provide information about drug-resistant strains if indicated and the importance of judicious use of antibiotics.
- Review sick day rules with patients who have diabetes.
- Explain adverse medication effects and s/s of complications to report.

Patient Population Considerations

Women (conception/pregnancy/lactation)
- Pregnant women with gestational diabetes who develop cellulitis should be monitored in the hospital for complications.

Geriatric
- Older patients with diabetes are at greater risk for hyperglycemic emergencies.

Pediatric
- Use cephalexin 25 mg/kg/dose (max 500 mg) PO TID for suspected mild staph or strep infection. Consider clindamycin 10 mg/kg/dose PO/IV (max 600 mg) for CA-MRSA, patients with a PCN allergic, or failure of prior therapy.

Referring Patients

- Surgical consult
- Infectious disease consult

Overview

- Contact dermatitis is an intermittent, pruritic, inflammatory condition that is from irritants (chemical, biologic or physical) or may be due to an IGE-mediated type I hypersensitivity reaction to allergens. (See atopic dermatitis.) See Figure 13.2.

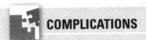

COMPLICATIONS

Acute: Anaphylaxis (atopy), secondary infection

Chronic: Chronic stasis dermatitis

Etiology

- Family and/or personal history of an allergic reaction to irritants
- Occupational exposure to an irritant
- History of atopic asthma, allergic rhinitis, hay fever, food allergy

Signs and Symptoms

- Pruritus, erythema, or maculopapular rash in distribution of exposure to an irritant.
- Lichenification can occur with chronic exposure to allergen or irritant.

Differential Diagnosis

- *HEM*: Cutaneous lymphoma
- *INT*: Eczema, seborrheic dermatitis, contact dermatitis photosensitivity reaction
- *Other*: DLE, autoimmune vasculitis

Diagnosis

Labs
- Clinical examination
- Bacterial culture if secondary infection is suspected

Additional Diagnostic Testing
- Biopsy if needed to rule out other conditions.
- Refer to an allergist for patch testing, if indicated.

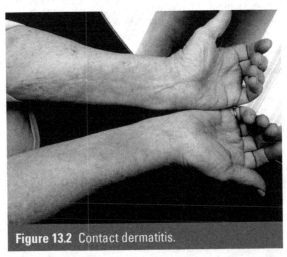

Figure 13.2 Contact dermatitis.

Source: Lyons, F., & Ousley, L. (2015). *Dermatology for the advanced practice nurse.* Springer Publishing Company.

Treatment and Management

Treatment Goals

- Relieve symptoms, protect skin from injury, implement environmental control measures, and avoid allergens and irritants.

Drug Treatment

- OTC routine care
  - Petrolatum healing ointment or equivalent topical as a barrier cream
  - Oatmeal lukewarm baths
  - Burow's solution topical soak
- Steroid management
  - Hydrocortisone 1% to 2.5% 2 to 3 times per day
    - *Pediatric*: 0.1% to 2.5% q12h, age <3 months—safety and efficacy are not established
  - Oral prednisone for severe cases
- Antihistamine management
  - Hydroxyzine 25 mg PO q6h to q8h (decrease frequency on advanced age)
    - *Pediatric*: Age <6 years 50 mg PO q6h divided doses; age >6 years 50 to 100 mg PO q6h divided doses
- Secondary infection—antibiotics
  - Mupirocin 2% to affected area q8h × 10 days
    - *Pediatric*: Age ≥3 months q8h × 10 days (reevaluate in 3–5 days if no response)

Interventions

- Review environmental control measures and refer patients to the National Eczema Association.
- Monitor for secondary infection and progression in atopic march.
- Reevaluate at periodic intervals to determine response to therapy and adjust as needed.
- Collaborate with allergists and dermatology for refractory moderate to severe disease.
- Monitor for acute food reactions (urticaria and anaphylaxis) in children.

Patient Education

- Provide counseling for tobacco cessation and avoidance.
- Teach patient to avoid irritants and allergens.
- Discuss daily therapy to prevent acute events.
- Review steps for Burow's solution and oatmeal bath.
- Teach patient and family s/s of anaphylaxis to seek attention in the ED.
- Teach the patient about medication adverse effects and symptoms to report.

Patient Population Considerations

Women (conception/pregnancy/lactation)

- Refer women who are pregnant with severe contact dermatitis to the obstetrician if steroids are indicated.

Geriatric

- The use of antihistamines for pruritus increases the risk of falls in geriatric patients.

Pediatric

- Twenty percent of pediatric patients experience allergic contact dermatitis, with prevalence rising with age.

Referring Patients

- Dermatology consult
- Allergy referral

HERPES ZOSTER (SHINGLES)

Overview

- Herpes zoster is a cutaneous eruption of vesicular lesions causes by dormant varicella virus from a prior chickenpox infection. Stressors reactivate varicella in the dorsal root ganglia; the virus migrates along the nerve to the integument triggering pain and lesion formation. The lesions follow the nerve distribution and do not cross the midline of the body. See Figure 13.3.
- The condition can last 14 to 21 days and can cause postherpetic neuralgia that can persist.

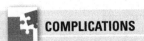

COMPLICATIONS

Acute: Encephalitis, Ramsey Hunt syndrome, neuropathy, disseminated herpes, secondary infection

Chronic: Chronic mucocutaneous candidiasis

Etiology

- Advancing age, immunosuppression by disease or treatment
- Prior chicken pox infection

Signs and Symptoms

- *Preeruptive phase*: Paresthesia or pain is reported at the site; may be confused with a stroke, sciatica, or MI symptoms; fever and myalgia; itching
- *Eruptive phase*: Patchy erythema with vesicles along the dermatome; lymphadenopathy may also be present
- Vesicular evolution and crusting
- Postherpetic neuralgia is diagnosed when pain persists more than 30 days after the last lesion crusted.

Differential Diagnosis

- *CV*: MI in the preeruptive phase
- *INT*: Bacterial infection, contact dermatitis, coxsackievirus, allergic dermatitis, HSV, poison ivy, varicella
- *NEURO*: Stroke in the preeruptive phase

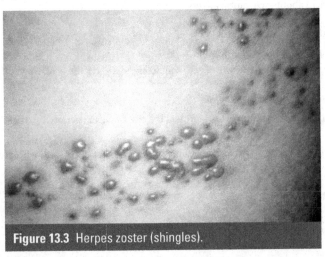

Figure 13.3 Herpes zoster (shingles).

Source: Centers for Disease Control and Prevention.

Diagnosis

Labs
- Diagnosis made by clinical examination
- Tzanck smear
- PCR testing in immunoincompetence or pregnancy

Additional Diagnostic Testing
- MRI with myelopathy

Treatment and Management

Treatment Goals
- Prevent infection transmission, limit progression, and control symptoms.
- Ophthalmic involvement requires a referral.

Drug Treatment
- *Prescribe antiviral therapy*: Acyclovir 800 mg PO 5 times per day for 7 to 10 days.
- *Prescribe therapy to minimize pain:*
  - Consider oral prednisone 40 to 60 mg daily for 1 week.
  - Offer capsaicin topical or lidocaine transdermal for pain.
  - Consider ATC acetaminophen with low-dose narcotics for breakthrough pain.
    - NSAIDs are preferred if no risk for harm.
  - Add TCAs or anticonvulsant for neuropathy.

> **)) ALERT**
>
> **Secondary Prevention of Shingles**
> Administer VZIG following exposure to active zoster case if patient is at risk for severe disease and complications within 96 hr.

Interventions
- Provide wet to dry Burow's solution dressings to lesion 4 to 6 times per day and offer calamine lotion in between for pruritus.
- Reevaluate at periodic intervals to determine response to therapy and adjust as needed.

Patient Education
- Review lesion care and discuss the course of the disease. Explain that adherence to antiviral therapy may prevent the development of postherpetic neuralgia.
- Teach patient and family s/s of systemic infection to seek attention in the ED.
- Teach patients about medication adverse effects and symptoms to report.

Patient Population Considerations

Women (conception/pregnancy/lactation)
- Pregnant women should avoid contact with patients who have herpes zoster.

Geriatric
- If the patient is immunosuppressed, initiate contact and airborne precautions and rule out disseminated disease.

Pediatric
- There is a decline in pediatric herpes zoster due to the benefit of routine varicella vaccination.

Referring Patients

- Dermatology consult
- Infectious disease consult

HIDRADENITIS SUPPURATIVA

Overview

- HS is a chronic, progressive skin disease of apocrine gland–bearing skin, causing multiple boils under the skin, otherwise referred to as acne inversa. Keloids, scars, and contracture are characteristic of this disorder, occurring due to follicular occlusion.

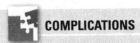 **COMPLICATIONS**

Acute: Pain, polyarthritis, infection, and sepsis
Chronic: Immobility from contractures

Etiology

- Exact etiology unknown, genetic factors may be present
- Menses
- *Frequent comorbidities:* Anxiety, depression, DM, PCOS, metabolic syndrome
- Cigarette smoking
- Onset as early as 11 years

Signs and Symptoms

- Erythema with painful boils under the skin of axilla, groin, buttocks, and breast that tunnel and rupture
- Discharge

Differential Diagnosis

- *INT:* Actinomycosis, erysipelas, granuloma, nocardiosis
- *PULM:* Blastomycosis
- *Other:* Cat scratch fever, chlamydia

 ALERT

Prompt identification and referral indicated to discuss initiation of biologic therapy to slow disease progression and prevent immobility.

Diagnosis

Labs

- CBC
- Elevated ESR
- Serum electrophoresis
- Skin lesion culture for secondary infection

Additional Diagnostic Testing

- Ultrasound of hair follicles

Treatment and Management

Treatment Goals

- Reduce recurrence, slow disease progression, and treat painful lesions.

Drug Treatment

- Prescribe clindamycin 1% solution/gel twice daily for 12 weeks.
- Consider tetracycline 500 mg orally twice daily for 4 months

Interventions

- Screen for comorbidities and treatment when present.
- If HTN is present, consider spironolactone to provide additional hormonal support.
- If BPH is present, consider finasteride to provide additional hormone support.

CLINICAL PEARL

Refer to Dermatology

- HS is staged according to Hurley tool. Patient may be prescribed intralesional therapy, or biologic therapy by dermatologist.
- Primary care manages metabolic comorbidities.

- Identify and treat secondary infections.
- Monitor response to therapy.

Patient Education

- Counsel on smoking cessation and encourage weight reduction, hygiene, loose clothing, and laser hair removal.
- Review triggers and discuss avoiding excessive heat and encouraging exercise with swimming.
- Discuss interventions to manage scarring to improve self-image.

Patient Population Considerations

Women (conception/pregnancy/lactation)

- Women may experience a reduction in symptoms during pregnancy.

Geriatric

- Complications of immobility can place geriatric patients at greater risk for complications; DVT, pneumonia, and so on.

Pediatric

- HS may manifest after puberty.

Referring Patients

- Dermatology consult

IMPETIGO

Overview

- Impetigo is an acute bacterial infection of the skin contracted through contact with an infected person or items they may have touched. See Figure 13.4.
- It may be bullous or nonbullous.

Etiology

- *Staphylococcus aureus, Streptococcus pyogenes*
- Congregate setting
- Warm, humid weather
- Contact sports, impaired integument, eczema

> **COMPLICATIONS**
>
> ***Acute***: Cellulitis, sepsis, glomerulonephritis
> ***Chronic***: CKD

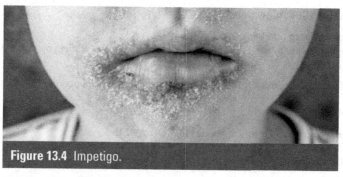

Figure 13.4 Impetigo.

Source: Centers for Disease Control and Prevention.

Signs and Symptoms

- Macule evolving into pustule with honey-crusted lesions to the affected skin with little edema or pruritus (abscess associated with CA-MRSA)
- Face and extremity most common distribution as well as sites of self-inoculation
- Mucous membrane bullae with adenopathy
- May report prior trauma to the area
- Recent exposure to someone infected

 ALERT

Prompt identification is indicated to minimize community outbreak in congregate settings.

Differential Diagnosis

- *INT*: Atopic dermatitis, candidiasis, chicken pox, contact dermatitis. erysipelas, herpes simplex, herpes zoster, scabies, *staphylococcal*-scalded skin syndrome
- *Other*: Drug reaction, infestation

Diagnosis

Labs
- Diagnosis made by clinical examination
- Wound culture of CA-MRSA suspected

Treatment and Management

Treatment Goals
- Prevent infection transmission, treat infection, and prevent complications.

Drug Treatment
- Prescribe uncomplicated local impetigo with topical mupirocin 3 times daily for 7 to 10 days in ages >2 months.
  - *Alternative*: Prescribe retapamulin 1% twice daily for 5 days in ages >9 months.
- Consider systemic medication if the infection is severe.
  - Prescribe cephalexin 25 to 50 mg/kg/d in divided doses twice daily for 10 days.
  - Prescribe cephalexin 250 to 500 mg PO 4 times daily in adults for 10 days.
- Consider clindamycin or doxycycline or TMP-SMX if CA-MRSA is suspected.

Interventions
- Clean wound bed and remove crusts using standard and contact precautions.
- Monitor response to therapy.

Patient Education
- Counsel patients and caregivers in hand hygiene to avoid transmission.
- Demonstrate gentle cleansing and removal of crusts

Patient Population Considerations

Women (conception/pregnancy/lactation)
- Instruct pregnant women to avoid contact with patients who have impetigo.

Geriatric
- Caution older patients with impetigo to avoid peers who are immunocompromised because of its infectivity.

Pediatric
- Impetigo most commonly occurs in young children ages 2 to 5 years.

Referring Patients

- Dermatology consult
- Infectious disease consult

PSORIASIS

Overview

- Psoriasis is a chronic, autoimmune skin disease of the epidermis. Hyperproliferation of keratocytes due to increased cytokine activity and activated T cells during flares cause lichenification and plaque formation.
- Chronic inflammation may play a role in the development of psoriatic arthritis and other diseases.

Etiology

- Exact etiology unknown
- Genetic factors, family history
- *Environmental trigger*: Cold, trauma, infections, alcohol, and drugs
- Improved with sun exposure

Signs and Symptoms

- Scaly skin lesions with lichenification over flexor prominences, scalp, intergluteal clefts, and penis
  - *Positive Auspitz sign*: Punctate bleeding points with scale removal
- Pruritus
- Onycholysis and stippled nails and pitting
- Joint pain
- Precipitated by the sudden withdrawal of steroid or a trigger
- Ocular manifestation may appear like blepharitis

Differential Diagnosis

- *HEENT*: Atopic keratoconjunctivitis, blepharitis, dry eye disease, onychomycosis
- *HEM/ONC*: SCC
- *INT*: Atopic dermatitis, contact dermatitis, lichen planus, pityriasis alba, pityriasis rosea
- *MSK*: Gout, pseudogout, psoriatic arthritis, reactive arthritis
- *Other*: Drug reaction, syphilis

Diagnosis

Labs
- The diagnosis is made by clinical examination.

Additional Diagnostic Testing
- Skin biopsy, as indicated
- Joint x-ray

Treatment and Management

Treatment Goals
- Promote comfort and positive self-image, prevent infection, and prevent complications.

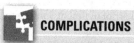

COMPLICATIONS

Acute: Secondary infection
Chronic: Psoriatic arthritis, possible lymphoma, ischemic heart disease, possible ulcerative colitis, MVP

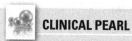

CLINICAL PEARL

Drugs Associated With Flares
Antimalarials, aspirin, beta blockers, botulinum toxin injections, Iodides

CLINICAL PEARL

Refer for Advanced Disease
Moderate to severe disease should be referred to dermatology for biologic therapy. Evidence of joint pain requires rheumatology referral.

Drug Treatment

- Manage mild disease with topical moisturizers, OTC topical steroids, and avoidance of triggers.
  - Apply thin layer of anthralin 0.5% to 1.2% daily to lesions to reduce hyperkeratinization.
    - Consider topical retinoids as an alternative.
  - Use calcitriol ointment 3 mcg/g to lesions in the morning and at night to prevent facial skin atrophy.
- Use an oral agent in a severe disease of 10 to 25 mg PO weekly.

Interventions

- Promote stress reduction, sun exposure, and trigger avoidance; refer for CBT as indicated.
- Monitor response to therapy.
- Assess for complications.

Patient Education

- *Counsel patients on strategies to promote skin integrity*: Moisturizers, coal tar products, oatmeal baths.
- Discuss stress and coping resources and provide referrals.

Patient Population Considerations

Women (conception/pregnancy/lactation)

- Recommend topicals as an option for women who are pregnant or breastfeeding.

Geriatric

- Caution older patients with impetigo to avoid peers who are immunocompromised because of its infectivity.

Pediatric

- A link has been made between psoriasis and strep infections in children. Ixekizumab has received approval for children ages 6 years and older.

Referring Patients

- Dermatology consult
- Ophthalmology consult
- Rheumatology consult

ROSACEA

Overview

- Rosacea is a chronic inflammatory disorder causing facial flushing, telangiectasia, papules, and pustules. Exacerbations of rosacea occur in response to triggers, such as sunlight, stress, and certain foods. As it progresses, the patient experiences persistent erythema, nodules, and pustules that can scar.

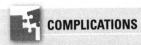 **COMPLICATIONS**

Acute: Ocular rosacea, anxiety, depression
Chronic: Scarring

Etiology

- Family history, immune response
- Mites
- *Presence of triggers*: Stress, alcohol, heat, cold, sunlight, exercise, spicy foods

Signs and Symptoms

- Erythema and flushing in response to a trigger
- Telangiectasia, papules, pustules, and nodules

Differential Diagnosis

- *ENDO*: Congenital adrenal hyperplasia, hypercortisolism, PCOS
- *INT*: Acneiform eruptions, acne maligna, acne conglobata, acne keloidalis nuchae, acne vulgaris, folliculitis, seborrheic dermatitis, steroid-induced dermatitis
- *Other*: SLE, sarcoidosis

Diagnosis

Labs
- Diagnosed by clinical examination.

Additional Diagnostic Testing
- Urine HCG before and during the administration of retinoids

Treatment and Management

Treatment Goals
- Reduce inflammation and bacterial colonization, prevent flares, and minimizing scarring.

Drug Treatment
- Topical antibiotics as the first-line agent
  - Metronidazole 1% topical daily
  - Topical erythromycin, metronidazole consideration
- Tretinoin 0.02% to 0.1%, pea-size amount at bedtime may be added if antibiotics are ineffective
- If all the abovementioned are ineffective, consider hormone therapy
- Spironolactone 50 to 200 mg PO daily in divided doses or oral contraceptive to suppress androgens
- Collaborate with dermatology if fulminant rosacea requires corticosteroids and oral retinoids

> 🔊 **ALERT**
>
> - Oral isotretinoin agents have been associated with depression and suicidality, as well as birth defects if taken when pregnant.
> - Review the risks and benefits of therapy and discuss strategies to seek consultation.

Interventions
- Monitor adherence to skin regimen.
- Monitor BMP for hyperkalemia in spironolactone therapy.

Patient Education
- Teach the patient to avoid triggers.
- Instruct the patient to avoid sunlight and apply liberal amounts of sunscreen with an SPF of 30.
- Discuss the risk and benefits of oral corticosteroids and retinoids in rosacea.
- Discuss interventions to manage scarring to improve self-image.

Patient Population Considerations

Women (conception/pregnancy/lactation)
- Oral contraceptives and aldosterone antagonists are effective adjuncts for women with acne. Preconception planning is critical in women of childbearing age. Oral retinoids should be avoided if planning pregnancy.

Geriatric
- Rosacea often affects older adults.

Pediatric
- Rosacea is uncommon in children.

Referring Patients

- Dermatology consult
- Endocrine consult

SCABIES

Overview

- Scabies is a skin infestation by mites that have buried and laid eggs triggering intense pruritus. Symptoms develop over a 4- to 8-week period. See Figure 13.5.

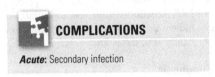

COMPLICATIONS

Acute: Secondary infection

Etiology

- *Human itch mite*: Sarcoptes scabiei
- Skin-to-skin contact with a person infected with scabies
- Household member, sexual partner
- Sharing clothing and bedding with a person with scabies

Signs and Symptoms

- Discrete pruritic papules and pustules in a linear pattern
- Burrows or thread-like elevations of the skin
- Can be in the interdigital space, dorsal feet, ankles, wrists, buttocks, and genitalia
- Frequently seen on trunk and back of children
- Can be nodular in appearance in children
- S/s of secondary infection and excoriation

Differential Diagnosis

- *INT*: Atopic dermatitis, contact dermatitis, eczema, folliculitis, lichen planus, pediculosis, psoriasis (guttate), pityriasis rosea, seborrhea dermatitis, sea bather's eruption, urticaria
- *MSK*: Gout, pseudogout, psoriatic arthritis, reactive arthritis
- *Other*: Drug reaction, insect bites, syphilis

Diagnosis

Labs

- Diagnosis made by clinical examination
- Skin scraping and microscopic exam for eggs, mites, and waste

Additional Diagnostic Testing

- Adhesive tape test

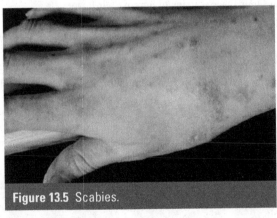

Figure 13.5 Scabies.

Source: Centers for Disease Control and Prevention.

Treatment and Management

Treatment Goals
- Eradicate mites, prevent infection, and prevent complications.

Drug Treatment
- Remove excess scales using warm soaks. If lesions do not remove easily, apply a keratolytic ointment to loosen the scales.
- Apply scabicidal agent such as permethrin cream 5% and remove as instructed.
- Demonstrate gentle cleansing and removal of crusts.
  - Only permethrin or sulfur ointment may be used in infants age 2 months and older.

Interventions
- Treat household members with scabicide.
- Promote stress reduction, sun exposure, trigger avoidance, and refer for CBT as indicated.
- Monitor response to therapy.
- Assess for the presence of complications.

Patient Education
- Counsel patients and caregivers to treat the entire household with scabicide, and to wash bedding and clothes in hot soapy water.
- Offer retreatment in 1 week and follow up in 2 weeks.
- Prescribe hydroxyzine or diphenhydramine PO PRN for pruritus.

Patient Population Considerations

Women (conception/pregnancy/lactation)
- Sulfur is an alternative topical agent considered safe during pregnancy.

Geriatric
- Norwegian scabies causes a severe form called crusted scabies, for which immunocompromised older adults are at greater risk. It has a larger population of mites and is more contagious.

Pediatric
- Crotamiton is approved for adult use only.

Referring Patients

- Dermatology consult

POP QUIZ 13.2

A 65-year-old female who has previously been vaccinated with the live virus for shingles asks if she should receive the new recombinant vaccine available now. She has a medical history of Graves' disease and a stroke.

What is the appropriate response?

SKIN CANCER

Overview

- Malignant transformation of the skin structures causes SCC, basal cell carcinoma, and melanoma. See Figure 13.6.
- SCC arises from actinic keratosis in keratinized epithelial cells. The slow-growing tumor usually develops on sun-exposed skin and can metastasize to the lung, bone, CNS, and liver.
- BCC arises from basal cells in the skin structure that grows slowly and rarely metastasizes. If left untreated, it metastasizes to the lung, bone, lymph nodes, and abdominal viscera.
- Melanoma arises from melanocyte in basal cells or existing nevi that spread vertically to allow for metastasis. It readily metastasizes to lymph nodes, lung, liver, brain, and bone with increased mortality.

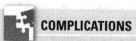

COMPLICATIONS

Acute: Anxiety
Chronic: Distant metastasis

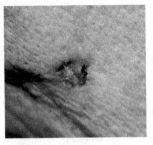

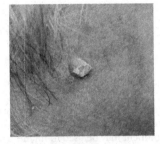

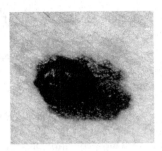

(A) Basal cell carcinoma   (B) Squamous cell carcinoma   (C) Melanoma

Figure 13.6 Skin cancers.

Source: A and C: Gawlik, K., Melnyk, B. M., & Teall, A. (2021). *Evidence-based physical examination.* Springer Publishing Company; (C): National Cancer Institute/Kelly Nelson, MD.

Etiology

- Family history, increasing age, fair skin, Celtic or Scandinavian ancestry, multiple nevi, freckling
- Cumulative exposure to UV light radiation
  - Extensive exposure to x-rays
  - Some industrial chemicals
  - Immunosuppression, hormones, burns

Signs and Symptoms

- *SCC*: Ulceration to a keratotic lesion that does not heal
- *BCC*: Enlarged nodule with a central depression and elevated border
- *Melanoma*: Change in an existing nevus or a new nevus meeting ABCDE criteria.

Differential Diagnosis

- *HEM/ONC*: Bowen's disease, BCC, cutaneous manifestations of neoplastic disease, lymphoma, malignant melanoma, SCC
- *INT*: Actinic keratosis, seborrheic keratosis, porokeratosis DLE, benign skin lesion, nevus

Diagnosis

Labs
- Clinical examination
- CBC may show pancytopenia of metastasis
- Elevated LDH and ESR with advanced disease
- LFTs, bilirubin to assess liver function

Additional Diagnostic Testing
- Full-depth biopsy by dermatology
- Chest CT chest MRI brain, PET scan for metastasis for staging if poorly differentiated

CLINICAL PEARL

Skin Cancer Screening

USPSTF makes no recommendations on frequency of skin cancer screening.

Individuals should assess their risks, engage in risk factor modification, and use shared decision-making with their provider regarding frequency of screening.

ALERT

ABCDE Criteria for Melanoma

A: Asymmetrical lesion

B: Border irregularity

C: Change in color or variegation noted

D: Diameter increase or >6 mm

E: Elevated skin lesion

Treatment and Management

Treatment Goals
- Treat according to the stage of cancer, prevent metastasis and recurrence, and modify risk factors.

Drug Treatment
- Managed by dermatology

Interventions
- Monitor response to therapy.
- Identify sites of metastasis.
- Encourage risk factor modification.

Patient Education
- Discuss the disease process and management.
- Review risk factor modification of sun exposure, x-rays, and certain chemicals.
- Teach patient to follow a low-fat diet, which may help prevent progression.

Patient Population Considerations

Women (conception/pregnancy/lactation)
- Review risk factors for melanoma with women of childbearing age and encourage risk factor modification. Skin cancer can be safely treated during pregnancy.

Geriatric
- Older adults have a higher burden of skin cancer due to their advanced age.

Pediatric
- Melanoma is the most common pediatric skin cancer. Obtain a family history of melanoma and reinforce risk factor modification.

Referring Patients

- Dermatology consult

TICK-BORNE DISEASES

Overview

- Tick-borne diseases occur from a tick bite, through which the tick transmits organisms that cause various acute infections (see Etiology). Tick bites are most likely to occur during the spring, summer, and fall seasons. Individuals bitten by a tick are at risk for bacterial, viral, and parasitic diseases.
- *Three ticks are responsible for most conditions*: the deer tick, Lone Star tick, and the American dog tick. The Lone Star tick is a trigger of alpha-gal syndrome causing anaphylaxis.
- The prevalence and geographic range of tick-borne diseases have increased and expanded.
- Ticks have developed improved survival with climate change and greater exposure to human populations with building and recreation in their indigenous areas.
- There are no vaccines for tick-borne disease.

 COMPLICATIONS

Acute: Sepsis, encephalitis, anaphylaxis, coinfection

Chronic: Neuropathy, disability

 ALERT

Primary Prevention of Tick-Borne Illness
- Avoid tall grasses in fields and forests.
- Wear a light-colored hat and a long sleeve shirt with pants tucked into socks if walking in wooded area or fields.
- Protect pets using an approved tick product.
- Use repellents or approved lotions to skin or clothing.
- Perform daily tick checks.

Etiology

- *Lyme disease*: *Borrelia burgdorferi*, *Borrelia mayonii*
- *Anaplasmosis*: *Anaplasma phagocytophilum*
- *Babesiosis*: A parasitic infection caused by *Babesia microti*
- *Ehrlichiosis*: *Ehrlichia chaffeensis* and *Ehrlichia ewingii*
- *Relapsing fever*: *Borrelia miyamotoi*
- *Tularemia*: *Francisella tularensis*
- *Rocky Mountain spotted fever*: *Rickettsia rickettsii*
- *Powassan virus disease*: Powassan virus
- *Rickettsiosis*: *Rickettsia parkeri*

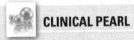 **CLINICAL PEARL**

The absence of a recalled tick bite does not exclude a tick-borne illness.

Signs and Symptoms

- Attached engorged tick or report of a recent tick bite
- *S/s of infection*: Fever, myalgia, HA, and gastrointestinal symptoms
- *CV symptoms*: Pericarditis, myocarditis, and arrhythmia
- *Neurological symptoms*: Bell's palsy, hearing loss, meningeal irritation, encephalitis, paresis, paralysis
- *GI symptoms*: Anorexia, jaundice, hepatosplenomegaly
- *MSK symptoms*: Joint pain, inflammation, arthralgia
- *INT symptoms*: Petechial rash, bull's-eye rash (may or may not be present; see Figure 13.7), urticaria, s/s of anaphylaxis when eating beef, pork, meat following a Lone Star tick bite

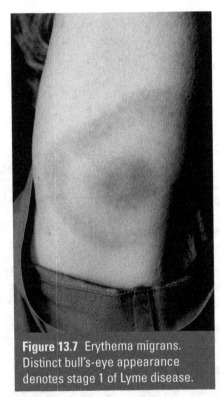

Figure 13.7 Erythema migrans. Distinct bull's-eye appearance denotes stage 1 of Lyme disease.

Source: Centers for Disease Control and Prevention.

Differential Diagnosis

- *CV*: Pericarditis, MI
- *GI*: Hepatitis, gastroenteritis
- *INT*: Atopic dermatitis, contact dermatitis, poison ivy, poison oak, urticaria
- *MSK*: Gout, pseudogout, psoriatic arthritis, reactive arthritis
- *NEURO*: Encephalitis, meningitis, Bell's palsy, stroke
- *Other*: RA flare, SLE, drug reaction, other insect bites, syphilis

Diagnosis

Labs

- Use a testing algorithm based on region
- Tick-borne disease antibodies serum panel and PCR testing to evaluate for Lyme, ehrlichiosis, anaplasmosis, babesiosis, tularemia
    - *Note*: There is a lag of 1 week for many tick-borne diseases antibodies to appear
- Spotted fever group antibody, IgG, IgM
- Peripheral smear for microscopic exam
- CBC may reveal thrombocytopenia, leukopenia, and hemolytic anemia
- BMP may reveal hyponatremia and rising azotemia
- Elevated LFTs and bilirubin may be present

Additional Diagnostic Testing

- Microscopic examination of blood
- *Parasite identification board card*: Affix removed tick to card
- Lumbar puncture after CT with neurological symptoms
- 12-lead EKG, echocardiogram

Treatment and Management

Treatment Goals

- Eradicate infection, treat symptoms, and prevent complications.

Drug Treatment

- Prescribe doxycycline for all suspected tick-borne diseases.
- Prescribe acetaminophen for fever and pain.

Interventions

- *Tick removal*: Use forceps to grasp the tick at the junction of attachment at the skin and smoothly remove in a continuous movement without squeezing the body of the tick.
- Provide supportive care and monitor response to therapy.

Patient Education

- Counsel patients on primary prevention strategies to avoid tick-borne illness.
- Counsel patients on an allergy action plan with alpha-gal syndrome.
- Teach patients to report s/s of complications and adverse medication effects.

Patient Population Considerations

Women (conception/pregnancy/lactation)

- Chloramphenicol may be prescribed in the presence of Rocky Mountain spotted fever and considered safe during pregnancy. It is ineffective in ehrlichiosis and anaplasmosis.

ALERT

Tick Bite Prophylaxis

Prescribe doxycycline 200 mg to patients >8 years as a single dose, if the following conditions are met:

a. Doxycycline is not contraindicated
b. The tick is and adult or nymph I. scapularis
c. The tick was attached for ≥36 hr
d. Lyme disease is common where the patient lives or has recently traveled
e. Prophylaxis can be started in 72 hr from tick removal

ALERT

Patients with acute cardiovascular, neurologic, or hepatorenal symptoms require immediate referral to the ED.

Geriatric

- There are no differences in the management of tick-borne disease in this population. However, tick-borne disease mimics other conditions frequently experienced by older adults, which may delay treatment and worsen course.

Pediatric

- The highest rate of tick infections occurs between the ages of 5 and 15 years.

Referring Patients

- Infectious disease consult
- Allergy consult

POP QUIZ 13.3

A 23-year-old male presents with right facial droop and a smooth forehead. He has no medical history. *His neurological examination:* Unremarkable except for CN V deficiency. *Musculoskeletal exam:* MAE, FROM, equal strength, no paranesthesia. Skin is tanned, warm, dry, no lesion. *Cardiovascular exam:* S1, S2 no rub with regular rate and rhythm. He explains that he woke up this morning with facial droop. He denies recent illness, injury, or insect bites, and reports recent travel to Cape Cod for camping. What is the most likely cause of this patient's symptoms?

TINEA INFECTION

Overview

- Tinea is a dermatophyte infection of the skin and nails caused by *Trichophyton, Microsporum, and Epidermophyton*. Sites of infection include scalp (capitus), groin (cruris), nails (unguium, or onychomycosis), feet (pedis), and skin lesions in areas other than scalp, groin, palms, or feet (corporis).

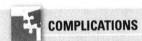

COMPLICATIONS

Acute: Secondary infection
Chronic: Chronic tinea infection

Etiology

- Exposure to a fungus in locker rooms, soil, poor hygiene, warm climate
- Immunosuppression, DM, malnutrition

Signs and Symptoms

- *Capitus:* Scaly scalp lesion with patchy alopecia
- *Corporis:* Ring-like pruritic rash with central clearing (See Figure 13.8.)

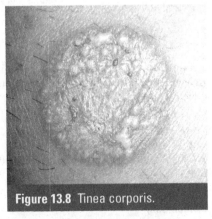

Figure 13.8 Tinea corporis.

Source: Gawlik, K., Melnyk, B. M., & Teall, A. (2021). *Evidence-based physical examination.* Springer Publishing Company.

- *Cruris*: Pruritic red rash with scale
- *Pedis*: Dry or moist scale
- *Unguium*: Opaque, yellowed, thickened nail

Differential Diagnosis

- *ENDO*: DM, hypercortisolism
- *HEM/ONC*: Cancer, myelosuppression, leukemia
- *INT*: Allergic dermatitis, candidiasis, seborrheic dermatitis, contact dermatitis,
- *REPRO*: STI, vaginosis
- *Other*: Acquired or inherited immunodeficiency, incontinence, HIV, medication-induced

Diagnosis

Labs

- Clinical examination
- KOH scraping reveals spores and pseudohyphae
- CBG testing and HgA1C testing with recurrent infections.
- Culture
- Baseline LFTs with systemic therapy

Additional Diagnostic Testing

- *Wood's light exam*: Nonfluorescent

Treatment and Management

Treatment Goals

- Prevent infection transmission, control contributing factors, treat infection, and heal skin injury.

Drug Treatment

- *Capitus*: Griseofulvin and topical antifungal point and selenium shampoo
- *Corporis*: Topical azole antifungal is first-line therapy. Topical steroids can be added for symptoms of pruritus.
- *Cruris*: OTC topical antifungal is the first-line therapy—prescribe systemic antifungal for persistent infection
- *Pedis*: Terbinafine and OTC foot powder
- *Unguium*: Topical efinaconazole if unable to tolerate systemic therapy; itraconazole PO 200 mg for 12 weeks for better nail penetration

Interventions

- Assess for the presence of systemic disease with frequent infections.
- Reevaluate at periodic intervals to determine response to therapy and adjust as needed.
- Monitor LFTs for systemic therapy.

Patient Education

- Discuss strategies to prevent infection transmission and risk factor modification to prevent recurrence or chronic infection.
- Teach patient and family s/s of systemic infection to seek attention in the ED.
- Teach patients about medication adverse effects and symptoms to report.

Patient Population Considerations

Women (conception/pregnancy/lactation)

- Antifungals considered first-line agents for women who are pregnant are clotrimazole, miconazole, and nystatin. Second-line agents are butenafine, ciclopirox, naftifine, oxiconazole, and terbinafine.
- Avoid econazole during the first trimester and use sparingly during the second and third trimesters.

Geriatric
- Monitor for contact dermatitis in older adults treated with topical antifungals for tinea pedis.

Pediatric
- Tinea infections are common in children.

Referring Patients

- Dermatology consult

URTICARIA AND ANAPHYLAXIS

Overview

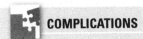

COMPLICATIONS

- *Urticaria* is a type I hypersensitivity skin response to allergens, cold, heat, or exercise. It is characterized by papules and wheals that are erythemic and pruritic. See Figure 13.9.

Acute: ARDS, AKI, ATN, hepatic failure, DIC, acute arterial thrombosis, and amputation.

  - Chronic urticaria is a skin disorder with wheals that wax and wane for more than 6 weeks.
  - *Anaphylaxis* is a life-threatening type I hypersensitivity reaction in response to high-risk allergens. In anaphylaxis, chemical mediators of inflammation cause systemic inflammation and increased capillary permeability of alveoli resulting in hypoxia and pulmonary congestion. Progressive capillary leaking cause hypotension and decreased tissue perfusion that cannot be corrected by the neurohormonal response.

Etiology

ALERT

- Personal history of asthma, eczema, allergic rhinitis, allergic dermatitis

Anaphylaxis Triggers

- Personal history of allergy to drugs, food, medications, insects, occupational agents

Insect stings, IV contrast, antibiotics, medications such as aspirin and NSAIDs, latex, and foods such as peanuts, eggs, wheat, soy, and red meat in alpha-gal syndrome

- Experienced a rash or angioedema with prior exposure to an antigen
- Family history or personal history of anaphylaxis

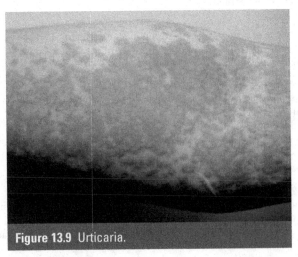

Figure 13.9 Urticaria.

Source: Courtesy of James Heilman, MD.

Signs and Symptoms

- Urticaria
  - Erythemic papules, wheals distributed in a pattern reflect contact or disseminated in ingested, inhaled, or injected allergen
  - Pruritus
- Anaphylaxis
  - Anxiety and apprehension after exposure to an allergen, progressing to AMS and LOC
  - Generalized urticaria, pruritus, flushed appearance, moving to cyanosis
  - Laryngospasm, audible wheeze, accessory muscle use, crackles
  - Chest pain, peripheral edema
  - Diarrhea and vomiting
  - Tachypnea, tachycardia, hypotension, and oxygen desaturation

Differential Diagnosis

Urticaria

- *CV*: Phlebitis
- *HEENT*: Angioedema, allergic dermatitis, contact dermatitis, chronic urticaria, drug eruption
- *Other*: Serum sickness, vasculitis

Anaphylaxis

- *CV*: Vasovagal reaction, cardiogenic shock, fulminant pulmonary edema
- *PULM*: Exacerbation of asthma/COPD, pulmonary embolism
- *HEENT*: Acute urticaria, angioedema, allergic dermatitis, contact dermatitis, chronic urticaria
- *HEM*: Malignancy
- *NEURO*: Anxiety, epilepsy, panic attack, stroke
- *Other*: Red man syndrome, monosodium glutamate poisoning, septic shock, transfusion reaction, viral exanthem, autoimmune disease flare

Diagnosis

Labs

- Urticaria—diagnosed by clinical examination
- Eosinophilia on CBC
- Elevated CRP
- RAST testing

Additional Diagnostic Testing

- Skin testing in the presence of a reaction to a high-risk allergen
- Lateral neck film with angioedema

Treatment and Management

Treatment Goals

- Protect from harm, treat urticaria, and prevent anaphylaxis.

Drug Treatment

- Prescribe diphenhydramine PO PRN for hives
- Consider a daily dose of nonsedating antihistamine and H2 antagonist, and or leukotriene antagonist daily
- Discharge patient with epinephrine injection pen
  - Adults and children weighing >25 kg (adult version)
  - Pediatric: Weight <5 kg: 0.01 mg/kg, 5 to 25 kg: 0.15 mg IM (junior version)

 ALERT

Collaborate with allergist in developing an allergy action plan based on degree of hypersensitivity.

If apprehensive with pruritus after exposure to a high-risk allergen, administer EpiPen and transfer to ED.

Interventions
- Monitor response to desensitization therapy.
- Monitor response to MAB if indicated.
- Prescribe allergy action plan individualized to patient needs.

Patient Education
- Review environmental control strategies to avoid triggers.
- Discuss daily therapy to prevent acute events.
- Explain the management of acute events using an allergy action plan.
- Teach patients about medication adverse effects and symptoms to report.

Patient Population Considerations

Women (conception/pregnancy/lactation)
- Anaphylaxis is a rare cause of neonatal mortality, with antibiotics as the most common trigger. Pregnant mother and baby need to be observed for 48 to 72 hr after an episode of maternal anaphylaxis.

Geriatric
- The presence of polypharmacology and comorbidities have a marked influence on the outcome of older adults.

Pediatric
- School-age children require an allergy action plan and medication with instructions at school. Ensure caregivers understand how to use an epinephrine injection pen and seek evaluation immediately.

Referring Patients

- Allergy consult

WOUNDS

Overview

- Wounds are a disruption to the structures of the skin and underlying tissue that may be acute or chronic. Wound healing progresses through stages of inflammation, proliferation, and maturation.
- Following hemostasis, increased vascular permeability permits neutrophils to eliminate bacteria and cellular debris. Inflammatory mediators, cytokines, growth factors, and prostaglandins form an exudate where fibroblasts synthesize collagen to lay down a matrix to stabilize the wound and set the stage for reepithelization. Deposition of granulation tissue and neovascularization occurs, fibrin framework matures, and the wound begins to contract and stabilize.

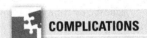

COMPLICATIONS

Acute: Pain, bleeding, infection
Chronic: Chronic wound infection, contractures

Types of Wounds
- *Skin lacerations and punctures*: Acute disruption to integument and underlying structures that may require closure to restore hemostasis and function.
- *High-risk wounds*: Chronic wounds that fail to progress through the stages of healing as expected and heal by secondary intention.
- *Bites (human, animal, and insect)*: Disrupt integument by tearing and puncturing tissue. Bites can introduce microorganisms that cause infection and sepsis. Venom from bites may trigger coagulopathy, neurotoxicity, systemic inflammatory response, and tissue necrosis.

- *Burns*: Destroy skin structures and underlying tissue. They are classified according to degree and depth in skin structures and underlying tissue and bone. Depending on the burn depth and body surface area, the patient is at risk for acute and systemic complications.

Etiology

- *Skin lacerations and punctures*: Trauma by sharp objects or blunt force as a result of intimate partner violence, self-harm, other-directed violence, motor vehicle crashes, recreational and sport activities, alcohol and substance use, machine operation, occupational hazards
- *High-risk wounds* (certain diseases, medications, and biopsychosocial conditions can result in infection, wound extension, and delayed healing):
  - *Disease*: Anemia, angiopathy, ASCVD, autoimmune disease, cancer, CKD, chronic venous insufficiency, cirrhosis, delirium, dementia, DM, eating disorder, HF, immunodeficiency, lymphedema, neuropathy, paralysis, paresis, peripheral arterial disease
  - *Medications*: Anticoagulants, antiplatelets, chemotherapy, corticosteroids, COX-2 inhibitors, immunosuppressants, NSAIDs, vasoconstrictors
  - *Environment*: Advanced age, alcoholism, excessive wound pressure, extensive wounds, homelessness, hyperglycemia, hypothermia, hypoxia, immobility, lack of social support and financial resources, obesity, protein-calorie malnutrition, radiation exposure, tobacco, substance abuse, vitamin A, C, and zinc deficiency
- *Bites*: Human, animal, and insect bites disrupt integument and increase the risk of concomitant infections, toxins, and allergic responses
- *Burns*: Thermal, chemical, electrical, radiation agents
  - Etiology of burns may compound the injury, causing inhalation injury, carbon monoxide poisoning, burn extension, arrhythmia, and systemic disease

Signs and Symptoms

- Lacerations and punctures
  - *Lacerations*: A tear in the skin structures, irregular in pattern and depth that may bleed excessively
  - *Punctures*: Circumscribed break in integument that extends into underlying tissue. Deeper, and bleed less
  - Both injuries can cause damage to underlying organs, disrupt circulation and/or nerve function distal to the injury
- High-risk wounds
  - *Ischemic*: Dry eschar and necrotic tissue
  - Purulent discharge
  - Increase in three-dimensional measurement with tunneling
  - Decreased distal pulses
  - Presence of a predisposing factor
  - S/s of a local and systemic infection may develop over time
- Bites
  - Bleeding, avulsed tissue, paresthesia, a decrease in ROM, foreign bodies, and debris
  - S/s of a local and systemic infection may develop over time
    - ○ *Human*: Superficial abrasions, laceration, tearing, avulsions, with bite mark impression
    - ○ *Dog*: Puncture, lacerations, nerve, muscle, and bone involvement

---

CLINICAL PEARL

Wound Assessment

History:
- Obtain time of onset, circumstances, mechanism of injury, degree of disability, immediate treatment provided at time of injury, associated symptoms, presence of progressive symptoms, current medical conditions and medications, tetanus status

Physical:
- Document location on body map, obtain photo, record the measurements, note the presence of foreign bodies, exudate, wound edges, and wound bed appearance

---

(continued)

Signs and Symptoms (*continued*)

- ○ *Cat*: Small punctures, abrasions, superficial lacerations
- ○ Brown *spider*: Erythemic papule with edema developing a central depression and necrosis over 72 hr
- Burns
  - Classify the type of burn; document location, mechanism, associated symptoms, and degree
    - ○ *Superficial burn*: Intact red epidermis with blanching erythema (first degree)
    - ○ *Partial thickness*: Red, moist wound bed with painful blisters (second degree)
    - ○ *Deep partial thickness*: Red, white dry, nonblanching erythema
    - ○ *Full thickness*: A black, white, dry wound that is painless (third degree)
  - Estimate BSA of the burn using the rule of nines or Lund–Browder chart in pediatrics (see Figure 13.10)

ALERT

Burn Center Referral
- Partial thickness >10% of BSA
- Burns involving face, hands, feet, perineum, major joints, circumferential, and genitals
- Inhalation injury
- Chemical and electrical burns
- Burned children in hospital without qualified personnel
- Third-degree burns in any age group
- Patients with comorbidity that could affect outcome and mortality

Differential Diagnosis

- Lacerations and punctures
  - *Other*: Abuse/neglect (child, elder), bites (animal, insect, human), body focused repetitive behavior, intimate partner violence, suicidality
  - High-risk wounds
  - *CV*: Peripheral arterial disease, venous stasis

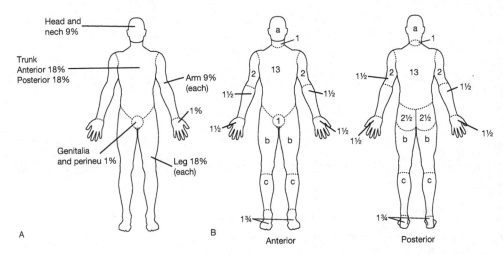

Relative percentage of body surfcace areas (%BSA) affected by growth

	0 yr	1 yr	1 yr	10 yr	15 yr
a— ½ of head	9½	8½	6½	5½	4½
b— ½ of 1 thigh	2¾	3¼	4	4¼	4½
c— 1½ of 1 lower leg	2½	2½	2¾	3	3¼

Figure 13.10 Estimating burns.

Source: U.S. Department of Health and Human Services: Radiation Emergency Medical Management. *Burn triage and treatment of thermal injuries in a radiation emergency.* https://www.remm.nlm.gov/burns.htm

- *HEM/ONC*: Malignancy
- *INT*: Cellulitis, SJS, TENS, erythema multiforme, CA-MRSA
- *Other*: Autoimmune vasculitis, diabetes, drug reaction, poisoning
- Bites
  - *NEURO*: Seizures, Tetanus
  - *MSK*: Osteomyelitis
  - *INT*: Cellulitis, tick-borne disease
  - *Other*: Abuse/neglect (child, elder)
- Burns
  - *CV*: Capillary leak syndrome
  - *PULM*: ARDS
  - *INT*: SJS, TENS, erythema multiforme
  - *Other*: Drug eruption

Diagnosis

Labs
- High-risk wounds
  - CBC for leukocytosis, leukopenia, or shift to the left
  - BMP to evaluate for azotemia, hyperglycemia
  - PT/INR to evaluate bleeding times
  - Serum albumin <3.5
  - HbA1c >7%
  - Wound cultures
- Bites
  - X-ray and wound culture
  - *Human*: Hepatitis profile, IGRA, HIV testing baseline, BMP, LFTs, CBC as a baseline for PEP therapy
  - *Brown spider*: CBC, BMP, PT/INR, U/A with signs of systemic toxicity in ED
- Burns
  - No labs indicated for uncomplicated burns in primary care
  - CBG testing with diabetes

Additional Diagnostic Testing
- Wound c/s and gram stain
- Plain x-ray, CT scan, and MRI or bone scan to evaluate high-risk wounds
- Biopsy to evaluate high-risk wounds
- Ankle-brachial index and arterial Doppler study to evaluate perfusion and refer to a vascular surgeon

Treatment and Management

Treatment Goals
- Prevent infection, promote wound healing, and prevent complications.

Drug Treatment
- Pain management
  - Acetaminophen PRN for pain
- Promote wound healing
  - Maintain BG, and prescribe vitamin C and zinc daily
- Reduce risk for infection
  - Silver sulfadiazine topical to burn BID
  - Ampicillin with clavulanic acid or doxycycline to human bites to hand or puncture wounds and dog bites

 ALERT

Clinical Decision Rules

Any patients with . . .
- ABCD problem
- Venom bites requiring antitoxin
- Avulsed tissue, deep puncture wound, multiple bites, foreign body or fractures, neurovascular compromise, tendon damage, urticaria
- CBG >250 mg dL
- S/s of infection and two qSOFA signs
- Deep burns

. . . require ED referral immediately.

(continued)

Drug Treatment (continued)

- Postexposure counseling for exposure to blood-borne pathogens in a human and animal bite
- Antitoxins and dapsone for brown spider bite
- Tetanus immunoglobulin IM if the last dose was administered over 5 years ago for any wound requiring cleansing

Interventions

- *Acute care: Elevation, immobilization, infection protection, compression with active bleeding, protect from further injury*: Lacerations and punctures
  - Achieve hemostasis, cleanse, and suture when necessary using local anesthesia.
    - ○ *Indications for primary closure*: Eliminate dead space, support hemostasis, reduce scarring support wound healing
- High-risk wounds
  - Manage electrolytes, BG, nutrition, and hydration.
  - Maintain euglycemia to promote wound healing.
  - Examine wound edges and for the need for debridement.
  - Collaborate with wound management with hyperbaric therapy.
- Bites
  - Irrigate the wound bed, remove any debris, and apply topical antimicrobial and dressing.
  - Do not close puncture wounds or wounds to hand.
  - Follow local regulations on reporting animal bites.
  - *Spider bites*: Cool compresses to stop necrosis.
- Burns
  - Evaluate in 1 week for burn extension and infection and ensure the patient protects from UV exposure.
  - Use compression and splinting to prevent contractures.

Patient Education

- Explain to the patient to avoid OTC aspirin and NSAIDs that can interfere with wound healing.
- Discuss risk factor modification to improve wound healing and prevent infections.
- Instruct in wound care and dressing.
- Teach s/s of infection and adverse effects to report.

Patient Population Considerations

Women (conception/pregnancy/lactation)

- Refer women who are pregnant to an obstetrician for additional follow-up.

Geriatric

- Older adults are at the most significant risk for infection. Arrange frequent follow-up.

Pediatric

- Avoid high-pressure irrigation in infants and young children due to the fragility of skin structures.

Referring Patients

- Refer facial injuries to plastic surgery.
- Refer insect bite with urticaria to allergy.
- Refer chronic wounds to enterostomal therapy and surgery.
- Refer patients with vascular insufficiency to vascular surgery.
- Refer patients with chronic wound infection and osteomyelitis to infectious disease.

 POP QUIZ 13.4

A 19-year-old college student presents to the walk-in clinic with a thermal burn to his left forearm and hand after falling into a lit charcoal barbeque. He has a history of DM type 1 on insulin glargine and insulin apart. *Vital signs*: BP 152/86, HR 122, RR, 16, T, 97.1°F (36.2°C), pain 10/10. CBG 251.

While attempting to remove the T-shirt that was wrapped around the burn, the nurse practitioner notices the smell of lighter fluid and that there is tissue adhered to the material. The wound bed appears moist and bright red. What is the priority intervention?

RESOURCES

Aneja, S. (2019). *Medscape: Irritant contact dermatitis.* https://emedicine.medscape.com/article/1049353-overview

Banasikowska, A. (2020). *Medscape: Rosacea.* https://emedicine.medscape.com/article/1071429-overview

Barret, J. (2018). *Medscape: Human bites.* https://emedicine.medscape.com/article/218901-overview#a3

Barry, M. (2019). *Medscape: Scabies.* https://emedicine.medscape.com/article/1109204-overview

Basta, P., Bak, A., & Roszkowski, K. (2015). Cancer treatment in pregnant women. *Contemporary Oncology, 19*(5), 354. https://doi.org/10.5114/wo.2014.46236

Becevic, M. (2018). USPSTF: Skin cancer screening recommendations. *Missouri Medicine, 115*(6), 517.

Berenguer, A., Couto, A., Brites, V., & Fernandes, R. (2013). Anaphylaxis in pregnancy: A rare cause of neonatal mortality. *BMJ Case Reports, 2013,* bcr2012007055. https://doi.org/10.1136/bcr-2012-007055

Campbell, R. L., Li, J. T., Nicklas, R. A., & Sadosty, A. T. (2014). Emergency department diagnosis and treatment of anaphylaxis: A practice parameter. *Annals of Allergy, Asthma & Immunology, 113*(6), 599–608. https://doi.org/10.1016/j.anai.2014.10.007

Cash, J. C., & Glass, C. A. (Eds.). (2019). *Adult-gerontology practice guidelines.* Springer Publishing Company.

Centers for Disease Control and Prevention. (2018a). *Shingrix recommendations.* https://www.cdc.gov/vaccines/vpd/shingles/hcp/shingrix/recommendations.html#summary-recommendations

Centers for Disease Control and Prevention. (2018b). *Parasites treatment: Suggested general guidelines.* https://www.cdc.gov/parasites/scabies/treatment.html

Centers for Disease Control and Prevention. (2019). *Tickborne diseases in the United States.* https://www.cdc.gov/ticks/tickbornediseases/

Centers for Disease Control and Prevention. (2020a). *Candida auris: Information for laboratorians and health care professionals.* https://www.cdc.gov/fungal/candida-auris/health-professionals.html

Centers for Disease Control and Prevention. (2020b). *Fungal diseases: Tinea.* https://www.cdc.gov/fungal/diseases/ringworm/health-professionals.html

Codina Leik, M. T. (2018). *Family nurse practitioner certification: Intensive review.* Springer Publishing Company.

Daley, B. (2020). *Medscape: Wound care.* https://emedicine.medscape.com/article/194018-overview

Gawlik, K., Melnyk, B. M., & Teall, A. (2021). *Evidence-based physical examination.* Springer Publishing Company.

Habashy, J. (2019). *Medscape: Psoriasis.* https://emedicine.medscape.com/article/1943419-overview.

Hayward, K., Cline, A., Stephens, A., & Street, L. (2018). Management of herpes zoster (shingles) during pregnancy. *Journal of Obstetrics and Gynecology: The Journal of the Institute of Obstetrics and Gynaecology, 38*(7), 887–894. https://doi.org/10.1080/01443615.2018.1446419

Helm, T. (2019). *Medscape: Irritant contact dermatitis.* https://emedicine.medscape.com/article/1049216-overview

Herchline, T. (2019). *Medscape: Cellulitis.* https://emedicine.medscape.com/article/214222-overview

Janninger, C. (2020). *Medscape: Herpes zoster.* https://emedicine.medscape.com/article/1132465-overview/

Janvanoic, M. (2020). *Medscape: Hidradenatis suppurativa.* https://emedicine.medscape.com/article/1073117-overview

Kaul, S., Yadav, S., & Dogra, S. (2017). Treatment of dermatophytosis in elderly, children, and pregnant women. *Indian Dermatology Online Journal, 8*(5), 310–318. https://doi.org/10.4103/idoj.IDOJ_169_17

Kim, B. (2020). *Medscape: Acute dermatitis.* https://emedicine.medscape.com/article/1049085-guidelines

Laube, S., & Farrell, A. M. (2002). Bacterial skin infections in the elderly: Diagnosis and treatment. *Drugs & Aging, 19*(5), 331–342. https://doi.org/10.2165/00002512-200219050-00002

Layton, A. M. (2016). Top ten list of clinical pearls in the treatment of acne vulgaris. *Dermatologic Clinics, 34*(2), 147–157. https://doi.org/10.1016/j.det.2015.11.008

Lewis. L. (2019). *Medscape: Impetigo.* https://emedicine.medscape.com/article/965254-overview\

Lyons, F., & Ousley, L. (2015). *Dermatology for the advanced practice nurse.* Springer Publishing Company.

Mustafa, S. (2018). *Medscape: Anaphylaxis.* https://emedicine.medscape.com/article/135065-overview

National Eczema Society. (n.d.). *Allergy and eczema: Information for healthcare professionals.* https://eczema.org/information-and-advice/

National Institutes of Health. (2020). *DailyMed: Absorica LD.* https://emedicine.medscape.com/article/1069804-overview

Otani, M. (2017). Treatment of *Tinea pedis* in elderly patients using external preparations. *Medical Mycology Journal, 58*(2), J35–J41. https://doi.org/10.3314/mmj.17.003

Patel, V. M., Schwartz, R. A., & Lambert, W. C. (2017). Topical antiviral and antifungal medications in pregnancy: A review of safety profiles. *Journal of the European Academy of Dermatology and Venereology, 31*(9), 1440–1446. https://doi.org/10.1111/jdv.14297

Perkins, A. (2018). *Medscape: Animal bites in the emergency room.* https://emedicine.medscape.com/article/768875-overview#a5

Perng, P., Zampella, J. G., & Okoye, G. A. (2017). Management of hidradenitis suppurativa in pregnancy. *Journal of the American Academy of Dermatology, 76*(5), 979–989. https://doi.org/10.1016/j.jaad.2016.10.032

Rao, J. (2020). *Medscape: Acne vulgaris.* https://emedicine.medscape.com/article/1069804-overview

Richard, H. (2020). *Medscape: Cutaneous candidiasis.* https://emedicine.medscape.com/article/1090632-overview#a5

Sheridan, R. (2018). *Medscape: Initial evaluation and management of the burn patient.* https://emedicine.medscape.com/article/435402-overview#a1

Siegfried, E. (2017). *Dermatology advisor: Neonatal acne (acne – neonatal and infantile).* https://www.dermatologyadvisor.com/home/decision-support-in-medicine/dermatology/neonatal-acne-acne-neonatal-and-infantile/

Silverberg, N. (2019). *Medscape: Pediatric contact dermatitis.* https://emedicine.medscape.com/article/911711-overview#:~:text=Allergic%20contact%20dermatitis%20may%20affect%20as%20many%20as,rates%20of%20allergic%20contact%20dermatitis%20on%20the%20face

Sorenson, M., Quinn, L., & Klein, D. (2019). *Pathophysiology: Concepts of human disease* (1st ed.). Pearson Education.

Spencer, J. (2020). *Medscape: Actinic keratosis.* https://emedicine.medscape.com/article/1099775-overview#:~:text=Actinic%20keratosis%20%28AK%29%20is%20a%20UV%20light%E2%80%93induced%20lesion,with%20malignant%20potential%20to%20arise%20on%20the%20skin

Temple, S. (2018). *Medscape: Tickborne diseases.* https://emedicine.medscape.com/article/786652-overview

Uray, I. P., Dmitrovsky, E., & Brown, P. H. (2016). Retinoids and rexinoids in cancer prevention: From laboratory to clinic. *Seminars in Oncology, 43*(1), 49–64. https://doi.org/10.1053/j.seminoncol.2015.09.002

U.S. Department of Health and Human Services: Radiation Emergency Medical Management. (2021). *Burn triage and treatment of thermal injuries in a radiation emergency.* https://www.remm.nlm.gov/burns.htm

Weinmann, S., Naleway, A. L., Koppolu, P., Baxter, R., Belongia, E. A., Hambidge, S. J., Irving, S. A., Jackson, M. L., Klein, N. P., Lewin, B., Liles, E., Marin, M., Smith, N., Weintraub, E., & Chun, C. (2019). Incidence of herpes zoster among children: 2003–2014. *Pediatrics, 144*(1), e20182917. https://doi.org/10.1542/peds.2018-2917

14

PSYCHIATRIC CONDITIONS

ABUSE

Overview

- Abuse is physical, sexual, emotional, financial maltreatment, or neglect that can affect an individual during their life span.
- Abusers can be intimate partners (IPV), caregivers at home or in other care settings, or supervisors/peers in the community, school, or workplace.
- The abuser exhibits aggression to exert power and control. Isolation, neglect, intimidation, threats, and leveraging relationships with others against the abuse are common features.
- NPs are mandatory reporters for child abuse under CAPTA according to individual state guidance.

Etiology

- *Internal factors*: Family history, age, female gender, physical dependency, personal history of substance use disorder, dementia, impaired communication, prior abuse, or adverse childhood experiences; low level of education, or socioeconomic status
- *External factors*: Presence of a firearm, or abuser history of substance use disorder, psychopathology, or sociopathy
- *Adverse events*: Unemployment/underemployment, financial stress, pregnancy, violence, or partnering with or entrusted to an abuser who experienced abuse as a child or has aggressive traits or risk factors for committing violence or maltreatment of others

COMPLICATIONS

Acute: Injury (intentional or nonintentional emotional or physical trauma and homicide), suicidality, forced displacement

Secondary Injury: Anxiety, depression, grief, system-induced retraumatization

Chronic: Anxiety, depression, PTSD, stress-induced exacerbation of medical disease/disorder

CLINICAL PEARL

Targeted Prevention/Screening
- Screen using a valid screening tool to improve the likelihood of detecting abuse according to age, relationships, and circumstances.
- Conduct screening in private setting, face to face, using direct questioning supported by use of an instrument to assist detection.
- Perform screening on initial presentation and ongoing at repeated intervals to increase the likelihood of detection.

Signs and Symptoms

- *Physical*: Injury that is not consistent with the history provided, multiple injuries at various stages of healing, injuries consistent with assault
- *Sexual*: Oral injury, labial/vaginal/anal trauma, pressure injury on bony prominences, presence of an STI; evidence of physical assault may or may not be present
- *Emotional*: Anxiety, depression symptoms, impaired concentration; separation anxiety or school refusal in a child; delay in seeking treatment for an injury; signs of withdrawal or agitation
- *Neglect*: Failure to thrive, poor hygiene, pest infestation, untreated or fictitious medical conditions, subtherapeutic or toxic medication levels

Differential Diagnosis

- *ENDO*: Hypercortisolism, hyperparathyroidism, thyroid disease
- *GI*: Cirrhosis
- *HEM/ONC*: Bone marrow failure, coagulopathy, immunodeficiency, hemophilia, pathological fracture of metastasis, thrombocytopenia
- *INT*: Capillary hemangiomas, congenital dermal melanocytosis, epidermolysis bullosa, phytophotodermatitis, senile purpura, steroid purpura, SJS, urticaria pigmentosa
- *MSK*: Osteogenesis imperfecta, primary or secondary osteoporosis
- *NEURO*: Eating disorder, cerebral thrombosis, failure to thrive, advanced dementia, Bloch–Sulzberger syndrome, depression, subdural hematoma, suicide
- *REPRO*: Lichen sclerosis
- *Other*: Cupping to neck and back, substance use disorder, drug eruption, falls, injury of alternative etiology

Diagnosis

Labs

- U/A, HCG
- Forensic testing according to the type of abuse
- Baseline CMP, CBC, LFTs, amylase, lipase, HIV screen, RPR, hepatitis profile as a baseline in the presence of sexual assault
- *Serology to rule out the alternative cause*: Serum Ca, phos, toxicology screen, alcohol level, serum drug levels as indicated

Additional Diagnostic Testing

- Imaging studies according to injury type

Treatment and Management

Treatment Goals

- Establish a therapeutic alliance to achieve safety, provide trauma-informed care, and report abuse according to standards of practice.

CLINICAL PEARL

- Hospitalization is considered for patients who are extremely ill, who are experiencing complications, or who require refeeding. Otherwise, treatment is outpatient.

Drug Treatment

- Prescribe tetanus toxoid if the last vaccination was >5 years earlier.
- Prevention of pregnancy, STI, and blood-borne disease is important in cases of sexual assault.
  - Prescribe HIV prophylaxis.
  - Prescribe metronidazole immediate release PO 2 g, and hepatitis B vaccination, if the hepatitis vaccine is naïve.
  - Prescribe ceftriaxone IM for exposure to gonorrhea.
  - Prescribe azithromycin PO for exposure to chlamydia.
  - Prescribe levonorgestrel as pregnancy prophylaxis.
  - Prescribe analgesics according to the pain scale if the trauma is present.

Interventions

- Gain trust with the patient to reduce feelings of shame and stigma and encourage the patient to verbalize as needed.
- Screen the patient for suicidal ideation and prepare for admission if present.

ALERT

Abuse Protocol for Emergencies

- Ensure that forensic examination is completed by credentialed HCP and preserve forensic evidence.
- Collaborate with patient advocate, social worker, and appropriate community advocacy agency according to policy to ensure a safe plan for discharge and follow-up.

- Provide a safe environment, separate the patient from the abuser, and initiate the reporting process and notification of authorities according to agency policy.
- Evaluate the emotional status of the patient and discuss follow-up for definitive treatment with psychotherapy.
- Treat injuries according to protocol.

Patient Education
- Explain that any type of abuse could trigger the development of PTSD, negative feelings, anxiety, and depression that could increase the need to self-medicate.
- Discuss s/s to report and the importance of follow-up.
- Review the safety plan and emergency contacts and identify a code to use with supportive friends or family to help them get out of a difficult situation.
- Instruct in medication therapy and s/s to report.

Patient Population Considerations

Women (conception/pregnancy/lactation)
- The CPG from the ENA recommend the HITS, WAST, PVS, and AAS, as tools that can be used in clinical settings.

Geriatric
- According to NCEA, the NP must defer to a competent patient to determine their care. The NP cannot report elder abuse on behalf of a competent adult who wishes to decline services from APS.

Pediatric
- Employ a screening tool such as PedHITSS or CTSPC to detect abuse. Suspect abuse if there is a decline in developmental function or a failure to thrive.

Referring Patients

- Social services, CPS, APS according to state guidance
- Victim advocacy groups
- Psychotherapy consult
- Psychiatry consult

ALCOHOL USE DISORDER

Overview

- Alcohol use disorder is a substance abuse disorder involving a psychological and physiologic dependence on alcohol that can be mild, moderate, or severe.
- Alcohol stimulates opiates, GABA, glutamate, serotonin, and dopamine. Excessive sedation from ingestion can result in acute alcohol intoxication that places the patient at risk for harm and trauma.
- With long-term use, the CNS experiences excitability. Abrupt withdrawal of alcohol which can lead to delirium tremens, which can be fatal.
- Long-term use leads to the development of multisystem disease and increased mortality.

 COMPLICATIONS

Acute: Alcohol intoxication with coma, DTs, hepatic encephalopathy, stroke, trauma from falls, violence and car crashes, suicide

Chronic: Alcoholism, Wernicke–Korsakoff syndrome, cardiomyopathy, hepatitis, cirrhosis, GI bleeding, PUD, pancreatitis, chronic disability, cancers (esophagus, liver, breast, head, and neck), vitamin deficiency (A, C, B_1, B_3, B_6, B_9, B_{12}), disability

Etiology

- *Internal factors*: Genetics, personal history of untreated anxiety, depression, schizophrenia, bipolar disorder
- *External factors*: Familial influences, social influences
- *Adverse events*: Emotional or physical trauma, lack of social support

Signs and Symptoms

- *Acute intoxication*: Slurred speech, blackouts, inappropriate behavior, impaired judgment, poor coordination
- *Alcohol withdrawal*: Diaphoresis, tremor, restlessness, HA, agitation, anxiety, fever, seizures following alcohol withdrawal
- *Chronic alcoholism*: Asterixis, confusion, ophthalmoplegia, hepatosplenomegaly, s/s of chronic complications

Differential Diagnosis

- *ENDO*: Adrenal insufficiency, delirium, hypoglycemia, hyperglycemia, parathyroid disorders, SIADH
- *GI*: Nonalcoholic liver disease
- *HEM*: Paraneoplastic syndrome of cancer
- *NEURO*: ALS, dementia, GBS, MS, normal pressure hydrocephalus, Parkinson's disease, stroke, tumor, or mass
- *Other*: Substance use disorder, toxins, poisoning, opportunistic infection, sepsis

 CLINICAL PEARL

Assess for comorbid conditions associated with alcohol use disorder
- Anxiety disorder
- Bipolar disorder
- Depression
- Panic disorder
- PTSD
- Insomnia

Diagnosis

Labs
- U/A and toxicology screen
- Blood alcohol level >300 mg/dL in acute intoxication
- *Presence of alcohol biomarkers*: EtG, Peth, CDT, LFTs, MCV
- CMP, CBC, LFTs, amylase, lipase to evaluate for the presence of complications and assess baseline renal and hepatic function

Additional Diagnostic Testing
- Pulse oximetry

Treatment and Management

Treatment Goals
- *Rehabilitation*: Establish therapeutic alliance to achieve safety, reduce cravings for alcohol, and support the patient in achieving sobriety and minimize acute/chronic complications.

 ALERT

Refer acute alcohol withdrawal to the ED immediately.
- Withdrawal onset is 6 to 36 hr after last drink.
- Seizures can occur between 6 and 48 hr.
- Hallucinations begin 12 to 48 hr.

CIWA protocol will be initiated to prevent DTs.

Drug Treatment
- Prescribe naltrexone to decrease cravings and relapses.
- Prescribe acamprosate to maintain alcohol abstinence.
- Consider topiramate or gabapentin if the patient does not respond to naltrexone or acamprosate.
- Consider disulfiram (aldehyde dehydrogenase inhibitor) to decrease the number of drinking days.
- Consider antidepressant medications for comorbid anxiety and or depression.
- Consider beta blockers, clonidine, or phenothiazines as an alternative to support sobriety.

Interventions

- Assess for substance use disorder, tobacco use, and comorbid mental health disorders.
- Monitor hepatorenal function when initiating and monitoring response to pharmacologic agents.
- Hospitalize patients with a history of DTs or significant comorbidity.
- Refer to Alcoholics Anonymous and encourage participants to achieve long-term sobriety.
- Consult social services for community resources.

Patient Education

- Discuss the diagnosis of alcohol use disorder, its management, and complications.
- Review psychological and behavioral therapy to assist in alcohol abstinence.
- Encourage participation in AA and refer family members to Al-Anon.
- Teach patient s/s of adverse medication effects to report.

Patient Population Considerations

Women (conception/pregnancy/lactation)

- Instruct women of childbearing age of the risks associated with exposing the fetus to alcohol and its effect on CNS development. Do not use pharmacologic treatments in pregnant or breastfeeding women with alcohol use disorder. Treat acute alcohol withdrawal with benzodiazepines.

Geriatric

- Perform medication reconciliation with geriatric patients diagnosed with alcohol use disorder. Polypharmacology increases their risk for injury and alerts the HCP to refer to community resources for intervention.

Pediatric

- Use the CRAFFT screening tool to identify at-risk behaviors with alcohol use disorder in adolescence.

Referring Patients

- Psychotherapy consult
- Social services
- Psychiatry consult

ANXIETY

Overview

- Anxiety is a disorder characterized by excessive worry and apprehension in response to a real or perceived threat as a result of fear conditioning.
- Conditioned stimuli trigger the locus coeruleus to release NE stimulating the hippocampus–amygdala complex to activate the HPA axis which releases cortisol and catecholamines. The exposure creates stored memories in the complex that are responsible for stronger, automatic response in future exposures. The conditioned responses bypass the prefrontal cortex and conscious thought, which can mediate the response. Additional neurotransmitters (5-HT, GABA, glutamate, DA) are involved in neural firing and extinction.
- Anxiety may lead to GAD or specific anxiety disorders named by their triggers or response, such as separation anxiety, social anxiety, panic disorder, and agoraphobia. *Note:* OCD and PTSD are not anxiety disorders.

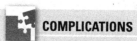 **COMPLICATIONS**

Acute: Suicidality, substance use disorder, MDD

Chronic: PDD, disability

Etiology

- *Internal factors*: Genetics, personal history
- *External factors*: Family, stimulant-abuse, prescribed sympathomimetics
- *Adverse events*: Medical conditions, negative or stressful life events, lack of social support, low socioeconomic status

Signs and Symptoms

- Hyperventilation, palpitations, diaphoresis, crying, chest pain, dizziness, dissociation, depersonalization, verbalizations of fear
- Hypertension, tachypnea, tachycardia, paresthesia
- Specific triggers may or may not be present.

Differential Diagnosis

- *CV*: Paroxysmal atrial fibrillation, SVT, MI, HF, MVP, cardiogenic shock
- *ENDO*: Hypoglycemia, hyperthyroidism, hypercortisolism, pituitary disorders
- *HEM*: Anemia and folate deficiency, vitamins B_{12} or D deficiency, IDA
- *NEURO*: Encephalopathy, conversion reaction, delirium tremens, dementia, essential tremor
- *PULM*: Exacerbation of asthma or COPD, allergy
- *Other*: Toxins, stimulants

Diagnosis

Labs:
- U/A and toxicology screen
- CMP, LFTs to rule out hepatorenal and metabolic/endocrine cause
- CBC to rule out infection
- TSH to rule out thyroid and additional testing based on PE

Additional Diagnostic Testing
To rule out medical causes:
- 12-lead EKG, cardiac profile, and chest x-ray with chest pain
- Pulse oximetry and peak flow with dyspnea

Treatment and Management

Treatment Goals
- Establish a therapeutic alliance to achieve safety and reduce the severity of distress to a mutually agreed-upon goal for quality of life.

Drug Treatment
- *Initial treatment for adults*:
  - Prescribe SSRI or SNR in adults. Titrate every 7 to 14 days.
  - Consider second-generation TCA, SNRI, NDRI as an alternative.
  - Consider clonazepam or buspirone as second-line therapy.
- *Initial treatment for adolescents (following titration)*:
  - Augment therapy with an additional antidepressant medication.

ALERT

Agents That Can Induce Anxiety

Cocaine, alcohol, cannabis, caffeine, amphetamines, hallucinogens, sympathomimetics, anesthesia, analgesics, levothyroxine, insulin, antihistamines, antiparkinsonians, antipsychotics, anticholinergics, corticosteroids

CLINICAL PEARL

Anxiety is a manifestation of many medical disorders. Exclude disorders based on comprehensive examination before attributing a diagnosis to a symptom.

ALERT

Screen for Comorbid Depression

Screening for adults: Use PHQ-2 or PHQ-9 screening instrument (or other).

Screening for <18 years: No recommended tool. Consider Beck Depression inventory or PHQ-2 or PHQ-9.

Interventions

- Employ CAMS care therapy approach in patients with comorbid depression.
- Provide information for suicide prevention hotline with 24-hr access.
- Offer CBT as a first-line intervention with medication to adults.
  - If ineffective, consider ACT and mindfulness as second-line therapy.
- Encourage regular physical exercise or yoga as an adjunct to medication and therapy.
- For treatment resistance or suicidality, consult with the psychiatrist.
  - Admit patients to an inpatient facility if they are a danger to themselves or others, refractory anxiety is severe, or the patient cannot care for themselves.
  - Offer cranial electrotherapy stimulation for treatment-resistant anxiety to complement medication and therapy.
  - Offer transcranial magnetic stimulation to patients with comorbid OCD.

Patient Education

- Instruct the patient to contact the suicide prevention hotline with suicidal ideation, if indicated.
- Discuss the diagnosis of anxiety and its management and complications.
- Explain that CBT cognitive restructuring and exposure therapy is the preferred method to interrupt fear-producing thoughts.
- Encourage a Mediterranean diet to support brain health and stabilize neurotransmitters.
- Teach the patient not to stop medications abruptly to avoid antidepressant discontinuation syndrome.

Patient Population Considerations

Women (conception/pregnancy/lactation)

- Discuss with women of childbearing age the potential effects of intrauterine exposure to high dose SSRIs. Explain that it may contribute to SGA <3 percentile, prematurity, and suboptimal breastfeeding.

Geriatric

- Consider prescribing paroxetine, escitalopram, or sertraline for anxiety in older adults. Use caution in prescribing benzodiazepines with SSRI and SNRI due to increased risk of falls.

Pediatric

- Offer CBT to children and adolescents. Consider computer-based CBT or evidence-based programs such as "coping cat."

Referring Patients

- Psychotherapy
- Psychiatry consult for treatment-resistant anxiety

DEPRESSION

Overview

- Depression is a mood disorder characterized by sadness, apathy, and anhedonia.
- It can lead to PDD and MDD which increase the risk of suicidality.
- Availability and regulation of neurotransmitters (CNS 5-HT, NE, DA, BDNF, and glutamine) contributes to the development of depression. Structural and functional abnormalities in the brain can contribute to depression.

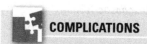

COMPLICATIONS

Acute: Suicidality, psychotic depression

Chronic: Persistent depressive disorder, disability

Etiology

- *Internal factors*: Genetics, personal history, anxiety disorder
- *External factors*: Substance abuse, prescribed medications
- *Adverse events*: Medical conditions, recent loss, negative life events, lack of social support

Signs and Symptoms

- Apathy, anhedonia, low mood (irritability in children), and hopelessness that persists over days
- Insomnia, hypersomnia, fatigue, impaired concentration
- Appetite or weight change (failure to thrive in children)
- Psychomotor retardation
- Recurrent thoughts of suicide
- Decreased interest in activities and decline in school performance in children and adolescence
- Somatic complaints

CLINICAL PEARL

Cultural Competence
The presentation of depression may be different in individuals based on their culture.

Differential Diagnosis

- *CV*: CHF, MI
- *ENDO*: Adrenal, thyroid disease, parathyroid disease, DM, electrolyte disturbance
- *GI*: Cirrhosis, inflammatory bowel disease
- *HEM*: Anemia and folate deficiency, vitamins B_{12} or D *deficiencies*, IDA
- *NEURO*: Bipolar disorder, schizophrenia, stroke, dementia, TBI, neurodegenerative diseases, mass lesions, epilepsy, encephalitis, T cell lymphoma, AIDS-related dementia
- *PULM*: COPD
- *Other*: Chronic autoimmune disorders, grieving, medication-induced depression, substance abuse

ALERT

Medications That Can Induce Depression
Beta blockers, immune-modulating, antiparkinson agents, anticonvulsants, antipsychotics, sedatives, isotretinoin

Polypharmacology in the geriatric population should be reviewed carefully.

Diagnosis

Labs:

- Clean catch U/A and toxicology screen
- CMP, LFTs to rule out hepatorenal and metabolic/endocrine cause
- CBC, folate, vitamin B_{12}, vitamin D, and ferritin to rule out anemia, infection, and nutritional deficiency
- TSH to rule out thyroid cause and additional thyroid function testing based on physical exam
- RPR, HIV

Additional Diagnostic Testing

- CT, MRI of the brain to rule out organic causes

ALERT

USPSTF Screening Recommendations
Screening for adults: Use PHQ-2 or PHQ-9 screening instrument (or other).

Screening for <18 years: **No recommended tool.** Consider Beck Depression inventory or PHQ-2 or PHQ-9.

Treatment and Management

Treatment Goals

- Establish a therapeutic alliance to achieve safety; determine the therapeutic setting, milieu, and mutually agreed-upon goals for quality of life; prevent relapse and ensure treatment adherence.

ALERT

Serotonin syndrome: Excess serotonin caused by overuse or interaction of serotonergic drugs that can trigger life-threatening event if left untreated

- Early signs are myoclonus, tremor, akathisia, AMS, fever, and tachycardia progressing to rigidity and seizures.
- Discontinue all SSRI, SNRI, TCAs, MAOI, NDRI) and administer dantrolene or benzodiazepine.
- Admit to hospital for observation.

Drug Treatment
- Initial treatment
  - *Adults*: Prescribe antidepressants in addition to psychotherapy with initial treatment: SSRI, SNRI, mirtazapine (TeCA), or bupropion (NDRI). Titrate every 7 to 14 days to achieve a therapeutic effect.
    - ○ Treat mild tremors associated with SSRI or SNRI with a beta blocker.
    - ○ Consider St. John's Wort as monotherapy as an alternative if the patient prefers.
  - *Geriatric*: Prescribe paroxetine, escitalopram, or sertraline.
    - ○ Consider second-generation TCA, SNRI, NDRI as an alternative. If currently taking MAOI, wait 14 days before starting the new medication.
  - *Adolescents*: Prescribe fluoxetine as the first-line SSRI.
    - ○ Do not use clomipramine, imipramine, mirtazapine, paroxetine, or venlafaxine.
- *If the patient does not meet the outcomes following titration*:
  - Augment medication with an additional antidepressant medication from an alternative class.

ALERT

Adverse Medication Effects

There is an increased risk of suicidality with SSRI medications in patients younger than age 24 years.

Interventions

SUICIDE SCREENING
- Suicide screening should be performed at each visit in all settings using a validated tool.
- *The ASQ Tool is a scripted four-question suicide risk screening tool asking*:
  1. In the past few weeks, have you wished you were dead?
  2. In the past few weeks, have you felt that you or your family would be better off if you were dead?
  3. Have you had thoughts about killing yourself?
  4. Have you ever tried to kill yourself?
  - If the answer to any of the questions in the ASQ Tool is no, the screening is complete.
  - If the answer is yes to any question, or the patient does not respond, then the patient is asked: *Are you having thoughts of killing yourself now?*
    - ○ If the patients answer yes, or the patient does not respond, the patient is placed on one-to-one observation and requires a full safety and mental health evaluation. If the patient answers no, safety evaluation is performed in conjunction with a full mental health evaluation. All patients receive resources for a suicide hotline.
- Employ CAMS care therapy approach in patients with suicidal risk to reduce suicidal ideation.
- Provide contact information for suicide prevention hotline available 24 hr per day.

OTHER INTERVENTIONS
- Encourage regular physical exercise or yoga as monotherapy or as an adjunct to medication.
- Offer bright light therapy for patients with seasonal affective disorder.
- Consider acupuncture as an adjunct to behavioral therapy and or medication.
- For treatment resistance or suicidality, consult with a psychiatrist.
  - Admit patients to an inpatient facility if they are a danger to themselves or others, depression is severe, or the patient cannot care for themselves.
  - Offer esketamine nasal spray in consultation with psychiatry in a clinical setting for patients experiencing suicidal ideation or treatment-resistant depression in adults.
  - Offer TMS with or without ketamine for treatment-resistant depression after the failure of one class of medications.
  - Offer ECT to patients who do not respond to drug therapy, are psychotic, or are suicidal.
  - Consider VNS for adult patients who have failed to respond to at least four adequate medication and/or ECT.

Patient Education
- Provide contact information for the suicide prevention hotline if suicidal thoughts occur.
- Refer to counseling for CBT.
- Discuss the diagnosis of depression and its management and complications.
- Reinforce the importance of exercise and exposure to sunlight.
- Encourage a Mediterranean diet to support brain health and stabilize neurotransmitters.
- Teach the patient not to stop medications abruptly to avoid antidepressant discontinuation syndrome.

Patient Population Considerations

Women (conception/pregnancy/lactation)
- American Academy of Pediatrics and the American College of Obstetricians and Gynecologists recommend screening all postpartum women for depression.

Geriatric
- Offer group-CBT, ITP, reminiscence therapy to geriatric patients with or without SSRI, SNRI, or NDRI (consider falls risk when prescribing agents).
- Consider problem-solving therapy in the geriatric patient with impaired cognition.

Pediatric
- Offer CBT to children and CBT, ITP-A in adolescence.
- Consider offering fluoxetine to adolescents with depression as initial therapy in combination with counseling.

Referring Patients
- CBT therapy consult
- Psychiatry consult

POP QUIZ 14.1

A 19-year-old female presents to the primary care provider's office with complaints of apathy, fatigue, anhedonia, and suicidal thoughts. She reports a 10-lb unintentional weight loss since starting back at college 6 weeks ago and difficulty concentrating. What is the most likely diagnosis?

EATING DISORDERS

Overview

- Anorexia, bulimia nervosa, and binge eating disorder are characterized by distorted body image and the following:
  - *Anorexia:* Restriction of nutritional intake to a level below the body's energy requirements due to fear of weight gain
  - *Bulimia nervosa:* Repeated binge eating episodes and purging (exercise, vomiting, laxatives) that occur one or more times a week for at least 3 months
  - *Binge eating disorder:* Recurrent episodes of binge eating without purging
  - *Anorexia binge–purge subtype:* Restricted intake with BP
- Comorbid anxiety, depression, insomnia has been observed.

COMPLICATIONS

Acute: Hypoglycemia, arrhythmia, MI, AKI, refeeding syndrome, protein calorie malnutrition, pathologic fractures, encephalopathy, suicide

Chronic: Starvation, impaired cognition, hypothyroidism, HF, pancytopenia, osteoporosis, renal colic, amenorrhea, infertility, miscarriage

Etiology

- *Internal factors*: Genetics, female gender, early feeding difficulties, personal history of untreated anxiety/depression; impulsivity in BED or BN
- *External factors*: Familial and peer remarks, social stigma, cultural expectations
- *Adverse events*: Stressful events, emotional, sexual, or physical trauma

Signs and Symptoms

- Low BMI
- Orthostatic hypotension, dysrhythmia, murmur, s/s of HF, edema, acrocyanosis
- Difficulty concentrating, HA, irritability, dizziness, social withdrawal, obsessiveness
- Amenorrhea, hair loss, dry skin, parotid enlargement, Russell's sign
- Pharyngeal irritation, dental caries, GI bleeding, constipation

CLINICAL PEARL

Targeted Prevention/Screening
- Use of social learning theory, group CBT, media literacy, and cognitive dissonance with groups of adolescents and young women, like "The Body Project."
- Addresses cultural influences on body image from media to identify strategies to challenge the pressures.

Individual screening with online NEDA tool

www.nationaleatingdisorders.org/screening-tool

Differential Diagnosis

- *ENDO*: Panhypopituitarism, hyperthyroidism, osteoporosis, SLE, malignancy
- *GI*: Gastric outlet obstruction, DM, achalasia, celiac sprue, irritable bowel syndrome, IBS
- *PSYCH*: Body dysmorphic disorder, avoidant restrictive food intake disorder, OCD, anxiety/depression, substance abuse

Diagnosis

Labs

- Scale weight and calculate BMI (BMI <16 is severe, <15 extreme)
- CMP (alkalosis with vomiting and acidosis with laxative abuse, decreased, K^+, Mg, Ca, Na, Phos), azotemia with dehydration
- Serial cardiac enzymes with chest pain
- CBC for pancytopenia
- ESR to eliminate immune-mediated disorders
- Vitamins D and B_{12}, iron, folate (decreased in nutritional anemia)
- Serum albumin and protein, cholesterol (elevated in starvation)
- TSH
- FOBT for patients with bulimia
- U/A, toxicology screen, HCG

Additional Diagnostic Testing

- Eating disorder screening tool
- Pulse oximetry and vital signs (monitor for HR <40, SBP <90 mmHg)
- Chest x-ray to rule out pneumomediastinum from excessive vomiting
- 12-lead EKG with chest pain; assess for the presence of bradycardia, ST-T wave changes due to ischemia or potassium disturbance, and prolonged QT interval
- Echocardiogram to evaluate valves and ejection fraction.

ALERT

Acute arrhythmia, MI, HF, bleeding, AKI may occur with eating disorders.

Refer patient with acute respiratory, cardiac, or gastrointestinal bleeding, or starvation to ED immediately.

Treatment and Management

Treatment Goals
- *Outpatient*: Establish therapeutic alliance to achieve safety, restore a healthy eating pattern, and obtain scale weight in gown weekly (1–2 lb per week).
- Minimize acute/chronic complications.

Drug Treatment
- Prescribe vitamin D3 with or without calcium to correct deficiencies.
- Prescribed folic acid, vitamin B_{12}, and iron replacement with vitamin C if anemia is present.
- Consider SSRI, fluoxetine, for bulimia, or olanzapine for anorexia.
- Consider lisdexamfetamine or acamprosate for binge eating without purging.
- Consider melatonin replacement for nighttime binge eating.

Interventions
- Gain trust with the patient to reduce feelings of shame and stigma.
- Discuss eating disorders and refer for psychological therapy.
- Family-based treatment is strongly recommended in anorexia and bulimia.
- CBT or DBT is preferred in binge eating disorder.
- CBT and CRT are helpful for use in anorexia while IPT therapy can be useful in bulimia and binge eating.
- Collaborate with nutrition consult for refeeding strategy (1,000–1,900 cal/d) and monitor electrolytes at days 3 and 6, then weekly thereafter, and for the development of edema and HF.

CLINICAL PEARL

Hospitalization is considered for extremely ill patient with complications or when refeeding is required. Otherwise, treatment is outpatient.

Patient Education
- Discuss eating disorders, their pathophysiology, and their complications. Refer to the NEDA website (www.nationaleatingdisorders.org) for information and tools. Provide parents or caregivers with the NEDA toolkit and evaluate their understanding.
- Teach patients about medication adverse effects to report.
- Incorporate support system into a relapse prevention plan and reinforce a sense of hope for the future.

Patient Population Considerations

Women (conception/pregnancy/lactation)
- Patients with a personal history of eating disorders have increased risk for complications of SGA, hydration, cardiac arrhythmias, gestational diabetes. Encourage patients of childbearing age to discuss family planning with their gynecologist and consult a nutritionist. Participation in individual therapy and a support group may be helpful.

Geriatric
- Eating disorders can arise in older adults especially if there is a personal history of an untreated eating disorder and new stressors such as an empty nest, death of a spouse or child, or disability.

Pediatric
- Include parents in history taking and examine feeding difficulties that may be present. In school-age children, monitor for SBP <80, orthostatic hypotension, body fat <10%, or intractable vomiting.

Referring Patients

- Nutrition consult
- Psychotherapy consult
- Dental consult for patients who purge
- Psychiatry consult

POP QUIZ 14.2

A 26-your-old female presents to the primary care office complaining of palpitations. Her scale weight indicates that she lost 40 lb. since her last visit a year ago, placing her BMI at 14. What testing should be ordered for this patient?

INSOMNIA

Overview

- Insomnia is a sleep disorder of impaired sleep initiation, maintenance, or consolidation of light, deep, or REM sleep. It can be acute or chronic and affects the quality and quantity of sleep. Insomnia can cause daytime somnolence; fatigue can contribute to developing new health considerations (anxiety, depression) or worsen existing health conditions.
- Cortisol, estrogen, melatonin, GABA, and progesterone play a role in insomnia.

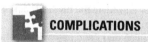

COMPLICATIONS

Acute: Daytime somnolence, learning problems, injury, anxiety, depression

Chronic: Obesity, substance use disorder

Etiology

- *Internal factors:* Genetic predisposition, advancing age, BPH, chronic pain disorders, female gender, hormonal changes HF, CKD, COPD, asthma, neurological disorders, anxiety/depression, PTSD, SUD, AUD, schizophrenia, bipolar disorder
- *External factors:* Stimulants, tobacco, alcohol, benzodiazepines, exercise before sleep, noise, warm temperatures, sunlight inadequate sleep hygiene
- *Adverse events:* Daytime stress, grieving, and loss

Signs and Symptoms

- Reports of difficulty getting to sleep, staying asleep, or is not rested when waking.
- Associated with anergia, daytime fatigue, difficulty concentrating, irritability, and reduced work performance.
- Compressive symptoms associated with reports of snoring, large neck size, mass, or goiter; enlarged tonsils, tongue, or low-lying palate.

Differential Diagnosis

- *ENDO:* Panhypopituitarism, hyperthyroidism, hypothyroidism, hypercortisolism
- *HEENT:* Obstructive sleep apnea
- *NEURO:* Restless leg syndrome, sleep apnea, anxiety, depression, periodic leg movement disorder, circadian rhythm disorder, fatal familial insomnia
- *Other:* Medication-induced insomnia

Diagnosis

Labs

- Diagnosed by clinical examination
- TSH to rule out thyroid dysfunction
- PRNP gene testing, if indicated, to rule out fatal familial insomnia

Additional Diagnostic Testing

- Pulse oximetry
- Sleep diary for 2 weeks
- Actigraphy with polysomnography

Treatment and Management

Treatment Goals

- Promote sleep hygiene, improve sleep quality, and reduce daytime impairment.

CLINICAL PEARL

Sleep Hygiene
- Avoid exercise, tobacco, stimulants, and eating before bedtime.
- Do not watch television in bed or take daytime naps.
- Reduce blue light, bright light, and noise.
- Go to bed at the same time every day. Leave the bed if you do not fall asleep within 20 min.
- Practice relaxation and mediation.
- Use sleep agonist, melatonin, for short intervals.

Drug Treatment

- Prescribe melatonin 0.5 to 5 mg at bedtime titrating for effect during course of CBT.
  - Do not exceed 12 mg. Long-term use is not well understood.

Interventions

- Manage or eliminate the medical cause for insomnia.
- Evaluate sleep diary and tailor behavioral plan to the individual.
- *Employ CBT to treat insomnia*: Cognitive therapy, relaxation therapy, stimulus control therapy, and sleep restriction therapy.

Patient Education

- Review strategies for sleep hygiene.
- Teach the patient about the adverse effects of melatonin to report.

Patient Population Considerations

Women (conception/pregnancy/lactation)

- Insomnia increases in the third trimester, aggravated by physical symptoms of leg cramps, GERD, and nocturia. Since there is an increased risk of comorbid depression, conduct a depression screen with reports of insomnia.

Geriatric

- Avoid prescription and OTC sleep aids in older adults that could impair mobility and increase the risk of falls.

Pediatric

- Pediatric insomnia is defined as sleep onset delay of more than 30 min, sleep less than 8 hr that occurs on three or more nights per week, and occur throughout infancy and childhood. It is more common in children with autism spectrum disorders, Down syndrome, restless leg syndrome, and epilepsy. Obstructive etiology should be explored as an alternative diagnosis.

Referring Patients

- Nutrition consult
- Psychotherapy consult
- Psychiatry consult

SMOKING CESSATION

Overview

Nicotine in tobacco causes a powerful addiction to nicotine that leads to nicotine use disorder and is the second leading cause of death worldwide. Smoking cessation is a therapeutic intervention to aid nicotine withdrawal and should be integrated into the plan at every clinical encounter when indicated. It integrates counseling, nicotine replacement therapy, non-nicotine pharmacology, or a combination of both. Tobacco and nicotine dependence frequently require repeated treatments.

Indications

- Nicotine dependence, although counseling should be provided to anyone who tries nicotine products

Treatment and Management

Treatment Goals
- Provide smoking cessation education, assist in developing an individualized quit plan, and provide resources for support.

Drug Treatment
- Prescribe nicotine replacement to reduce cravings and withdrawal symptoms.
  - Transdermal patch, spray, gum, lozenge, tablet, or inhaler titrated for daily nicotine use.
  - ACS recommends that e-cigarettes be avoided.
  - A long-acting nicotine patch can by combine with short-acting bolus (gum, inhaler, lozenge) is more effective than either alone.
- Consider adding second-line therapy to reduce cravings for nicotine.
  - Use bupropion or varenicline if creatinine clearance >30 mL/min
  - Consider nortriptyline up to 75 mg daily.
  - Consider clonidine if nicotine and antidepressants fail.

Interventions
- Refer the patient to a comprehensive smoking cessation program or application for support.
- Evaluate for cardiovascular side effects with nicotine replacement.
- Monitor therapeutic levels of nortriptyline (50–100 ng/mL), if in use.

Patient Education
- Discuss the adverse effects of nicotine on body systems.
- Reassure patients that nicotine dependence frequently requires repeated treatments and that every day of non-smoking improves their health and wellness.
- Discuss adverse medication effects to report.

Patient Population Considerations

Women (conception/pregnancy/lactation)
- Refer the pregnant patients to their obstetrician regarding the use of bupropion. It has been studied as a smoking cessation aid for pregnant women and is safe for use. Provide smoking cessation counseling to all women of childbearing age.

Geriatric
- Nicotine replacement products can be used in the geriatric population but should be prescribed in the lowest effective dose.

Pediatric
- Parental smoking is a major source of secondhand smoke in pediatrics that can cause childhood illnesses. Provide smoking cessation counseling to parents as part of the child wellness plan.

 POP QUIZ 14.3

A 56-year-old male presents to the primary care office with a history of anxiety, panic disorder, and major depressive disorder with a past hospital admission for suicidality. He is considering smoking cessation with nicotine replacement and an adjunct medication. He is currently prescribed sertraline 150 mg PO, propranolol 40 mg PO daily, and clonazepam 0.5 mg PO PRN for panic attacks. He appears anxious and remarks that his anxiety is elevated lately since starting to consider tobacco cessation. Which additional medication should be prescribed for the patient to aid in smoking cessation?

RESOURCES

American Cancer Society. (n.d.). *American Cancer Society position statement on electronic cigarettes.* https://www. cancer.org/healthy/stay-away-from-tobacco/e-cigarette-position-statement.html

American Psychiatric Association. (2006). Treatment of patients with eating disorders, American psychiatric association. *The American Journal of Psychiatry, 163*(Suppl 7), 4.

American Psychological Association. (2019). *Clinical practice guideline for the treatment of depression across three age cohorts.* https://www.apa.org/depression-guideline/guideline.pdf

Anxiety and Depression Association of America. (2015). *Clinical practice review for GAD.* https://adaa.org/ resources-professionals/practice-guidelines-gad

Barkley Burnett, L. (2018). *Medscape: Domestic violence.* https://emedicine.medscape.com/article/805546-overview

Batt, J. N. (2019). *Medscape: Anxiety.* https://emedicine.medscape.com/article/286227-overview

Berntstein, B. (2020a). *Medscape: Anorexia nervosa.* https://emedicine.medscape.com/article/2221362-overview

Berntstein, B. (2020b). *Medscape: Binge eating disorder.* https://emedicine.medscape.com/article/2221362-overview

Brown, K. M., & Malow, B. A. (2016). Pediatric insomnia. *Chest, 149*(5), 1332–1339. Elsevier. https://doi.org/10.1378/chest.15-0605

Cash, J. C., & Glass, C. A. (Eds.). (2019). *Adult-gerontology practice guidelines.* Springer Publishing Company.

Chawala, J. (2020). *Medscape: Insomnia.* https://emedicine.medscape.com/article/1187829-overview

Child Welfare Information Gateway. (2019). *Mandatory reporters of child abuse and neglect.* US Department of Health and Human Services, Children's Bureau. https://www.childwelfare.gov/topics/systemwide/laws-policies/statutes/manda/

Cochrane. (2004). *Does clonidine help smokers to quit?* https://www.cochrane.org/CD000058/TOBACCO_does-clonidine-help-smokers-to-quit

Codina Leik, M. T. (2018). *Family nurse practitioner certification: Intensive review.* Springer Publishing Company.

Duma, S. R., & Fung, V. S. (2019). Drug-induced movement disorders. *Australian Prescriber, 42*(2), 56–61. https://doi.org/10.18773/austprescr.2019.014

Emergency Nurses Association. (2018). *Clinical practice guideline: Intimate partner violence – for adult (18 and older) emergency department patients, how effective is screening and/or intervention for intimate partner violence.* https://www.ena.org/docs/default-source/resource-library/practice-resources/cpg/ipvcpg.pdf?sfvrsn=7ce56a4f_4

Giardino, A. (2017). *Medscape: Physical child abuse.* https://emedicine.medscape.com/article/915664-overview

Giustino, T. F., Ramanathan, K. R., Totty, M. S., Miles, O. W., & Maren, S. (2020). Locus coeruleus norepinephrine drives stress-induced increases in basolateral amygdala firing and impairs extinction learning. *The Journal of Neuroscience: The Official Journal of the Society for Neuroscience, 40*(4), 907–916. https://doi.org/10.1523/JNEUROSCI.1092-19.2019

Halverson, J. (2019). *Medscape: Depression.* https://emedicine.medscape.com/article/286759-overview

Hilty, D. (2020). *Medscape: Bulimia nervosa.* https://emedicine.medscape.com/article/286485-overview

Horowitz, L. M., Snyder, D. J., Boudreaux, E. D., He, J. P., Harrington, C. J., Cai, J., Claassen, C. A., Salhany, J. E., Dao, T., Chaves, J. F., Jobes, D. A., Merikangas, K. R., Bridge, J. A., & Pao, M. (2020). Validation of the ask suicide-screening questions (asq) for adult medical inpatients: A brief tool for all ages. *Psychosomatics, 61*(6), 713–722. https://doi.org/10.1016/j.psym.2020.04.008

Jobes, D. A., Au, J. S., & Siegelman, A. (2015). Psychological approaches to suicide treatment and prevention. *Current Treatment Options in Psychiatry, 2*(4), 363–370. https://doi.org/10.1007/s40501-015-0064-3. https://www.samhsa.gov/sites/default/files/psychological-approaches-to-suicide-treatment-and-prevention-10222015.pdf

Jordan, S., Davies, G. I., Thayer, D. S., Tucker, D., & Humphreys, I. (2019). Antidepressant prescriptions, discontinuation, depression, and perinatal outcomes, including breastfeeding: A population cohort Analysis. *PLOS ONE, 14*(11), e0225133–. https://doi.org/10.1371/journal.pone.0225133

Kirsch, D. L., Price, L. R., Nichols, F., Marksberry, J. A., & Platoni, K. T. (2014). Military service member and veteran self-reports of efficacy of cranial electrotherapy stimulation for anxiety, posttraumatic stress disorder, insomnia, and depression. *US Army Medical Department Journal,* 46–54.

Miller, M. A., Renn, B. N., Chu, F., & Torrence, N. (2019). Sleepless in the hospital: A systematic review of non-pharmacological sleep interventions. *General hospital psychiatry, 59,* 58–66. https://doi.org/10.1016/j.genhosppsych.2019.05.006

Mills, J. (2019). *Medscape: Elder abuse.* https://emedicine.medscape.com/article/805727-overview

Nanovskaya, T. N., Oncken, C., Fokina, V. M., Feinn, R. S., Clark, S. M., West, H., Jain, S. K., Ahmed, M. S., & Hankins, G. (2017). Bupropion sustained release for pregnant smokers: A randomized, placebo-controlled trial. *American Journal of Obstetrics and Gynecology, 216*(4), 420.e1–420.e9. https://doi.org/10.1016/j.ajog.2016.11.1036

National Eating Disorders Association. (n.d.a). *NEDS: Types of psychotherapy.* https://www.nationaleatingdisorders.org/treatment/types-psychotherapy

National Eating Disorders Association. (n.d.b). *NEDA toolkit for parents.* https://www.nationaleatingdisorders.org/sites/default/files/Toolkits/ParentToolkit.pdf

National Institutes of Health. (2019a). *Melatonin: What you need to know.* https://www.nccih.nih.gov/health/melatonin-what-you-need-to-kno

National Institutes of Health. (2019b). *National institute on alcohol abuse and alcoholism: Fetal alcohol exposure.* https://www.niaaa.nih.gov/publications/brochures-and-fact-sheets/fetal-alcohol-exposure

National Institutes of Health. (2020a). *DailyMed: Spravato esketamine hydrochloride solution.* https://dailymed.nlm.nih.gov/dailymed/drugInfo.cfm?setid=d81a6a79-a74a-44b7-822c-0dfa3036eaed

National Institutes of Health. (2020b). *National institute on alcohol abuse and alcoholism: Alcohol use disorder: A comparison between DSM–IV and DSM–5.* https://www.niaaa.nih.gov/publications/brochures-and-fact-sheets/alcohol-use-disorder-comparison-between-dsm

National Institutes of Health Research. (2019). *Using both nicotine patches and gum together improves the chances of quitting smoking* https://evidence.nihr.ac.uk/alert/using-both-nicotine-patches-and-gum-together-improves-the-chances-of-quitting-smoking/#:~:text=Using%20a%20nicotine%20patch%20together%20with%20a%20fast-acting,than%20lower%20dose%20ones%2C%20this%20NIHR-funded%20review%20suggests

Pisa, F. E., Reinold, J., Kollhorst, B., Haug, U., & Schink, T. (2020, June 22). Individual antidepressants, and the risk of fractures in older adults: A new user active comparator study. *Clinical Epidemiology, 12,* 667–678. https://doi.org/10.2147/CLEP.S222888. PMID: 32606992; PMCID: PMC7319507

Quellette, L., TenBrink, W., Gier, C., Shepherd, S., Mitten, S., Steinberger, M., & Jones, J. (2019). Alcoholism in elderly patients: Characteristics of patients and impact on the emergency department. *The American Journal of Emergency Medicine, 37*(4), 776–777. https://doi.org/10.1016/j.ajem.2018.08.061

Reus, V. I., Fochtmann, L. J., Bukstein, O., Eyler, A. E., Hilty, D. M., Horvitz-Lennon, M., Mahoney, J., Pasic, J., Weaver, M., Wills, C. D., McIntyre, J., Kidd, J., Yager, J., & Hong, S. H. (2018). The American Psychiatric Association practice guideline for the pharmacological treatment of patients with alcohol use disorder. *American Journal of Psychiatry, 175*(1), 86–90. https://doi.org/10.1176/appi.ajp.2017.1750101

Schaeffer, J. (2016). *Elder eating disorders: Surprising new challenge.* https://www.todaysgeriatricmedicine.com/news/exclusive_0409_03.shtml

Shakil, A., Day, P., Chu, J., Woods, S., & Bridges, K. (2018). PedHITSS: A screening tool to detect childhood abuse in clinical settings. *Family Medicine, 50*(10), 763–769. https://doi.org/10.22454/FamMed.2018.778329

Shepardson, R. L., Kosiba, J. D., Bernstein, L. I., & Funderburk, J. S. (2019). Suicide risk among veteran primary care patients with current anxiety symptoms. *Family Practice, 36*(1), 91–95. https://doi.org/10.1093/fampra/cmy088

Smyka, M., Kosińska-Kaczyńska, K., Sochacki-Wójcicka, N., Zgliczyńska, M., & Wielgoś, M. (2020). Sleep problems in pregnancy-a cross-sectional study in over 7000 pregnant women in Poland. *International Journal of Environmental Research and Public Health, 17*(15), 5306. https://doi.org/10.3390/ijerph17155306

Sorenson, M., Quinn, L., & Klein, D. (2019). *Pathophysiology: Concepts of human disease* (1st ed.). Pearson Education.

Thompson. W. (2020). *Medscape: Alcoholism.* https://emedicine.medscape.com/article/285913-overview

U.S. Department of Health and Human Services. (2017). *Administration for community living: Elder abuse and prevention.* https://acl.gov/programs/protecting-rights-and-preventing-abuse/elder-justice

15

PEDIATRIC AND ADOLESCENT REVIEW

NORMAL GROWTH AND DEVELOPMENT

Overview

Knowledge of physical development milestones and key cognitive–behavioral stages improves understanding of children and adolescents and facilitates clinical encounters in all levels of illness prevention. Emphasis should be placed on identifying deviations from normal findings in each of these areas to improve clinical decision-making.

Developmental Monitoring

One out of every four young children is at moderate to high risk for a developmental, behavioral, or social delay. Healthcare providers can engage caregivers and parents to participate in developmental monitoring to assist in communicating concerns about their child's growth and development. The CDC's "Learn the Signs. Act Early" program maintains printable checklists and a downloadable "Milestone Tracker" application to improve early identification of concerns and communications with the healthcare provider. The materials aid healthcare providers in the referral process for early intervention. The app is available for free in iOS and Android app stores.

Tables 15.1 and 15.2 outline physical and cognitive/psychosocial developmental milestones.

Developmental Screening

Clinical assessment of development milestones, social determinants of health, and maternal depression are integrated into regular well visits. Tools for performing screening by providers are compiled in the "Compendium of Screening Measures for Children" published by HHS (link in Sources section of this chapter), and additional AAP screening tools and education is locations on the AAP's website.

Recommendations

- Developmental and behavioral screening at ages 9, 18, and 30 months (American Academy of Pediatrics)
- Autism spectrum screening (18 months and 24 months)

 POP QUIZ 15.1

The nurse practitioner examines a 3-month-old infant for a well-care visit in the primary care office. The posterior fontanelle in not yet closed and the infant is unable to sit upright at 90 degrees unassisted. What is the significance of these findings?

Table 15.1 Physical Development Milestones

Age	Physical Development Milestones

Infant (birth to 1 year)	**Birth to 1 month**
	• *Physical*
	  • Head circumference increases 1–1.5 cm/mo.
	  • *Weight:* Regain birth weight in 2 weeks.
	    • Fat percentage is 13% at birth.
	    • Body water 70% at birth.
	• Sucking, rooting, and grasping reflexes are present.
	• *Milestones:* Brings hand to mouth, holds hand in fist, moves head from side to side when prone, follows object moved in an arc, turns toward familiar voices, focuses on a face.
	
	2–4 months
	• *Physical*
	  • Head circumference increases 1–1.5 cm/mo, posterior fontanelle closes.
	  • *Weight:* Gains 5–7 oz per week, eats 2 oz./lb./d.
	• *Milestones:* Moro reflex fades, smiles, raises head 45 degrees, holds objects in hand, follows object 180 degrees, can hold head midline with some bobbing when sitting.
	
	4–6 months
	• *Physical*
	  • Head circumference increases 1–1.5 cm/mo.
	  • *Weight:* Double birth weight in 5–6 months, eats 1.5 oz/lb./24 hr. Introduces new foods (rice cereal, vegetables, fruits).
	• *Milestones:* Most inborn reflexes gone. Sits with support, no head lag when sitting, rolls from prone to supine at 4 months and supine to prone at 6 months. Will drop an object to reach for another object, listens intently to voices, recognizes people at a distance.
	
	6–8 months
	• *Physical*
	  • Head circumference increases 1–1.5 cm/mo.
	  • *Weight:* Gains 3–5 oz/wk; growth rate slows in second half.
	• *Milestones*
	  • Sits unsupported. Bears some weight. likes to bounce, begins pincer grasp, transfer objects hand to hand. Holds own bottle. Shows excitement in anticipation play. Plays peekaboo. Responds to own name and being told no; babbles.
	  • Teeth begin to erupt at 6–10 months.
	
	8–10 months
	• *Physical*
	  • Steady growth rate.
	• *Milestones*
	  • Crawls and pulls self to standing by 10 months. Stands holding onto things. May say "Ma" or "Da" to anyone. Picks up objects. Uses pincer grasp well.
	  • More anxious about separation from parents. Develops a sense of object permanence.
	
	10–12 months
	• *Physical*
	  • Brain 70% of adult size; head circumference equals chest circumference.
	  • *Weight:* Triples birth weight at 12 months, at 1 cm/mo.
	    • Fat percentage is 25% at 12 months.
	    • Body water 61%.
	  • Six teeth.
	• *Milestones:* Stands alone, plays patty cake, and cruises furniture. May walk a few steps. Drinks from a cup. Places objects in containers through holes. Uses "Mama" and "Dada" appropriately. Claps and waves bye-bye. Speaks several words. Can hold a crayon.

Age	Physical Development Milestones
Toddler **(1–3 years)**	• *Physical* • Head circumference increases 3.5 cm increase over 3 years • *Weight:* Quadruple weight by 2 years. • All teeth by 2.5 years. • *Milestones* • *18 months:* Can speak 10 words, make a tower of four cubes, can climb stairs holding on and walks well; object permanence is fully developed, and searches for missing things; resolves separation anxiety when they understand that the missing parent will return. • *18 months to 2 years:* Recognizes gender identity. • *2 years:* Understands the concept of time and has a vivid imagination; can throw tantrums to express frustration. • *2.5 years:* Makes two- to three-word sentences and a tower of seven cubes; climbs stairs without help; handles spoon well; turns single pages of books; verbalizes need for potty. • *3 years:* Uses plural in language and counts to 10. Copies a circle. Dresses except for buttons and laces; feeds self; questions constantly; toilets self; plays interactively with other children.
Preschool **3–6 years**	• *Physical* • Head circumference increases 3.5 cm increase over 3 years. • *Weight:* Quadruple weight by 2 years, all teeth by 2.5 years. • *Milestones* • *4 years:* Can hop on one foot, dress self and wash face and hands; throws a ball overhand. • *5 years:* Catches the ball, dresses without assistance, knows four colors, draws a person in six parts, and copies a triangle. • *3–5 years:* Interest in fantasy play and have typical childhood fears; *Animism:* Giving life to inanimate objects; *Centration:* Only considers one aspect of a situation at a time.
School age **(6–12 years)**	• *Physical* • Brain 90% of adult size at age 7. • *Weight:* Gains 2 kg/yr. From age 2 through puberty, boys' weight > girls' weight. • *Milestones* • *6 years:* Can walk heel-toe, write name; can recite the alphabet, read by age 6 or 7; starts to develop intuition, sees consequences. • *7 years:* Can follow rules of a game, take turns. • Puberty may start in some girls as early as age 8; earlier onset is considered precocious puberty
Adolescent **(12–18 years)**	• *Physical* • *Growth spurt:* Boys ages 12–17, girls ages 9.5–13.5. • Protein and energy requirements decline in ages 15–18 years; boys 45.5 kcal/kg and girls 40 kcal/kg. • *Sexual maturation* • Tanner stages 1–4, boys 10–18 years: testes, pubic hair, lengthening of the penis, change in voice, growth spurt peak, axillary hair, facial hair. • Tanner stages 1–4, girls 8–16 years: breast budding, pubic hair, growth spurt, axillary hair, menarche, adult breast. • *Delayed puberty:* Refer to endocrinology. • *Boys:* No testicular enlargement by age 14 or more than 5-year lapse between initial and complete genital growth. • *Girls:* No breast development by age 13 years, menarche more than 3 years after the beginning of breast growth, no menses by age 16.

Table 15.2 Cognitive and Psychosocial Development

Age	Cognitive and Psychosocial Development

Infant (birth to 1 year)	*Erikson:* Trust versus mistrust
	• Trust in caregivers providing basic needs including comfort.
	  • Mistrust from basic needs not met.
	    • Have the caregiver hold the infant whenever possible during the exam.
	
	Piaget: Sensorimotor
	• Learns from movement and senses.
	  • Distract the infant with toys to complete tasks.
	
	Freud: Oral stage
	• Comfort from mouth
	  • Encourage breastfeeding, pacifier.

Toddler 1–3 years	*Erikson:* Autonomy versus shame
	• Sense of independence and control.
	  • Shame from criticism of lack of control (toileting).
	
	Piaget: Preoperational
	• Learns from exploration and develops language.
	  • Name objects during the examination.
	
	Freud: Anal stage
	• Gratified from the control of excretions.
	  • Reassure child and parents when toileting regresses during illness.

Preschool 3–6 years	*Erikson:* Initiative versus guilt
	• Initiates new activities and ideas. Becomes involved and busy.
	  • Accept the child's verbalizations of frustration and show empathy.
	    • Risk of lack of involvement or purpose from excessive criticism.
	
	Piaget: Preoperational
	• Continues to develop language and explore.
	• Cognition still developing. Confused about causality and feels responsible for causing illness.
	  • Offer explanations and explain that they are not responsible for the illness.
	
	Freud: Phallic stage
	• Initially identifies with the parent of the opposite sex, then with the same-sex parent.
	  • Include parents in assessment and planning.

School-age 6–12 years	*Erikson:* Industry versus inferiority
	• Takes on activities and focuses on accomplishment, develops self-worth and pride.
	  • Encourage the child to talk about activities and school.
	• Failure to meet individual or imposed benchmarks leads to feelings of inferiority.
	Piaget: Concrete operational
	• Mature thought develops as the child can manipulate objects.
	  • Provide clear instructions and details.
	Freud: Latency stage
	• Child values privacy and understanding the body.
	  • Preserve modesty in the exam, knock before entering the exam room.

Age	Cognitive and Psychosocial Development
Adolescent **12–18 years**	*Erikson:* Identity versus role confusion • Matures and establishes their sense of identity as they redefine peer group, family, and community. • Introduce shared decision-making in adolescence to engage the patient in self-health management. • Refer adolescent to peer support groups for health conditions. *Piaget:* Formal operational • Develops abstract thought with greater maturity. • Ask adolescent if they would like to come into the room alone first and invite parents afterward. *Freud:* Genital stage • Adolescents value genital function and relationships. • Provide resources on sexuality and protection from infection.

IMMUNIZATIONS

Overview

- The CDC maintains an updated schedule for children and adolescent vaccinations and catch-up schedules for children and adolescents 4 months through 18 years on their website at www.cdc.gov/vaccines/schedules/index.html. The most recent chart as of the date of this publication is shown in Exhibit 15.1.
- Also, providers can download the CDC vaccine app so that they have access to current information when prescribing vaccines. Family education materials are available online for printing.
- Toolkits to help providers improve performance in achieving vaccination benchmarks are available. The Immunization Action Coalition has educational resources for providers www.immunize.org. IAC provides a collection of presentations to facilitate immunization at www.immunize.org/resources/res_powerpoint.asp.
- The AAP has established best practices to improve vaccination rates and reduce errors to meet the National Vaccine Advisory Committee standards. Their resources can be accessed at www.aap.org/en-us/advocacy-and-policy/aap-health-initiatives/immunizations/Pages/Immunizations-home.aspx.

 POP QUIZ 15.2

The nurse practitioner reviews the immunization requirements for a 6-year-old child who has not received any vaccinations since the hepatitis B vaccine at birth and requires catch-up vaccinations. The child has not developed any childhood infections protected by vaccine nor is the patient high risk. What principles for immunization should be applied in this situation?

Exhibit 15.1 Recommended Child and Adolescent Immunization Schedules for Ages 18 Years or Younger, United States, 2020.

Vaccine	Birth	1 mo	2 mos	4 mos	6 mos	9 mos	12 mos	15 mos	18 mos	19–23 mos	2–3 yrs	4–6 yrs	7–10 yrs	11–12 yrs	13–15 yrs	16 yrs	17–18 yrs
Hepatitis B (HepB)	1st dose	← 2nd dose →			←————— 3rd dose —————→												
Rotavirus (RV): RV1 (2-dose series), RV5 (3-dose series)			1st dose	2nd dose	See Notes												
Diphtheria, tetanus, acellular pertussis (DTaP <7 yrs)			1st dose	2nd dose	3rd dose		←— 4th dose —→					5th dose					
Haemophilus influenzae type b (Hib)			1st dose	2nd dose	See Notes		← 3rd or 4th dose → See Notes										
Pneumococcal conjugate (PCV13)			1st dose	2nd dose	3rd dose		←— 4th dose —→										
Inactivated poliovirus (IPV <18 yrs)			1st dose	2nd dose	←————— 3rd dose —————→							4th dose					
Influenza (IIV)					Annual vaccination 1 or 2 doses						Annual vaccination 1 or 2 doses		Annual vaccination 1 dose only				
or Influenza (LAIV4)											Annual vaccination 1 or 2 doses		Annual vaccination 1 dose only				
Measles, mumps, rubella (MMR)					See Notes		←—— 1st dose ——→					2nd dose					
Varicella (VAR)					See Notes		←—— 1st dose ——→					2nd dose					
Hepatitis A (HepA)							2-dose series, See Notes										
Tetanus, diphtheria, acellular pertussis (Tdap ≥7 yrs)														Tdap			
Human papillomavirus (HPV)							See Notes							See Notes			
													*	1st dose			
Meningococcal (MenACWY-D ≥9 mos, MenACWY-CRM ≥2 mos, MenACWY-TT ≥2 yr)							See Notes							1st dose		2nd dose	
Meningococcal B																See Notes	
Pneumococcal polysaccharide (PPSV23)													See Notes				

Legend:
- Range of recommended ages for all children
- Range of recommended ages for catch-up immunization
- Range of recommended ages for certain high-risk groups
- Recommended based on shared clinical decision-making or *can be used in this age group
- No recommendation/ not applicable

Source: https://www.cdc.gov/vaccines/schedules/downloads/child/0-18yrs-combined-schedule-bw.pdf.

RESOURCES

American Academy of Pediatrics. (2017). *American academy of pediatrics: Screening time.* https://screeningtime.org/star-center/#/

Ball, J. W., Bindler, R. C., Cowen, K., & Shaw, M. R. (2017). *Principles of pediatric nursing: Caring for children* (7th ed.). Pearson.

Centers for Disease Control and Prevention. (2020a). *Child development: Developmental monitoring and screening.* https://www.cdc.gov/ncbddd/childdevelopment/screening.html

Centers for Disease Control and Prevention. (2020b). *Immunizations schedules for health care providers.* https://www.cdc.gov/vaccines/schedules/hcp/index.html

Ezeanolue, E., Harriman, K., Hunter, P., Kroger, A., & Pellegrini, C. (2019). General best practice guidelines for immunization: Best practices guidance of the advisory committee on immunization Practices (ACIP). *National Center for Immunization and Respiratory Diseases.* https://www.cdc.gov/vaccines/hcp/acip-recs/general-recs/intro.pdf

Graber, E. (2019). *Merck manual: Introduction to growth and development. Professional version.* https://www.merckmanuals.com/en-ca/professional/pediatrics/growth-and-development/introduction-to-growth-and-development

U.S. Department of Health & Human Services. (2014). *Birth to 5: Watch me thrive. A compendium of Screening measures for young children.* https://eclkc.ohs.acf.hhs.gov/sites/default/files/pdf/screening-compendium-march2014.pdf

16

GERIATRIC REVIEW

FRAILTY

Overview

- Frailty in gerontology describes an older adult patient who has lost their ability to respond to stressors due to a loss of physiologic reserve across multiple systems.
- Older adults who are frail present with weakness, weight loss, muscle atrophy, and immobility. Anergia and exercise intolerance is evident. They may have difficulty dressing, toileting, or feeding themselves.
- Multiple comorbidities are exacerbated with any stress. Associated cognitive impairment, depression, and withdrawal interferes with the patient's self-determination. Frailty is more common in women, in those who are prescribed polypharmacology, and in patients who are in a lower socioeconomic class.
- Progression to frailty syndrome increases the risk of complications of immobility, falls, hospitalization, and death.

Prevention and Screening

- As the population ages, effective screening and early intervention for patients at higher risk for frailty is necessary.
- The use of objective screens for cognition, depression, and frailty (such as the frailty phenotype or index) is critical.
- Self-reporting of unintentional weight loss, slower walking, fatigue on most days, muscle weakness, poor endurance alerts the clinician of high risk for frailty and requires further inquiry.
- Early intervention with rehabilitation may prevent or delay the onset of frailty.
- Employ frailty prevention strategies in patients who are newly diagnosed with diseases associated with the onset of frailty.

Treatment and Management

- Treatment for frailty is focused on reducing progressive decline by health behavior intervention. Emphasis on exercise (balance, flexibility, resistance, and endurance) and nutrition (protein and micronutrient supplementation) may be helpful.
- Resilience can be improved with support from a patient-centered care team tailored to provide individualized care. Medication reconciliation to identify agents that contribute to frailty and exploring alternatives is an effective pharmacological intervention. The current study of biologic agents to reverse sarcopenia are ongoing. Without intervention, the patient requires placement in a long-term care facility, where progressive decline can ensue.

COMPLICATIONS

CV: Coronary ischemia, advanced heart failure, arrhythmia, DVT, PE, chronic venous insufficiency, critical limb ischemia, orthostatic hypotension

GI: Aspiration, GERD, anorexia ileus, fecal impaction, malnutrition, incontinence

GU: UTI, Renal colic, AKI, electrolyte disturbance, renal insufficiency

HEM: Nutritional anemias, cancers, immunosuppression, and infection

INT: Thrush, impaired mucus membranes, decubitus ulcers, perineal candidiasis, fragile skin

MSK: Osteoporosis, pathologic fractures, trauma from falls

NEURO: Anxiety, chronic confusion, dementia, depression, weakness, social isolation, sleep disturbance, sundowning, stroke, subdural hematoma from falls

PULM: Atelectasis, pneumonia, frequent respiratory infections

POLYPHARAMCOLOGY AND GERIATRIC PATIENTS

Overview

- Polypharmacy is defined as regular use of at least five medications.
- Many chronic diseases require medications from multiple classes in its therapeutic management. Geriatric patients with more than one chronic health condition would most likely exceed five medications.

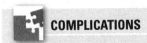

COMPLICATIONS

Acute: Delirium, somnolence, fatigue, toxicity, bleeding, arrhythmia

- Healthcare providers are held to quality metrics that may require additional medications to meet outcomes. With informatic alerts and triggers suggesting the use of a medication, the provider may feel time-pressured to prescribe the medication without perceiving the risk of polypharmacology. The problem would be compounded when older adult patients see more than one specialist.
- Patient factors can contribute to polypharmacology as well. Some patients have been conditioned to treat problems with medication and some care settings are accustomed to prescribing them.
- Polypharmacology can lead to devastating health consequences and can become a financial burden to patients who are in a lower socioeconomic status.
- The Joint Commission's requirement for medication reconciliation has not corrected this public health concern.

Preventions and Screening

- Primary prevention of disease and secondary detection of conditions before symptoms would delay the onset of illness or reduce its severity, thus reducing the need for initiating additional medications.
- Use of Beers screening tool or STOPP and START can reduce falls, complications of polypharmacology, and reduce cost and adverse drug events.

DELIRIUM

Overview

- Delirium is a condition of neurologic dysfunction with features of psychiatric abnormalities that can easily be confused with psychosis or dementia.
- It is seen frequently in older adults but can occur at any age.
- When present, the clinician excludes all reversible causes, such as sepsis or complications of an existing chronic health condition.

Sundowning

- Sundowning may be a confounding variable in the presentation of delirium in an older adult patient. Sudden change in behavior that develop daily as the day progresses should be investigated for a syndrome commonly referred to as "sundowning."
- Sundowning is delirium as a person becomes more tired toward the end of the day. It is associated with neuropsychiatric syndromes such as dementia and Alzheimer's disease.
- The exact etiology is unknown, but it is believed to be a combination of environmental stressors and biologic disease. There may be a circadian rhythm disorder.

Etiology

- Dementia is the greatest risk factor for the onset of delirium
- Pain syndromes
- Increased intracranial pressure from bleeding, hydrocephalus, or mass

- Hypoxia from airflow limitation or impaired gas exchange due to fluid, inflammation, infiltrate, masses, atelectasis, or effusion
- Ischemia from decreased tissue perfusion (stroke, MI, PAD), decreased cardiac output (hypovolemia, hemorrhage or pulmonary edema), sepsis
- Capillary leak syndrome, uremia, electrolyte disturbance, dilutional hyponatremia, hepatic encephalopathy, hyperglycemia, hypercortisolism, paraneoplastic syndrome
- Anticholinergic excess, medications, poisoning, toxins

Signs and Symptoms

- Change in arousal, sensorium, or behavior that may be of sudden onset or insidious, become progressively worse
  - Neurologic changes associated with a specific time in afternoon or evening is referred to as sundowning.
- Additional symptoms of change in consciousness, dysarthria, dysphasia, hallucinations, motor disturbance, tremor, asterixis, seizure may occur.

Differential Diagnosis

- *NEURO*: Brain lesion, dementia, depression, hydrocephalus, Huntington's disease, intracranial hemorrhage, Parkinson's disease, psychosis, seizure disorder, stroke
- *CV*: Aneurysm rupture, myocardial infarction, pulmonary edema
- *ENDO*: Hyperglycemic emergency, hyperparathyroidism, hypoadrenalism, hypoglycemia, hypothyroidism, pituitary disorders, SIADH
- *GI*: Hepatic encephalopathy
- *GU*: Dehydration, uremia
- *HEM*: Coagulopathy, DIC, hemorrhage, sepsis
- *Other*: Lactic acidosis, medication adverse effects, overdose, poisoning vitamin deficiency (thiamine and cobalamin)

Diagnosis

Labs

- POC lab diagnostic testing includes pulse oximetry, vital signs, CBG testing, and 12-lead EKG. If CBG <70 mg dL treat for hypoglycemia and investigate its cause.
- Examination for a source of infection if 2 qSOFA signs are present is warranted.
- *If the patient is stable, and can tolerate hydration and nutrition, you can continue to investigate for the underlying cause of delirium; otherwise transfer to the ED immediately.*
- Obtain CMP, Ca, Phos, Mg, LFTs with bilirubin, CBC, TSH, drug levels as indicated.
- Obtain vitamin B$_{12}$, folate, thiamine, RPR, VDRL, ESR, HIV.

 ALERT

If the patient is experiencing hypoxia, ischemia, decreased cardiac output, has s/s of infection and 2 qSOFA signs, has stroke signs, 2-point drop in Glasgow coma scale, or hypoglycemia refractory to treatment, suspected poisoning, alcohol overdose, or toxicity transfer to the ED immediately.

Additional Diagnostic Testing

- Perform medication reconciliation to identify agents that may have contributed.
- Assessment instruments for delirium and dementia can be used to obtain an objective measure for comparison.
- Use the ADEPT tool (www.acep.org/patient-care/adept) to assess, diagnose, evaluate, prevent, and treat. The ADEPT tool includes a mini-cog assessment. Consider using an agitation inventory to assess baseline and evaluate outcomes.

Treatment and Management

- Protect the patient from harm, treat the underlying cause, and reverse the delirium.

Nonpharmacological Therapy

- Maintain patient safety and protect from falls or harm. Do not prescribe restraints for the patient. Employ the least restrictive method to keep the patient safe.
- Treat pain, nausea, and constipation that may be aggravating agitation.
- Instruct staff to reduce environmental sensory stimuli as reasonably possible but have sensory aids such as glasses and hearing aids available.
- Limit use of noisy devices, procedures, and intravenous and urinary catheterization.
- Prescribe interventions to decrease agitation such as music therapy, art therapy, aromatherapy, and reminiscence therapy.
- *Instruct staff to promote sleep hygiene*: Eliminate caffeine, promote exercise earlier in the day. Eliminate excessive noise in afternoon. Consider aroma therapy and music therapy during this period.

Pharmacological Therapy

- Prescribe melatonin 5 mg PO in the evening to promote sleep.
- Refer to psychiatry regarding use of melatonin agonists and cholinesterase inhibitors.

ESSENTIAL TREMOR

Overview

- Essential tremor is a common neurological movement disorder of unknown etiology that may be neurodegenerative in origin. Tremor is aggravated with activity, emotional stress, fatigue and resolves with rest and sleep. The patient denies paresthesia, symptoms that get progressively worse, or associated motor problem that would be seen in neurodegenerative disorders. There are no dystonic features.
- Reflexes are normal and there is no flaccidity, weakness, spasticity, or rigidity consistent with lower or upper motor neuron disease.

Etiology

- Exact cause is unknown
- Family history

Signs and Symptoms

- Tremor in upper extremity that increased when attempting to perform motor activities
- May progress to both upper extremities and head
- Can become pronounced over time, interfering with self-care, feeding, motor function and work
- Increases with anxiety, hunger, fatigue, and changes in temperature

Differential Diagnosis

- *NEURO*: Brain lesion, cerebellar tremors, dystonia, movement disorders, Parkinson's disease, psychogenic tremor
- *GI*: Hepatic disease
- *GU*: Renal disease
- *ENDO*: Hyperthyroidism, hypocalcemia, hyponatremia, hypoparathyroidism
- *HEM*: Leukemia

- *Other*: Medication adverse effects (anticonvulsants, antidepressants, beta agonists, lithium, methylxanthines, neuroleptics, thyroid replacement hormone) drug withdrawal, substance abuse, Wilson's disease

Diagnosis

Labs

- Exclusion of neurologic, electrolyte, endocrine, or metabolic causes should be excluded by BMP, CA, Mg, LFTs, TSH, and toxicology screen for substances and medications as indicated.

Additional Diagnostic Testing

- Imaging is not indicated unless it is a new acute symptom or neurodegenerative disorders are considered. MRI and head CT will be normal.

Treatment and Management

POP QUIZ 16.1

- Prescribe propranolol 10 mg PO once daily 30 min before needed effect on motor performance.
- Teach patient to avoid excess caffeine or stimulant before events requiring motor performance.
- Refer to neurology if additional intervention is required.

An 85-year-old male who is newly admitted to a skilled nursing facility has developed agitation during dinner. What should the nurse practitioner prioritize?

RESOURCES

Alagiakrishnan, K. (2019). *Medscape: Delirium.* https://emedicine.medscape.com/article/288890-overview#a1
Bernabei, R., Martone, A. M., Vetrano, D. L., Calvani, R., Landi, F., & Marzetti, E. (2014). Frailty, physical frailty, sarcopenia: A new conceptual model. *Studies in Health Technology and Informatics, 203*, 78–84.
Burke, D. (2018). *Me3dscape: Essential tremor.* https://emedicine.medscape.com/article/1150290-overview
Campins, L., Camps, M., Riera, A., Pleguezuelos, E., Yebenes, J. C., & Serra-Prat, M. (2017). Oral drugs related with muscle wasting and Sarcopenia. A review. *Pharmacology, 99*(1-2), 1–8. https://doi.org/10.1159/000448247. Epub 2016 Aug 31. PMID: 27578190
Cash, J. C., & Glass, C. A. (Eds.). (2019). *Adult-gerontology practice guidelines.* Springer Publishing Company.
Cesari, M., Fielding, R., Bénichou, O., Bernabei, R., Bhasin, S., Guralnik, J. M., Jette, A., & O'Mahony, D. (2020). STOPP/START criteria for potentially inappropriate medications/potential prescribing omissions in older people: Origin and progress. *Expert Review of Clinical Pharmacology, 13*(1), 15–22. https://doi.org/10.1080/175 12433.2020.1697676
CGA Toolkit. (n.d.). *Frailty phenotype screen.* https://www.cgakit.com/fr-1-frailty-phenotype
Codina Leik, M. T. (2018). *Family nurse practitioner certification: Intensive review.* Springer Publishing Company.
Evans, N. (2016). *Sundowning: Phenomenology, pathophysiology, and treatment approaches.* https://www.psychiatryadvisor.com/home/topics/neurocognitive-disorders/alzheimers-disease-and-dementia/sundowning-phenomenology-pathophysiology-and-treatment-approaches/
Halli-Tierney, A. D., Scarbrough, C., & Carroll, D. (2019). Polypharmacy: Evaluating risks and deprescribing. *American Family Physician, 100*(1), 32–38.
Hsiao, C. Y., Shu-Li, C. H. E. N., Hsiao, Y. S., Huang, H. Y., & Shu-Hui, Y. E. H. (2020). Effects of art and reminiscence therapy on agitated behaviors among older adults with dementia. *Journal of Nursing Research, 28*(4), e100. https://doi.org/10.1097/jnr.0000000000000373
Kojima, G., Liljas, A., & Iliffe, S. (2019). Frailty syndrome: Implications and challenges for health care policy. *Risk Management and Healthcare Policy, 12*, 23–30. https://doi.org/10.2147/RMHP.S168750
Landi, F., Pahor, M., Rodriguez-Manas, L., Rolland, Y., Roubenoff, R., Sinclair, A. J., Studenski, S., Travison, T., & Vellas, B. (2015). Pharmacological interventions in frailty and sarcopenia: Report by the international conference on frailty and sarcopenia research task force. *The Journal of Frailty & Aging, 4*(3), 114–120. https://doi.org/10.14283/jfa.2015.64
Lundger, G. (2018). *Medscape: Is sarcopenia inevitable as we age?* https://www.medscape.com/viewarticle/901654
Norris, C. M., & Close, J. C. (2020). Prehabilitation for the frailty syndrome: Improving outcomes for our most vulnerable patients. *Anesthesia & Analgesia, 130*(6), 1524–1533. https://doi.org/10.1213/ANE.0000000000004785

Puts, M., Toubasi, S., Andrew, M. K., Ashe, M. C., Ploeg, J., Atkinson, E., Ayala, A. P., Roy, A., Rodríguez Monforte, M., Bergman, H., & McGilton, K. (2017). Interventions to prevent or reduce the level of frailty in community-dwelling older adults: A scoping review of the literature and international policies. *Age and Ageing, 46*(3), 383–392. https://doi.org/10.1093/ageing/afw247

Shenvi, C., Kennedy, M., Austin, C. A., Wilson, M. P., Gerardi, M., & Schneider, S. (2020). Managing delirium and agitation in the older emergency department patient: The ADEPT tool. *Annals of Emergency Medicine, 75*(2), 136–145. https://doi.org/10.1016/j.annemergmed.2019.07.023

Uchmanowicz, I., Jankowska-Polańska, B., Wleklik, M., Lisiak, M., & Gobbens, R. (2018). Frailty syndrome: Nursing interventions. *SAGE Open Nursing, 4*, 2377960818759449. https://doi.org/10.1177/2377960818759449

Uchmanowicz, I., Młynarska, A., Lisiak, M., Kałużna-Oleksy, M., Wleklik, M., Chudiak, A., & Gobbens, R. (2019). Heart failure and problems with frailty syndrome: Why it is time to care about frailty syndrome in heart failure. *Cardiac Failure Review, 5*(1), 37. https://doi.org/10.15420/cfr.2018.37.1

17

POP QUIZ ANSWERS

CHAPTER 2

Pop Quiz 2.1

Prescribe duloxetine if depression is confirmed by quantitative measures to improve mood and pain management in comorbid depression and osteoarthritic pain. Consider topical capsaicin and lidocaine application, individually or in combination, to complement medication. Explore nonpharmacologic strategies to improve pain management.

Pop Quiz 2.2

The clinician should suspect *Staphylococcus aureus*, which is a frequent cause of skin infection. It is prudent to consider CA-MRSA in circumstances where there is crowding, frequent skin contact, compromised skin, contaminated personal care items, and lack of cleanliness. Adolescents participating in contact sports are at high risk for CA-MRSA skin infections. Obtain a culture with incision and drainage with ultrasound guidance if needed. Prescribe oral clindamycin, trimethoprim/sulfamethoxazole, or a tetracycline (doxycycline or minocycline, or linezolid). Notify the health department for follow-up.

Pop Quiz 2.3

The patient is experiencing a hypertensive event. Exclude acute target organ damage. If asymptomatic, treat for severe uncontrolled hypertension and evaluate for secondary causes of hypertension and comorbid cardiovascular disease, thyroid dysfunction, hyperlipidemia, and diabetes. Prescribe an ACEI or ARB in view of prior gestational diabetes, instruct in BP monitoring, lifestyle modifications, and criteria to seek consultation. Avoid rapid lowering of blood pressure >20% and schedule follow-up in 1 to 2 weeks to evaluate effect and tolerance.

Pop Quiz 2.4

In the absence of ASCVD or CKD, determine if there is a compelling need to minimize hypoglycemia, weight gain, or cost. Prescribe an additional antidiabetic, such as a GLP-1 RA, which will promote weight loss. An SLGLT2I may also be considered.

Pop Quiz 2.5

The patient is exhibiting warning signs of gastric or gastroesophageal cancer, which requires prompt referral to a gastroenterologist for endoscopic examination and biopsy. Obtain CBC, CMP, and LFTs. The patient can discontinue famotidine.

Pop Quiz 2.6

Obtain a history and physical examination to exclude the presence of a respiratory infection or new respiratory irritant. Obtain a peak flow. If peak flow is 80% of personal best without SABA, review current GERD management. If there is no infection or irritants present, ensure lifestyle modifications for GERD are in use (truncal weight management, small meals with food abstinence for 3 hr before bedtime, head of bed elevated lying on left side during sleep, and avoidance of triggers). Advise patient to take her PPI 30 min before evening meal instead of the morning and evaluate response.

CHAPTER 3

Pop Quiz 3.1

Jaw claudication is highly predictive of neurovascular disorders such as temporal arteritis, migraines, and migrainous neuralgia; examination should exclude trigeminal neuralgia, cardiovascular, dental, autoimmune, or infectious causes. Perform a complete neurological exam to exclude stroke syndromes. Pay careful attention to the CN examination, especially CN V, to exclude neuralgia.

Pop Quiz 3.2

Facial weakness with a recent tick bite and viral syndrome in a young adult should be further explored for acute OM, Bell palsy, vitamin B_{12} deficiency, cholesteatoma, immune-mediated vasculitis, myasthenia gravis, parotid mass, peripheral and central demyelinating disorders, Ramsay–Hunt syndrome, tick-borne illness, trauma, and viral infection with HSV, CMV, EBV. It is critical to avoid cognitive bias and workup the most obvious cause as the only possible diagnosis.

Pop Quiz 3.3

The patient should be evaluated immediately in the ED for a stroke. Risk factors for stroke include age, HTN, PAD, and hyperlipidemia. Pertinent findings suggest MCA stroke. MCA stroke accounts for a large percent of thromboembolic strokes in clinical practice, although a hemorrhagic stroke cannot be excluded without CT of the head. Symptoms of a stroke may include contralateral hemiparesis and homonymous hemianopia. This stroke can lead to unilateral neglect, dysarthria, aphasia, apraxia, which may or may not be present. Do not administer aspirin or antiplatelets until CT is completed to rule out hemorrhage. The BP is elevated but does not require urgent intervention. Rapid reduction in BP can exacerbate cerebral ischemia. Do not administer antipyretics. Maintain the patient NPO, apply oxygen according to pulse oximetry, and prepare the patient for transfer to ED.

Pop Quiz 3.4

Resting tremors should be immediately evaluated as this likely indicates Parkinson's disease. You should have heightened concern when you notice a resting tremor on a general survey, especially in a patient who had TBI from military service. TBI has been implicated in increasing the incidence of PD. A change in behavior, resting tremor, and TBI history support further inquiry into PD. Medications (antipsychotics, antidepressants, prokinetics) are associated with medication-induced PD symptoms. Apathy and withdrawn behavior require careful evaluation for depression. Untreated PTSD can lead to self-harm. Compounded with a diagnosis of PD, the risk for self-harm is increased.

CHAPTER 4

Pop Quiz 4.1

The priority is to admit the patient to the hospital for immediate treatment. An unattended homebirth increases the likelihood that the newborn did not receive silver nitrate, erythromycin, or tetracycline ophthalmic ointment at birth. Copious secretions that are mucopurulent and crust in the first week after birth is gonococcal. Chlamydia is scant mucoid; HSV is nonpurulent discharge.

Pop Quiz 4.2

The most likely diagnosis is sensorineural loss in the right ear, and the patient should be referred to otolaryngology. Sensorineural loss can be caused by anterior cerebral artery occlusion, acoustic neuroma, aging (presbycusis), atherosclerosis, cochlear otosclerosis, CVVIII damage, drugs, frequent infections, Meniere's disease, meningitis, mumps, noise-induced (sound > 85–90 dB), and tumor. Inquire about the use of headphones for recreation and work, occupational exposure to loud noise and chemicals, past and present OTC and prescribed medications, and past infections.

Pop Quiz 4.3

Her use of daily steroids likely contributed to the bleeding, and daily NSAID use may have compromised her brief attempt at hemostasis. Her alcohol use exceeds daily recommendations and liver function tests may be evaluated in a follow-up. The BP is elevated and should be repeated in both arms according to AHA standards after bleeding is resolved. It is not contributing to the current bleeding. Do not apply a topical vasoconstrictor with hypertension present. Apply petroleum jelly to the nares to promote humidification. Anterior septal bleed should be referred to otolaryngology. Discharge with instructions to stop NSAIDs, nasal steroids, and to avoid strenuous activity, digital trauma, and hot showers. Instruct the patient to follow up with PCP for blood pressure.

Pop Quiz 4.4

The patient is exhibiting signs of acute rheumatic fever and should be referred to the ED immediately. The onset of rheumatic fever usually occurs about 2 to 4 weeks after strep pharyngitis. Complete a neurologic, cardiac, abdominal, and peripheral vascular exam with vital signs. A 12-lead EKG may also be performed, but transfer should not be delayed. The patient may have decreased cardiac output, myocardial ischemia, and requires evaluation in the ED.

CHAPTER 5

Pop Quiz 5.1

The priority assessment data should exclude the presence of s/s of pulmonary embolism and ensure that the patient is hemodynamically stable and is not hypoxic.

Pop Quiz 5.2

Routine CBG, UA, BMP, and CBC should be performed. Additionally, this patient has diabetes and is reporting polyuria, a symptom of hyperglycemia and UTI. These complications can have a devastating consequence of hyperglycemic emergencies and sepsis in patients with diabetes. Both HCTZ and diltiazem can increase BG, which can be determined quickly by point of care BG testing. Neuropathy can interfere with the perception of dysuria, which is a common finding in UTI. UA may indicate the presence of a UTI, which must be excluded.

Pop Quiz 5.3

Prioritize a 12-lead EKG. Female patients do not routinely complain of chest discomfort with ACS. The patient has a family history of CVHD and four risk factors for CVHD. HR of 59 is not consistent with the report of pain. STAT 12-lead EKG is a priority and transfer to the ED for evaluation of symptomatic bradycardia versus ACS. The patient is taking both an ARB and an NSAID, which is contradicted and may contribute to hyperkalemia. Potassium should be assessed to identify if hyperkalemia is a contributing factor to bradycardia but should not delay the transfer.

CHAPTER 6

Pop Quiz 6.1

Clubbing indicates that the patient has an underlying cardiopulmonary disease and is at higher risk for complications. Perform an exam to identify if hypoxia, ischemia, and decreased cardiac output are present. The patient has AF, which increases the risk of stroke and PE. In addition, the patient has a low-grade fever and may be experiencing infections such as acute bronchitis or pneumonia. Infections increase the risk of dehydration. The incidence of stroke increases with AF and dehydration. Carefully evaluate hydration status and perform a neurologic, respiratory, cardiac, and peripheral vascular examination. The presence of diabetes and possible infection increases the risk of a hyperglycemic state.

Obtain a stat CBG to determine if hyperglycemia is present. *Warning signs for admission*: A change in mental status, complaints of ischemic discomfort, pulse oximetry <90% on room air, peak flow <50%, RR >22, SBP <100 mmHg, CBG >250 mg/dL.

Pop Quiz 6.2

The patient is in respiratory distress. The physical exam findings of pleuritic chest pain, tachypnea, dullness to percussion, and crackles in the right lower low with egophony is consistent with right lower lobe pneumonia. It is aggravated by his history of cigarette smoking and the use of a cough suppressant. The patient is at risk for airflow limitation due to COPD and wheezing, respiratory failure, and sepsis. There is one qSOFA sign, which excludes septic shock at this time. Obtain a peak flow to determine if the patient is less than 50% to 80% PV and pulse oximetry on room air. Patients with a peak flow <50% or pulse oximetry that is <93% in a non-CO_2-retaining COPD and should be transported to the ED. If the peak >50% but <80% administer SABA and SAMA combined, obtain a chest x-ray and reevaluate.

Pop Quiz 6.3

The interpretation of the patient's tuberculin skin test is 12 mm of induration. The measurement of erythema is not included when classifying the results. A finding of 12 mm' induration is a positive finding in a person with high or intermediate risk for tuberculosis. Because the patient does not have any symptoms of TB, proceed with history taking using standard precautions and exclude a false-positive result.

CHAPTER 7

Pop Quiz 7.1

The student nurse practitioner should obtain a history of present illness that examines associated symptoms of the gastrointestinal and infectious state. Most importantly, inquiry and examination should include gynecological, genitourinary, in addition to gastrointestinal systems. When assessing a patient with symptoms of infection, question the patient if they had recent travel, exposure to food pathogens, vaccination against hepatitis, or recent contacts with patients who are sick. Every patient between the ages of 13 and 64 should be offered HIV testing, especially if they present with a fever. Every woman of childbearing age should be assessed for signs of pregnancy.

Pop Quiz 7.2

The etiology for acute pancreatitis includes environmental, disease, and medication risk factors. The patient's use of tobacco, alcohol, and medications are positive risk factors. Both antiretrovirals and antipsychotics can cause pancreatitis. Review the ED laboratory results to determine if a lipid panel was performed to rule out hypertriglyceridemia. Complete a metabolic profile with calcium and phosphorus to exclude hyperparathyroidism as a cause. Examine imaging results to identify if biliary disorders require additional investigation.

Pop Quiz 7.3

Differential diagnosis includes hepatitis B and C, HIV, NAFLD, biliary disorders, and ovarian cancer. The patient's presentation requires further examination of hepatic etiology, which could be infectious, medication-induced, or as a result of acute or chronic disease. Because most patients in her age group are not aware of their hepatitis B/C and HIV status, HIV testing should be offered, and the hepatitis profile performed to determine if acute hepatitis C or chronic hepatitis B/C is present. Disease risks include obesity, hypertension, and hyperlipidemia. This may be associated with the progression of nonalcoholic fatty liver disease. Biliary disorders may contribute to symptoms. The patient should also be examined for reproductive disorders. Vague symptoms could be associated with ovarian cancer, and a gynecological examination should be performed.

CHAPTER 8

Pop Quiz 8.1

The most likely diagnosis is pyelonephritis. Increased CVA tenderness with nausea, fever, and vomiting support pyelonephritis as the cause. The characteristics of the patient's pain can be genitourinary or gastrointestinal in origin. Obstructive nephropathy and acute abdomen should be excluded. The patient's pain is severe and could be contributing to hypertension and his BP should be retaken. Narcotic analgesia should be avoided until an acute abdomen is excluded. Transfer to the ED would be prudent for further evaluation.

Pop Quiz 8.2

The patient reports frequent UTIs over the past 6 months. "Recurrent UTIs" is defined as having more than three UTIs with two or more those occurrences within the past 6 months. It is important to get a sexual history in female patients to determine the frequency of sexual activity, hygiene, the number of sexual partners, and the use of spermicidal agents or mechanical barriers for contraception. Because all of the infections were diagnosed by urinalysis, a urine culture should be obtained. A gynecological exam and STI testing should be considered. Hyperglycemia and HIV infection are possible causes of recurrent infection. Perform HIV rapid testing, CBG, and HbA1c.

CHAPTER 9

Pop Quiz 9.1

Sick day rules for a patient with type 2 diabetes using an insulin pump and prescribed metformin include: Test BG more frequently (every 2–4 hr). Call HCP if BG levels >250 mg/d after correction insulin or there is persistent diarrhea or vomiting when taking metformin. Watch closely for dehydration from vomiting, diarrhea, or inadequate fluid intake. Dehydration can cause adverse effects of metformin and can be aggravated by hyperglycemia from illness. Continue basal and bolus insulin therapy. Maintain hydration with sugar-free drinks or low carbohydrate options unless hypoglycemia is present.

Pop Quiz 9.2

This patient has clinical manifestations of hyperthyroidism confirmed by TSH and free T4 and T3 levels. The next step is to determine the presence of Graves' disease by ordering a thyrotropin receptor antibody test. The presence of antibodies confirms Graves' disease.

CHAPTER 10

Pop Quiz 10.1

Interview the patient privately. UTIs are not common in adolescent males unless there are comorbid conditions or obstructive pathology. Urethritis secondary to sexual activity can contribute to the complaint. Sexual activity can be consensual or not. Adolescent males may be victims of sexual abuse and may not make their first outcry to a parent. They may not acknowledge abuse for decades. Therefore, it is imperative to create a safe environment and establish trust so that the adolescent can disclose sexual abuse if it occurred. Many adolescents have their first consensual sexual encounters between the ages of 15 and 19 years. A sexual history should be obtained to identify if STIs may be present.

Pop Quiz 10.2

The patient's age and HPI indicate that BPH may be at the cause of the complaints. Secondary UTI may be present but complicated due to bladder outlet obstruction. Referral to a urologist is indicated in the presence of BPH.

Pop Quiz 10.3

Refer to urology for evaluation for recurrent prostate cancer and assess for symptoms of metastasis to distant sites. The presence of a PSA level in a patient who is treated with brachytherapy for prostate cancer coupled with a high Gleason score should alarm the nurse practitioner to refer the patient to urology immediately. The PSA level after treatment should be close to zero, and elevations in PSA levels indicate cancer recurrence.

Pop Quiz 10.4

Scaling lesions of the breast can be dermatologic or oncologic in origin. While eczema can be a cause, oncological etiology requires further investigation and workup. Assess the patient's personal and genetic risk factors for breast cancer, squamous cell cancer, and personal history of fibrocystic changes. Actinic keratosis, squamous cell carcinoma, or Phyllodes tumor can manifest with scaling lesions. Paget's disease is a scaling lesion of the nipple and/or areola; it is not usually located near the bra strap.

CHAPTER 11

Pop Quiz 11.1

The serum ferritin is >100 which excludes IDA. The transferrin is <15% to 20% and GFR <60 which supports a diagnosis of anemia of chronic disease. Explain that the results need to be evaluated by a nephrologist and provide instruction in strategies for energy management while waiting to be seen.

Pop Quiz 11.2

An adolescent female who describes menses as heavy with associated symptoms of anemia requires an examination of signs and symptoms of nutritional anemia and chronic blood loss. Assess the patient about excessive bruising and frequent infections to eliminate myeloid dysplastic etiology. Ask the patient if they take any OTC agents or nutraceuticals that can increase bleeding. Assess the family and personal history to rule out coagulopathy or an inherited disorder of anemia. Examine the patient for petechiae and purpura. Note if there any symptoms of infection. Assess diet and for the presence of nutritional anemias; pallor, a systolic murmur, cheilitis, glossitis, koilonychia, pica, and orthostatic changes, and refer to hematology as needed. Assess pad saturation and the size of clots present in menses to gauge the severity of bleeding and consider gynecology referral.

Pop Quiz 11.3

Prepare to transfer the patient to the ED. Sickle cell anemia is characterized by painful vaso-occlusive events that can cause tissue organ damage and premature death. Acute chest syndrome is the second most common reason for hospitalization in a person with sickle cell disease. It may be related to ischemia of the lung and heart, fat embolism, myocardial infarction, and pneumonia. Obtain vital signs, stat 12-lead EKG, pulse oximetry, and provide supportive care before transfer.

CHAPTER 12

Pop Quiz 12.1

The patient is experiencing motor sensory disturbance to the upper extremities that should be evaluated for neurodegenerative disorders, cervical radiculopathy, and carpal tunnel syndrome. Carpal tunnel syndrome risk factors are present. However, the physical examination does not support it as the cause of the symptoms. In carpal tunnel syndrome, the paresthesia is on the palmer surface of the first to fourth digits, there is associated weakness, and a positive Tinel and Phalen sign. Symptoms are reproducible with the carpal compression test. In this patient, the decreased sensation and motor weakness exclude carpal tunnel syndrome as a likely cause. Neurodegenerative disease or radiculopathy is more likely. The motor or sensory weakness that begins in a glove and stocking pattern in the upper and lower extremities following an infection or vaccination needs to be further evaluated for a diagnosis of GBS. Obtain a history of systemic, arthritic, traumatic causes of cervical spine trauma that could lead to nerve root compression. Assess for the presence of a positive Spurling test to support the presence of radiculopathy. Assess for Lhermitte's sign to support the presence of multiple sclerosis and assess lower extremities for similar symptoms to support GBS as a possible cause.

Pop Quiz 12.2

A large inflamed great toe that is painful should be examined for trauma and broken integument. Increased warmth to the affected area and pain in the absence of signs of infection, insect bite, or injury is seen in gout and pseudogout.

Pop Quiz 12.3

An x-ray revealing penciling of the vertebrae is associated with severe osteoporosis. It may be caused by disorders such as Cushing disease, hyperparathyroidism, hyperthyroidism, renal failure, leukemia, multiple myeloma, and metastatic disease. The patient's medications are not associated with an increased risk for osteoporosis; thiazide diuretics are associated with improved bone strength. Considering that the patient has hypertension and BPH by history and is African American, renal failure should be carefully evaluated. The patient's age, race, and concurrent BPH, suggests referral to urology for evaluation for the presence of prostate cancer metastasis.

CHAPTER 13

Pop Quiz 13.1

Female patients with adult-onset acne should be evaluated for hyperandrogenism found in polycystic ovary syndrome. Late-onset acne in females with hirsutism and amenorrhea require an endocrine referral.

Pop Quiz 13.2

The CDC recommends that every person who has received the live vaccine should receive the recombinant zoster vaccination. The recombinant zoster vaccination is recommended for healthy adults who are immunocompetent and 50 years and older even if they received the live zoster vaccine in the past.

Pop Quiz 13.3

A patient who presents with facial droop and a smooth forehead is exhibiting signs of a cranial nerve palsy, the facial nerve, also called Bell's palsy. In endemic areas for tick-borne diseases, cranial nerve neuropathy may be seen in within weeks of the inoculation. Many patients will not recall being bitten by a tick nor have the classic bull's-eye rash. Patients who present with risk factors and evidence of early disseminated Lyme disease such as headache, fever, adenopathy, meningeal signs, neuropathy, should be evaluated for Lyme disease.

Pop Quiz 13.4

The patient with diabetes who has a thermal burn that involves the hand and is hyperglycemic should be managed by a burn center. While awaiting transfer, remove any circumferential garments items from the affected extremity and irrigate the burn wound bed to remove debris and accelerants that are contaminating the tissue and continuing the burning process. Apply saline-moistened gauze that is nonadherent after cleansing, elevate the extremity, and keep the hand in a position of function to preserve mobility and function.

CHAPTER 14

Pop Quiz 14.1

The patient is experiencing signs of an exacerbation of major depressive disorder with suicidal ideation. Signs associated with major depression include apathy, anorexia, anhedonia, low mood, weight change, fatigue, insomnia, hypersomnia, impaired concentration, and thoughts of suicide.

Pop Quiz 14.2

Unintentional weight loss resulting in extremely low BMI requires careful evaluation to rule out an endocrine, gastrointestinal, and psychiatric cause. Patients with profound weight loss, regardless of age, are at risk for cardiovascular events and should have a 12-lead EKG, complete metabolic profile with special attention to levels of potassium, magnesium, calcium, sodium, phosphorus, and BUN and creatinine especially when palpitations are present. Obtain serum albumin and total protein level for baseline. CBC should be evaluated for pancytopenia, and vitamins D, B_{12}, iron, and folate evaluated for nutritional anemia. Obtain a TSH, T3, and T4 to evaluate for hypermetabolic states and refer to endocrine. Establish trust and perform an eating disorder screen. A patient with extreme weight loss and palpitations would require medical stabilization and inpatient care.

Pop Quiz 14.3

Bupropion is an adjuvant antidepressant that can be combined with SSRI to reduce anxiety and is a second-line agent for tobacco cessation, reducing cravings. Nortriptyline 75 mg can be considered as an alternative if contraindications to bupropion are present. Clonidine has a hypotensive effect that will interact with propranolol.

CHAPTER 15

Pop Quiz 15.1

The findings are normal. The infant's fontanelle should begin to close between ages 2 and 4 months. Expect the infant to sit unsupported at age 6 to 8 months.

Pop Quiz 15.2

Follow the CDC's vaccine catch-up schedule. According to the CDC, administer recommended vaccines based on shared decision-making if the immunization history is incomplete or unknown. Use combination vaccinations when possible and reassure caregivers that several vaccines administered in one visit is safe. If vaccination doses were given at the valid age, do not restart or add doses to vaccine series regardless of the time that has passed since the valid vaccination. When a vaccine is not administered at the recommended age, administer at a subsequent visit. Refer to the CDC catch-up schedule: www.cdc. gov/vaccines/schedules/hcp/imz/catchup.html

CHAPTER 16

Pop Quiz 16.1

The first priority is to identify any urgent concerns: airway compromise, hypoxia, myocardial ischemia, pulmonary edema, or stroke, and obtain point of care BG to eliminate hypo/hyperglycemia, if indicated. While agitation can occur from exacerbation of medical illness, it can also occur from changes in settings, routines, stimulation, pain, or unmet needs such as incontinence, hunger, or dehydration. Reduce environmental stimuli and assess for the presence of contributing factors using a calm/positive tone and provide reassurance and reorientation. Monitor the patient's response to help isolate the cause.

APPENDIX: ABBREVIATIONS

5-HT	5-hydroxytryptamine receptor
A&O	alert and oriented
A1C	glycosylated hemoglobin
AA	alcoholic anonymous
AAA	abdominal aortic aneurysm
AANP	American Association of Nurse Practitioners
AANPCB	American Association of Nurse Practitioners Certification Board
AAP	American Academy of Pediatrics
AAT	alpha-1 antitrypsin deficiency
ABCD	airway, breathing, circulation, disability
ABCDE	aspirin and ACE inhibition, beta-blocker and blood pressure, cholesterol and cigarette smoking cessation, diet and diabetes management, education and exercise
ABG	arterial blood gas
ABI	ankle-brachial index
ABM	acute bacterial meningitis
ABR	auditory brainstem response
AC	air conduction
ACE	angiotensin converting enzyme
AChE	acetylcholinesterase
AChR	acetylcholine receptor
ACL	ATP citrate lyase
ACOG	American College of Obstetricians and Gynecologists
ACOS	asthma-COPD overlap syndrome
ACS	acute coronary syndrome
ACT	acceptance and commitment therapy
ACTH	adrenocorticotropic hormone
AD	advance directive
ADH	antidiuretic hormone
ADHD	attention deficit hyperactivity disorder
ADLs	activities of daily living
AF	atrial fibrillation
AFB	acid-fast bacillus
AGNP	adult-gerontology nurse practitioner
AHRQ	Agency for Healthcare Research and Quality
AI	anemia of inflammation
AICD	automatic implantable cardiac defibrillator
AIDS	acquired immunodeficiency syndrome
AKI	acute kidney injury
ALP	alkaline phosphatase
ALS	amyotrophic lateral sclerosis
AMS	altered mental state
AN	anorexia nervosa
ANA	antinuclear antibody
AN-BP	anorexia nervosa-binge purge subtype
ANCC	American Nurses Credentialing Center

APLA	antiphospholipid antibody syndrome
APOE4	apolipoprotein E4 gene
aPPT	activated partial thromboplastin
APS	adult protective services
AR	aortic regurgitation
ARB	angiotensin receptor antagonist
ARDS	acute respiratory distress syndrome
AS	ankylosing spondylitis
ASA	acetylsalicylic acid
ASCVD	atherosclerotic cardiovascular disease
ASD	acetylsalicylic acid
ASD	atrial septal defect
ASQ	Ask Suicide Screen Questions tool
ATC	around-the-clock
ATN	acute tubular necrosis
AUA-SI	American Urological Association Symptom Inventory
AUD	alcohol use disorder
AV	atrioventricular
AVM	arteriovenous malformation
BC	bone conduction
BCC	basal cell carcinoma
BCG	Bacillus Calmette–Guérin vaccine
BDNF	brain-derived neurotrophic factor
BE	bacterial endocarditis
BED	binge eating disorder
BEFAST	balance, eye change, facies asymmetric speech slurred, arms unequal, timing sudden
BG	blood glucose
BID	two times daily
BMD	bone mineral density
BMI	body mass index
BMP	basic metabolic profile
BN	bulimia nervosa
BNP	brain natriuretic peptide
BON	Board of Nursing
BOO	bladder outlet obstruction
BP	blood pressure
BPH	benign prostatic hypertrophy
BSA	body surface area
BUN	blood urea nitrogen
BZ	benzodiazepine
c/s	culture and sensitivity
C1	cervical vertebrae 1
C2	cervical vertebrae 2
C3	cervical vertebrae 3
C4	cervical vertebrae 4
C5	cervical vertebrae 5
C6	cervical vertebrae 6
C7	cervical vertebrae 7
C8	cervical vertebrae 8
Ca++	calcium
CABG	coronary artery bypass graft
CADASIL	cerebral autosomal dominant arteriopathy
CA-MRSA	community-acquired methicillin-resistant staphylococcus aureus
CAMS	Collaborative Assessment and Management of Suicidality

cANCA	antineutrophil cytoplasmic antibodies
CAP	community-acquired pneumonia
Cap	capillary
CAPTA	Child Abuse Prevention and Treatment Act
CAUTI	catheter associated urinary tract infection
CBC	complete blood count
CBG	capillary blood glucose
CBT	cognitive behavioral therapy
CCB	calcium channel blocker
CDAD	clostridium difficile associated diarrhea
CDC	Centers for Disease Control and Prevention
CDS	clinical decision support
CEA	carcinoembryonic antigen test
CGM	continuous glucose monitoring
CGRP antagonist	calcitonin gene-related peptide receptor antagonist
CHA_2DS_2-VASc	congestive heart failure, hypertension, age, diabetes, and previous stroke/transient ischemic attack (CHA_2DS_2); vascular disease (VASc, including peripheral arterial disease, preceding myocardial infarction, aortic atheroma))
CHD	congenital heart disease
ChEI	cholinesterase inhibitor
CHF	congestive heart failure
CIN	cervical intraepithelial neoplasia
CJD	Creutzfeldt–Jakob disease
CKD	chronic kidney disease
Cl	chloride
CMV	cytomegalovirus
CN I–XII	cranial nerve I–XII
CNM	certified nurse midwife
CNS	central nervous system
CNS	clinical nurse specialist
CO	carbon monoxide
CO_2	carbon dioxide
COMT	catechol-O-methyltransferase
COMT	catechol-O-methyltransferase
COPD	chronic obstructive pulmonary disease
CoQ10	coenzyme Q10
COX-1	cyclooxygenase-1
COX-2	cyclooxygenase-2
CPS	child protective services
CPT	common procedural technology
CrCl	creatinine clearance
CRE	carbapenem-resistant *enterobacteriaceae*
CRGP	calcitonin gene-related peptide
CRKP	carbapenem-resistant *Klebsiella pneumoniae*
CRNA	certified registered nurse anesthetist
CRP	C-reactive protein
CRPS	complex regional pain syndrome
CSF	cerebrospinal fluid
CT	computerized tomography
CV	cardiovascular
CV	cardiovascular
CVA	costovertebral angle
CVD	cardiovascular disease
CVHD	cardiovascular heart disease

CVI	chronic venous insufficiency
DA	dopamine
dB	decibel
DBP	diastolic blood pressure
DBT	dialectical behavioral therapy
DCIS	ductal carcinoma in situ
DDAVP	desmopressin acetate
DES	diethylstilbestrol
DEXA	dual energy x-ray absorptiometry
DHT	dihydrotestosterone
DIC	disseminated intravascular coagulation
DKA	diabetic ketoacidosis
DLE	discoid lupus erythematosus
DM	diabetes mellitus
DMARD	disease modifying anti-rheumatic drugs
DNA	deoxyribonucleic acid
DOAC	direct oral anticoagulants
DOE	dyspnea on exertion
DOH	Department of Health
DOT	Direct observed therapy
DPP-4	dipeptidyl peptidase IV
DRE	digital rectal examination
DTR	deep tendon reflexes
DTs	delirium tremens
DVT	deep vein thrombosis
DVT/PE	deep vein thrombosis/pulmonary embolism
EBP	evidence-based practice
EBV	Epstein–Barr virus
ECHO	echocardiography
ECOG	Eastern Cooperative Oncology Group
ECT	electroconvulsive therapy
ED	emergency department
EDD	expected date of delivery
EEG	electroencephalogram
EF	ejection fraction
eGFR	estimated glomerular filtration rate
EKG	electrocardiogram
EMB	ethambutol
EMG	electromyography
ENDO	endocrine
ENT	ears, nose, throat
EOM	extraocular movement
EpiPen	epinephrine autoinjector
EPN	emphysematous pyelonephritis
ER	extended release
ERCP	endoscopic retrograde cholangiopancreatography
ESA	erythropoiesis-stimulating agents
ESR	erythrocyte sedimentation rate
ESRD	end-stage renal disease
F	Fahrenheit
FDA	Food and Drug Administration
FFP	fresh frozen plasma
FISH	fluorescent in situ hybridization
FNP	family nurse practitioner

FOBT	fecal occult blood test
FROM	full range of motion
G6PDD	glucose-6-phosphate dehydrogenase deficiency
GABA	gamma-aminobutyric acid
GABHS	group A beta hemolytic streptococci
GAD	generalized anxiety disorder
GBS	Guillain–Barré syndrome
GCA	giant cell arteritis
GCS	Glasgow coma scale
GDM	gestational diabetes
GERD	gastroesophageal reflux disease
GFR	glomerular filtration rate
GI	gastrointestinal
GINA	Global Initiative for Asthma
GLP-1 RA	glucagon-like peptide-1 receptor agonist
GPCOG	General Practitioner Assessment of Cognition
GU	genitourinary
GYN	gynecological
H & P	history and physical
H2	histamine 2
HA	headache
HAI	hospital-acquired infection
HA-MRSA	hospital-acquired methicillin-resistant *Staphylococcus aureus*
HCC	hepatocellular cancer
HCG	human chorionic gonadotropin hormone
HCO_3	bicarbonate
HCP	healthcare provider
HCT	hematocrit
HCTZ	hydrochlorothiazide
HDL	high-density lipoprotein
HEENT	head, eyes, ears, nose, throat
HELLP	hemolysis, elevated liver enzymes, and low platelet count
HEM	hematology/oncology
Hep A	Hepatitis A vaccine
HEPA	High-Efficiency Particulate Air
Hep B	Hepatitis B vaccine
HF	heart failure
Hg	hemoglobin
HbA1C	glycosylated hemoglobin
HgB	hemoglobin
HHS	hyperosmolar hyperglycemic state
Hib	*Haemophilus influenzae* type b
HIPAA	Health Insurance Portability and Accountability Act
HIV	human immunodeficiency virus
HNPCC	hereditary nonpolyposis colorectal cancer
HOB	head of bed
HPA	hypothalamic–pituitary–adrenal axis
HPI	history of present illness
HPV	human papillomavirus
HR	heart rate
hr	hours
HRS	hepatorenal syndrome
HS	hidradenitis suppurativa
HSV	herpes simplex virus

Ht	heart
HTN	hypertension
I&D	incision and drainage
I/O	Intake and output
IBD	inflammatory bowel disease
IBS	irritable bowel syndrome
ICH	intracranial hemorrhage
ICP	intracranial pressure
ICS	inhaled corticosteroid
ID	Infectious diseases
IDA	iron deficient anemia
IDSA	Infectious Diseases Society of America
IgA	immunoglobulin assay
IgE	immunoglobulin E
IgM	immunoglobulin M
IGRA	interferon-gamma release assay
IM	intramuscular
INH	isonicotinyl hydrazide
INT	integument
IOP	intraocular pressure
IPC	intermittent pneumatic compression
IPV	intimate partner violence
IR	intermediate release
ITP	interpersonal psychotherapy
IUD	intra-uterine device
IV	intravenous
IVDA	IV drug abuse
IVIG	intravenous immunoglobulin
JVD	jugular vein distension
K+	potassium
KOH	potassium hydroxide
KUB	kidneys, ureter, bladder
L1	lumbar vertebrae 1
L2	lumbar vertebrae 2
L3	lumbar vertebrae 3
L4	lumbar vertebrae 4
L5	lumbar vertebrae 5
LABA	long-acting beta agonist
LACE	licensure, accreditation, certification, and education
LADA	latent autoimmune diabetes
LAMA	long-acting muscarinic antagonist
LBBB	left bundle branch block
LCIS	lobular carcinoma in situ
LDH	lactic acid dehydrogenase
LDL	low density lipoprotein
LET	leukocyte esterase
LFTs	liver function tests
LH:FSH	luteinizing hormone-follicular stimulating hormone
LH-RH	luteinizing hormone-releasing hormone
LLE	left lower extremity
LLL	left lower lobe
LLQ	left lower quadrant
LMN	lower motor neuron
LMWH	low molecular weight heparin

LTRA	leukotriene receptor antagonist
LUE	left upper extremity
LUTS	lower urinary tract symptoms
LVH	left ventricular hypertrophy
MAB	monoclonal antibodies
MAE	moves all extremities
MAO-BI	monoamine oxidase type B inhibitor
MAO-I	monoamine oxidase inhibitor
MCHC	mean cell hemoglobin concentration
MCV	mean corpuscular volume
MDD	major depressive disorder
MDI	metered dose inhaler
MDRHI	multidrug resistant *Haemophilus influenzae*
MELAS	mitochondrial encephalomyopathy, lactic acidosis, and stroke-like episodes
MEN2	multiple endocrine neoplasia type 2
MenACWY	meningococcal conjugate vaccine, quadrivalent
MenB	meningococcal serogroup B vaccine
mg	milligram
Mg	magnesium
mg/d	milligram/day
mg/dL	milligram/deciliter
mg/kg	milligram/kilogram
MI	myocardial infarction
MMSE	mini mental status exam
MNT	medical nutrition therapy
MOA	mechanism of action
MOH	medication overuse headache
MOOC	massive open online course
MPTP	1-methyl-4-phenyl-1,2,3,6-tetrahydropyridine
MRA	magnetic resonance angiography
MRCP	magnetic resonance cholangiopancreatography
MRI	magnetic resonance imaging
MRSA	methicillin-resistant *Staphylococcus aureus*
MS	multiple sclerosis
MSK	musculoskeletal
MSM	men who have sex with men
MSSA	methicillin-sensitive *Staphylococcus aureus*
MVI	multivitamin
MVP	mitral valve prolapse
Na	sodium
NAAT	Nucleic Acid Amplification Test
NAFL	nonalcoholic fatty liver disease
NASH	nonalcoholic steatohepatitis
NE	norepinephrine
NEDA	National Eating Disorders Association
NEURO	neurological
NMDA	*n*-nitrosodimethylamine
NP	nurse practitioner
NPI	National Provider Identifier
NPO	nothing by mouth
NRDI	norepinephrine–dopamine reuptake inhibitor
NSAIDs	nonsteroidal anti-inflammatory drugs
NSCLC	non–small cell lung cancer
NSR	normal sinus rhythm

NTG	nitroglycerin
NYHA	New York Heart Association
O_2 SAT	oxygen saturation
OA	osteoarthritis
OAB	overactive bladder
OBC	oral birth control
OCD	obsessive–compulsive disorder
OE	otitis externa
OGTT	oral glucose tolerance test
OM	otitis media
OME	otitis media effusion
OT	occupational therapy
OTC	over-the-counter
PACE	programs for all-inclusive care
PAD	peripheral arterial disease
PANDAs	pediatric autoimmune neuropsychiatric disorders associated with streptococcal infections
Pap	Papanicolaou
PCA3	prostate cancer antigen 3
PCI	percutaneous coronary intervention
PCN	penicillin
PCOS	polycystic ovarian syndrome
PCR	polymerase chain reaction
PCV13	pneumococcal conjugate vaccine
PD	Parkinson's disease
PDA	patent ductus arteriosus
PDD	persistent depressive disorder
PE	pulmonary embolism
PEFR	peak flow rate
PEP	post exposure prophylaxis
PERRLA	pupils equal, round, and reactive to light and accommodation
PET	positron emission tomography scan
pH	potential hydrogen
PHN	postherpetic neuralgia
PHOS	phosphorus
PID	pelvic inflammatory disease
PKD	polycystic kidney disease
PLLR	Pregnancy, Lactation, Reproductive Labeling Rule
PMI	point of maximal impulse
PMR	polymyalgia rheumatica
PNU	pneumonia
PO	oral
POC	point-of-care
PPD	purified protein derivative
PPE	personal protective equipment
PPI	proton pump inhibitor
PPSV23	Pneumococcal polysaccharide vaccine
PPT	partial thromboplastin
PR	per rectum
PRBC	packed red blood cells
PrEP	pre-exposure prophylaxis
PRN	as needed
PSA	prostatic-specific antigen
PSGN	post-streptococcal glomerulonephritis
PT	physical therapy

PT/INR	prothrombin time/international normalized ratio
PTNS	percutaneous tibial nerve stimulation
PTSD	posttraumatic stress disorder
PTT	partial thromboplastin time
PTU	propylthiouracil
PUD	peptic ulcer disease
PULM	pulmonology
PV	predicted value
PVR	post void residual
q	every
QSEN	Quality and Safety in Educating Nurses
qSOFA	quick SOFA score for sepsis
RA	rheumatoid arthritis
RAAS	rein angiotensin aldosterone system
RAI	radioactive iodine
RAS	renin angiotensin system
RAST	radioallergosorbent test
RBC	red blood cell
re	regarding
REMS	Risk Evaluation and Mitigation Strategy
REPRO	Reproductive
RH	rhesus factor
RIF	rifampin
RLE	right lower extremity
RLL	right lower lobe
RMSF	spotted fever
ROM	range of motion
RPR	rapid plasma reagin
RR	respiratory rate
RSV	respiratory syncytial virus
RUE	right upper extremity
RUQ	right upper quadrant
RZV	recombinant zoster vaccine
s/s	signs and symptoms
S1	sacral vertebrae
SABA	short-acting beta agonist
SAD	social anxiety disorder
SAGE	Self-Administered Gerocognitive Examination
SAMA	short-acting muscarinic antagonist
SBP	systolic blood pressure
SC	subcutaneous
SCC	squamous cell carcinoma
SCI	spinal cord injury
SCLC	small cell lung cancer
SERM	selective estrogen receptor modulators
SGA	small for gestational age
SGLT2I	sodium-glucose cotransporter 2 inhibitor
SIADH	syndrome of inappropriate antidiuretic hormone
SL	sublingual
SLE	systemic lupus erythematosus
SMBG	self-monitoring of blood glucose
SMX	sulfamethoxazole
SMZ	sulfamethoxazole
SNRI	serotonin norepinephrine reuptake inhibitor

SQ	subcutaneous
SSI	surgical site infection
SSRI	serotonin reuptake inhibitor
Staph	staphylococci
STEMI	ST elevation myocardial infarction
STI	sexually transmitted infections
SU	sulfonylurea
SUD	substance use disorder
T	temperature
T cell	T lymphocytes
T1	thoracic vertebrae 1
T2	thoracic vertebrae 2
T3	triiodothyronine
T3	thoracic vertebrae 3
T4	thoracic vertebrae 4
T4	thyroxine
T5	thoracic vertebrae 5
T6	thoracic vertebrae 6
T7	thoracic vertebrae 7
T8	thoracic vertebrae 8
T9	thoracic vertebrae 9
T10	thoracic vertebrae 10
T11	thoracic vertebrae 11
T12	thoracic vertebrae 12
TAGVHD	tissue associated graft versus host disease
TB	tuberculosis
TBI	traumatic brain injury
TCA	tricyclic antidepressant
Tdap	tetanus–diphtheria vaccine
TeCA	tetracyclic antidepressant
TEE	transesophageal echocardiography
Temp	temperature
TG	triglycerides
TIA	transient ischemic attack
TIBC	total iron-binding capacity
TID	three times daily
TLS	tumor lysis syndrome
TM	tympanic membrane
TMJ	temporomandibular joint
TMS	transcranial magnetic stimulation
TMX-SMZ	trimethoprim-sulfamethoxazole
TN	trigeminal neuralgia
TNF	tumor necrosis factor
TR	tricuspid regurgitation
TSH	thyroid-stimulating hormone
TST	tuberculin skin test
TT	thrombin time
TTH	tension type headache
TTP	thrombotic thrombocytopenic purpura
TURP	transurethral resection of the prostate
TWIST	testicular workup for ischemia and suspected torsion
TZD	thiazolidinediones
U/A	urinalysis
UAB	underactive bladder

UCG	urine chorionic gonadotropin
UFH	unfractionated heparin
UMN	upper motor neuron
UO	urinary output
URI	upper respiratory infection
USPSTF	United States Preventive Services Task Force
UTI	urinary tract infection
UV	ultraviolet
VDRL	Venereal Disease Research Laboratory
VNS	vagus nerve stimulation
VQ	pulmonary ventilation/perfusion
VRSA	vancomycin-resistant Staphylococcus aureus
VS	vital signs
VSD	ventricular septal defect
VZIG	varicella-zoster immune globulin
VZV	varicella-zoster virus
WBC	white blood cell
WGT	weight
WPW	Wolff–Parkinson–White
yr	years
ZV	zoster vaccine
ZVL	live zoster vaccine

INDEX

Printed in the United States
by Baker & Taylor Publisher Services